# OVERVIEW-MAP KEY

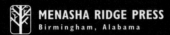

**MENASHA RIDGE PRESS**
Birmingham, Alabama

# 60 HIKES WITHIN 60 MILES

# NEW YORK CITY

INCLUDING
Northern **NEW JERSEY**,
Southwestern **CONNECTICUT**,
and Western **LONG ISLAND**

THIRD EDITION

CHRISTOPHER AND CATHERINE BROOKS

# 60 HIKES WITHIN 60 MILES: NEW YORK CITY

Copyright © 2013 by Christopher and Catherine Brooks
All rights reserved
Printed in the United States of America
Published by Menasha Ridge Press
Distributed by Publishers Group West
Third edition, fourth printing 2022

Library of Congress Cataloging-in-Publication Data

Brooks, Christopher, 1959–
   60 hikes within 60 miles, New York City : including northern New Jersey,
southwestern Connecticut, and western Long Island / Christopher and Catherine
Brooks. — Third edition.
      pages cm
   Includes index.
   ISBN-13: 978-0-89732-714-5; eISBN: 978-0-89732-715-2
   ISBN-10: 0-89732-714-4
1.   Hiking—New York Region—Guidebooks. 2.   New York Region—
Guidebooks. I. Brooks, Catherine. II. Title. III. Title: Sixty hikes within
sixty miles, New York City.
   GV199.42.N64B76 2013
   796.5109747—dc23

                                          2013012579

Editor: Ritchey Halphen
Cover design: Scott McGrew
Cartography: Christopher and Catherine Brooks, Scott McGrew
Text design: Steveco International
Cover and interior photos: Christopher and Catherine Brooks
Proofreader: Julie Hall Bosché
Indexer: Ann Cassar / Cassar Technical Services

**MENASHA RIDGE PRESS**
An imprint of AdventureKEEN
2204 First Avenue South, Suite 102
Birmingham, Alabama 35233
menasharidge.com

## DISCLAIMER

This book is meant only as a guide to select trails in the New York City area and does not guarantee hiker safety—you hike at your own risk. Neither Menasha Ridge Press nor Christopher and Catherine Brooks are liable for property loss or damage, personal injury, or death that may result from accessing or hiking the trails described in this guide. Be especially cautious when walking in potentially hazardous terrains with, for example, steep inclines or drop-offs. Do not attempt to explore terrain that may be beyond your abilities. Please read carefully the introduction to this book, as well as safety information from other sources. Familiarize yourself with current weather reports and maps of the area you plan to visit (in addition to the maps provided in this guidebook). Be cognizant of park regulations, and always follow them. While every effort has been made to ensure the accuracy of the information in this guidebook, land and road conditions, phone numbers and websites, and other information can change from year to year.

# TABLE OF CONTENTS

# DEDICATION

*To those people inspired with the vision to set this precious space aside. And those enlightened hikers, bikers, and riders with the grace to tread the land lightly.*

# ACKNOWLEDGMENTS

Like the many trees, shrubs, and ground cover that compose a forest, a number of people have been involved in the successful completion of this book. We would like to thank the following for helping to inspire this work and nurture it along:

Catherine's parents, Jan and Liliane, taught her the importance of respecting nature. They loved to stroll through fields and forests, they planted many a tree and fed the birds that came to roost in them, and they made sure that their five daughters had a spacious backyard in which to play.

Likewise, Christopher's parents, Patricia and Lester, introduced him to the delights of the wide-open woods. Some of his earliest, fondest memories are of family outings to Ward Pound Ridge, where Chris, barely able to walk, roamed the forest floor, gathering fiddlehead ferns for the family meal. His brothers, too, inspired him with the desire to spend as much of his free time outside as possible.

We would like to thank our eight nephews and nieces for their willingness to accompany us on several of these hikes. Their enthusiasm, stamina, and determination to go wherever the trail led allowed us to see the hikes from many different, insightful perspectives.

Without the selfless efforts of trail volunteers, venturing into the wilds would be a considerably different—and more taxing—experience. While they all deserve our gratitude, we would like to send a special thank-you to the New York–New Jersey Trail Conference, which has been highly active in developing and maintaining a vast network of paths in this region.

We are grateful to all of the people who took the time to answer our questions about their respective domains. Likewise, we extend our thanks to the many hikers we have encountered on the trail, our readers and other outdoors enthusiasts, who have offered suggestions and shared their insights. One in particular, Channan Willner of the New York Public Library, has been especially generous in his trail observations and hiking advice.

And finally, special recognition is due to Ritchey Halphen, our editor at Menasha Ridge Press, and the rest of the team in Birmingham, for their invaluable support and encouragement throughout the production of this book.

—Christopher and Catherine Brooks

# FOREWORD

Welcome to Menasha Ridge Press's *60 Hikes within 60 Miles,* a series designed to provide hikers with the information they need to find and hike the very best trails surrounding metropolitan areas.

Our strategy is simple: First, find a hiker who knows the area and loves to hike. Second, ask that person to spend a year researching the most popular and very best trails around. And third, have that person describe each trail in terms of difficulty, scenery, condition, elevation change, and other categories of information that are important to hikers. "Pretend you've just completed a hike and met up with other hikers at the trailhead," we told each author. "Imagine their questions, and be clear in your answers."

Experienced hikers and writers, Christopher and Catherine Brooks have selected 60 of the best hikes in and around the New York City metropolitan area. From the rugged beauty of the challenging Sterling Ridge Trail to a coastal trek on the Sandy Hook Peninsula, the Brookses provide hikers (and walkers) with a great variety of outings—and all within roughly 60 miles of New York City.

As much to free the spirit as to free the body, let these hikes elevate you above the urban fray.

**All the best,**
**The Editors at Menasha Ridge Press**

# ABOUT THE AUTHORS

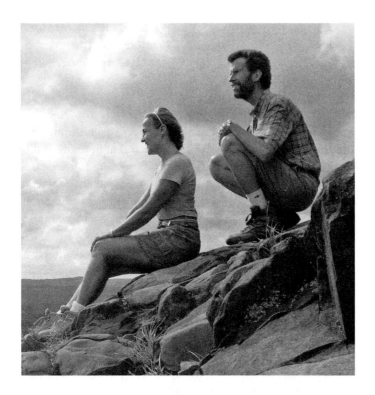

**Christopher Brooks** brings to *60 Hikes within 60 Miles: New York City* more than two decades of writing experience. In addition to a five-year stint as contributing editor at *Market Watch* (a sister publication to *Wine Spectator*) and 14 years as contributing editor and columnist at Hearst's *Country Living*, his many credits include *Family Circle, The Christian Science Monitor, Cigar Aficionado,* the *Chicago Tribune,* the *International Herald Tribune, USA Today,* and *Diversion.* A graduate of Wesleyan University, Christopher also contributes food-related stories to *The New York Times*—a subject that goes well with hiking, he claims.

**Catherine Brooks,** née Van der Maat, spent her childhood in Belgium, delving often into the forests around Brussels while raising rabbits and roosters as pets. Her enjoyment of nature falls under a large umbrella of passions, including birding, mycology, and botany. With a university degree in languages, Catherine started her career as an interpreter-translator. Later, she went to work for a United States–based multinational corporation, with marketing responsibilities spread over six European countries. A professional photographer, she has had her images published in *Backpacker* and many other magazines.

Together, the Brookses wrote the California half of Frommer's *The Unofficial Guide to the Best RV and Tent Campgrounds in California and the West* and have teamed up to write restaurant reviews for *Westport* and *New Canaan–Darien & Rowayton* magazines. They have hiked the Appalachian, Pacific Crest, and Inca Trails and have extensively explored the United States, Mexico and South America, Europe, Asia, and northern Africa. As a unit, they are fluent in five languages, one or another of which occasionally facilitates the interpretation of cryptic trail maps and oblique signposts.

# PREFACE

Congratulations! What you have in your hands (either physically or digitally) is the very latest hiking guide to the New York region. It's the third edition of *60 Hikes within 60 Miles: New York City,* with numerous new hikes, updated classics, revised trail descriptions, freshly drawn maps, and more.

If you already possess either or both of the previous editions of this book, you're in for a special treat: not only have we revised many of the great hikes in those books, we've added several new outings that are sure to satisfy even the most adventurous of souls. Hikes to the eagle's nest pinnacle of Anthony's Nose, and deep into the boggy dales of the Angle Fly Preserve. Far forays beyond Bennett's Pond to the ruin of Charles Ives's summer cabin, and short romps back in history, to the Revolutionary War winter camp at Jockey Hollow. These hikes, along with such new additions as Fahnestock's Catfish Pond Loop, Harriman's Seven Hills circuit, Hook Mountain, and others, are so rugged, or remote, or little-known, or jaw-droppingly beautiful, we're confident you'll soon list them among your favorites, too.

Sure, to make room for the new entries, we had to toss aside some earlier listings. Rest assured that we put a great deal of thought into which hikes to delete, and we removed only those that had, over time, become degraded by overuse, or failed, after repeat visits, to deliver the desired "Wow!" effect. Meanwhile, in holding on to some of the old classics, like the jaunts at Bear Mountain, Black Rock, Fishkill Ridge, Wawayanda, Norvin Green, Ramapo Mountain, Schunemunk, Sterling Ridge, and more, we've tweaked the routes and, in many cases, added to their overall distance, thus providing you with tours that go farther, showcase more, and last longer.

Putting all the write-ups together, we've provided you with nearly 400 miles of outdoor fun and excitement—400 miles in

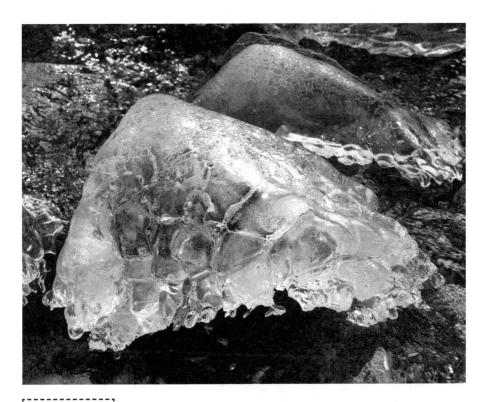

Ice-covered rocks

which to escape, week after week, for a few hours at a time, from the modern world. Many of these hikes, 21 in all, are easy enough underfoot to be ideal for young children, and we've identified 21 that we feel sure your dog will enjoy. For those occasions when a heartier excursion is desired, you'll have your pick among 23 hikes that are greater than 8 miles in length, and 4 that clock in at more than 12 miles (with several others that may easily be extended). Distance, of course, doesn't necessarily equate to quality (or heartiness), and all of the longer treks listed in this book may be shortened using cutoff trails. But in case you *do* feel like losing yourself in the woods for an afternoon, or the entire day, you'll find plenty of options here for doing just that. And if you're an über-hiker, someone who likes to push his or her physical endurance to the limit, we have a special category just for you: the "Iron Leg" Hikes, each of which features a cumulative elevation gain of more than 2,500 feet—or twice the height of the Empire State Building!

All in all, we think this book is better, and not just better than the first and second editions: we feel it's better than all the other hiking guides out there. Ultimately, though, it's your call. So go ahead and try out the hikes in this book; we feel so confident you'll agree, we're already looking forward to hearing your comments when next we meet up, out there on the trail.

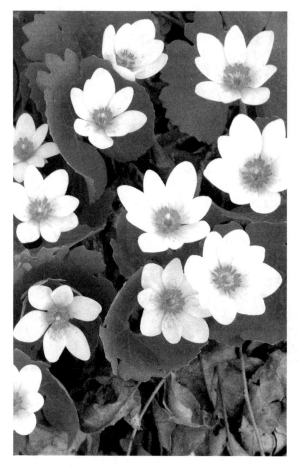

Bloodroot

You will also find in this edition GPS coordinates to help you locate each and every trailhead. Our publisher requested this information, and frankly, we're of two minds regarding it. On the one hand, it bears the faintest reek of a marketing gimmick, as something of little value beyond its use as a plug on the back cover of the book. Few hikers worth their salt tablets, after all, will require GPS data to find the trailhead. On the other hand, even experienced trail-hounds may find themselves, on occasion, baffled by an unexpected intersection, or an absent side trail, or some other debacle that leaves them in doubt as to which path to take. In an attempt to anticipate such moments, we have inserted GPS coordinates into the narratives at those junctures we believe to be particularly nettlesome. You probably won't require them, and, in all candor, we'd prefer for you to leave your GPS at home rather than allowing it to distract you from the unexpected thrills of being out in nature. Indeed, for many of us, a great part of the pleasure we feel in taking to the woods is derived from the very act of getting away from the gadgetry of modern life.

While we're on the subject of taking to the woods, it may interest you to know how we set about selecting the hikes in this book. First, we decided that only walks in natural settings would make the cut, thus excluding with one blow city parks, botanical gardens, and arboretums. No question, such open spaces serve a useful purpose within a metropolitan environment, but most are already quite well known and would simply be filler in a guide like this. Similarly, to our minds, the surface of a trail should be grounded in the natural world. Many excellent hikes briefly overlap macadam, but those that are paved from start to finish were dropped from consideration. Then there are the "rails to trails" paths and other long, level, linear treks. We're all for greenways like the Old Croton Aqueduct, but too often they feel like bicycle freeways, and hiking loses its allure when you are jarred out of peaceful reveries by the need to dodge speeding objects hurtling down the track. So those, too, were eliminated.

What was left over, you wonder? Plenty. It is no secret that this is one of the richest cultural centers on the planet. What we have been delighted to discover during our peregrinations is that the New York area is no less blessed with an increasing number of stellar hikes. Admittedly, in the end we did have trouble settling on 60 hikes. The difficulty arose from the limit; we might easily have given you a volume of 70, 80, or even 90 hikes (hence the additional tips in the Nearby Activities sections), but that book would have had a different title. Instead, we restricted ourselves to a minimal number of hike profiles per park, even though many, like Bear Mountain–Harriman, Wawayanda, Stokes, High Point, and Ward Pound Ridge (to name a mere handful), deserve to have several of their superb trails featured. No matter; once you go there and get your feet wet, you'll soon be venturing out on your own, discovering other exciting treks.

It is customary in a preface to include remarks relating to the history of the region. Rather than bore you, though, with too many words about stuff we all should know anyway, we decided to leave the history lesson up to you, in the form of fieldwork. Would you like to see where indigenous peoples lived long ago? Several of these hikes, including Devil's Den and Ramapo–Ringwood, showcase Paleolithic rock shelters. Care to learn about some of the first settlers on Long Island? Caleb Smith Full Circuit and Connetquot State Park are great starting points. Do you have an interest in the Revolutionary War period? There are connections at Morristown's Jockey Hollow, Sourland Mountain, and Sterling Forest, to name just three. And in Wawayanda and Westchester Wilderness you will find a link (albeit a tenuous one) to the Civil War. Curious about how the Big Apple roared back to life after the Great Fire of 1835? Look for the answers at Clay Pit Ponds. Then there is the question of how the city and its harbor were defended against the possibility of foreign attack during the Cold War and before. Sandy Hook and Hartshorne Woods provide an insight into that. On the other hand, if your taste flows more toward social history than bellicose matters, the historic mines of the Black River Trail and Norvin Green, the Leatherman's Cave at Ward Pound Ridge, and the abandoned lunatic asylum at Sunken Meadow should all make your short list. And for that fin de siècle sense of a golden era coming to an end, the ruins at Muttontown and Hudson Highlands are among the most expressive and atmospheric we've seen. A small slice of history surrounded by the beauty of the backwoods is about as sweet a classroom as there is. Best of all, the only tests you are likely to face concern stamina, and how long a wait you will have to endure until the next outing.

At one time or another we have all heard it said that when it comes to hitting the wilderness, the West is best. Well, after spending months at a time on the trails in the West, from the Rocky Mountains on out to the coast, we've arrived at a simple conclusion: it's not true. Why sugarcoat what we should be yodeling

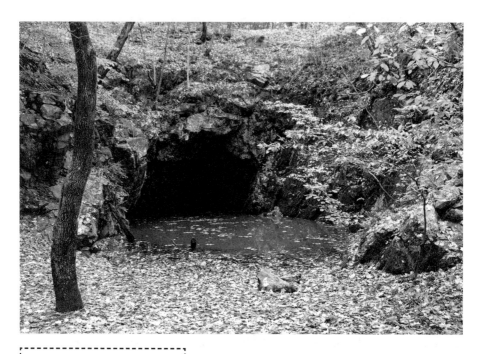

Norvin Green's Blue Mine (Hike 38)

from the crest of Storm King Mountain? The New York City region has some of the best hiking trails in the country, maybe even the world. True, there are no killer mountains out here, no death-defying climbs to nosebleed altitudes. But then, we don't have to schlep 10-plus miles just to see a different kind of cactus. Our woods and lowlands and granite-graced mountains are so rich in beauty and rife with diversity that it doesn't require a marathon trek to fill our souls with the sweet honey of nature. Sure, our Eastern peaks are lower than those in the Sierra Nevada range and the Cascades, but for better views than what you will find atop Anthony's Nose or Fishkill Ridge, you'll have to hire a blimp.

Oddly enough, as ever more houses are shoehorned into the region, New York has become an even better place in which to hike, not because of the influx of people, but rather as a reaction to it. Recognizing the imperative to preserve whatever remains of large blocks of open space, grassroots conservationists have waged determined and sustained drives, resulting in the creation of a number of great parks in recent years. We have included a handful of those in this volume—preserves so diverse, and of such head-turning beauty, that we feel certain you will want to visit them again and again. But don't take our word for it . . . go see for yourself with a hearty scramble along the densely forested trails of Angle Fly Preserve (established in 2006) and a quiet stroll by the pastoral pond at Weir Farm (1990, Connecticut's first—and only—national park). Have your binoculars handy for those far-reaching vistas from atop the "Hill of Pines," at Bennett's Pond State

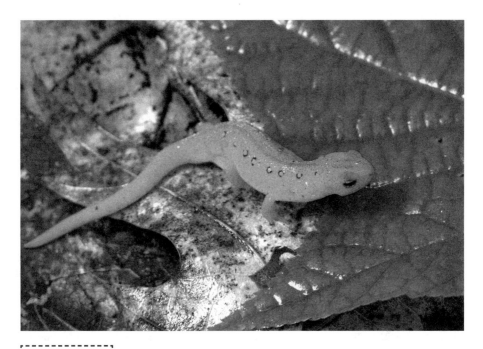

Red-spotted newt

Park (2002), and for the great birding along the water at Nissequogue River State Park (1999). You probably won't require an energy bar during the peaceful ramble by the streams, swamps, and granite bluffs of Westchester Wilderness (2001), but an extra apple or pack of trail mix will be a welcome restorative after the exhilarating climbs up Sterling Ridge (2000) and Turkey and Pyramid Mountains (1987, with preservation efforts ongoing).

As conservation campaigns continue, additional parks will no doubt be established. Already, there has been much excitement over the creation of a Meadowlands preserve, with 8,400 acres tucked into its borders. This park has canoe rentals, boat tours, miles of hiking trails (some of which traverse scenic swamps and a rambling riverside), even an environmental center—all within view of Manhattan and easily accessed via Exit 16 off the New Jersey Turnpike. Then there is the new Highlands Trail, stretching west from the Hudson River all the way to the Delaware Water Gap. Even though volunteers have yet to finish the entire 150-mile path, it has already been designated by the Rails-to-Trails Conservancy as a Millennium Legacy Trail, one of only 50 such treks nationwide. We have gamboled along parts of this route and found that it incorporates some of the most wild and wonderful land between the Big Apple and Pennsylvania. This truly is a magnificent time to be a hiker.

Some of the trails included in this guide are all but impassable when snow covers the ground. Most, however, are still navigable and take on a lustrous appearance when in the icy grip of winter. Sight lines are clearer, hitherto-hidden rock formations rise into high relief, streams magically become more beautiful than Waterford crystal, and animal tracks in the snow reinforce just how abundantly our woodlands teem with wildlife. You may not be able to see as much in summer, but the long days and warm, humid weather lend a pleasurable lassitudinousness to an excursion, transforming the outing from a brisk march to one that is more pensive, seemingly pregnant with possibilities. Most of our black-bear sightings have occurred when it was so uncomfortably sticky that the beasts couldn't be bothered to duck into hiding. There are a number of dark, densely forested swamp and river hikes included in this book that you will find enticingly cool and welcoming when the streets and sidewalks are sizzling. Autumn means leaf-peeping, and we know of no better place to enjoy the annual fall foliage displays than deep in our New York–area woods. There is an invigorating sharpness to the air, most biting bugs are gone, and animals tend to be more visible as they engage in a final, frantic foraging for wild nuts and seeds. Autumn is also hunting season, a sport that is permitted in many of the parks listed in these pages. We suggest you call ahead to confirm when and where such activities are taking place. Then there is spring, our favorite time to be out, to witness nature renewing itself. With streams and rivers running high, the tiny spearlike tips of skunk cabbage are among the first greens to surface from the soft ground. Soon, though, the entire forest, great swaths of swampland, and sandy stretches of pine barrens all erupt in a kaleidoscope of colorful flowers. Simultaneously, migratory birds return, contributing a chatty insouciance to the realm as they build their nests and defend their territory.

Spring also marks the return of bugs, and two varieties, ticks and mosquitoes, merit special attention. Deer ticks, which are a little larger than a poppy seed in their nymph stage, are known for transmitting Lyme disease, while mosquitoes are the vector for West Nile virus. Neither of these concerns should inhibit you from lacing up your boots and setting off on the trail. We have met more people who have caught Lyme by lolling about in their own backyard than from any backwoods adventure. Basically, if you wear light-colored clothing, check yourself regularly for ticks, and lather on a DEET-rich insect repellent (especially around the ankles, wrists, and neck), you'll be more likely to bump into Donald Trump out in the forest than come down with Lyme disease. Bug spray also wards off mosquitoes, giving you added insurance against West Nile virus. (And keeping your dog on a leash will help minimize its exposure to parasites, too.)

If you plan to spend a fair amount of time out in the woods—and we hope that you do—consider investing in an **Empire Passport** ($65; **nysparks.com /admission/empire-passport**) or a **New Jersey State Park Pass** ($50; **tinyurl.com/nj parkshop**). For a set fee, both programs permit unlimited day-use admission to nearly all New York and Garden State parks. Westchester County provides a discount on park-admission fees through a similar plan for its residents ($60; **parks.westchester gov.com/park-passes**). And in those parks where fishing is allowed, you will need to purchase a license.

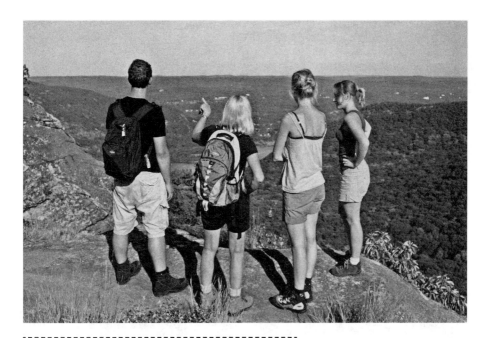

Hikers enjoy a view of Hudson Valley from Butter Hill (Hike 23).

Finally, while we have made every effort to be accurate in our trail maps and descriptions, the best bet is to rely wherever possible on the park or preserve's own map and information. Most organizations now have their trail systems posted on the Internet, and many of those maps are downloadable. Even so, remember that conditions change over time and it is always prudent before visiting a park to contact its authorities for the latest trail information. Trees fall, causing paths to be rerouted. Hurricanes and other extreme weather events can drastically change the landscape, leading to trail closures. Erosion from equestrians and bikers alters the appearance of intersections. Right-of-ways and easements are revoked, forcing the creation of new connector trails. We apologize in advance should you encounter any such circumstance. Remember, though, that these sorts of challenges are but a small part of the thrill and pleasure of a few hours or a day spent in the woods. And in the most densely populated area of the country, where else but in the woods can you find yourself both alone and totally at home?

# 60 HIKES BY CATEGORY

| HIKE CATEGORIES | | | |
|---|---|---|---|
| 1–4 miles | 4–8 miles | 8–12 miles | 12+ miles |
| birding hotspots | children's delight | dog's paradise | |
| **DIFFICULTY** | | | |
| E = easy | M = moderate | S = strenuous | |
| I = "Iron Leg" (+2,500 ft. elevation gain) | | | |

| REGION<br>Hike Number/Hike Name | page number | 1–4 miles | 4–8 miles | 8–12 miles | 12+ miles | birding hotspots | children's delight | dog's paradise |
|---|---|---|---|---|---|---|---|---|
| **NEW YORK: EAST OF THE HUDSON RIVER** | | | | | | | | |
| 1 Angle Fly Amble | 14 | | M | | | ✓ | | |
| 2 Anthony's Nose Ascent | 19 | | S | | | | | |
| 3 Butler Outer Loop Trail | 24 | E | | | | | ✓ | ✓ |
| 4 Fahnestock Catfish Loop | 29 | | E | | | | | |
| 5 Fahnestock Greater Hidden Lake Tour | 34 | | | M | | | | |
| 6 Fahnestock Wilderness Trail | 40 | | | | SI | | | |
| 7 Fishkill Ridge Trail | 45 | | SI | | | | | |
| 8 Hudson Highlands Breakneck Ridge Loop | 51 | | | SI | | | | |
| 9 Mianus River Gorge Trail | 58 | | E | | | | ✓ | ✓ |
| 10 Pelham Bay Islands Loop | 63 | E | | | | | ✓ | ✓ |
| 11 Rockefeller Medley | 68 | | | M | | | ✓ | ✓ |
| 12 Teatown Triple | 73 | | M | | | | ✓ | ✓ |
| 13 Ward Pound Ridge Star Loop | 78 | | M | | | | ✓ | ✓ |
| 14 Westchester Wilderness Walk | 83 | | M | | | | ✓ | ✓ |
| 15 Westmoreland Grand Tour | 90 | | M | | | | ✓ | |

| REGION<br>Hike Number/Hike Name | | page number | 1–4 miles | 4–8 miles | 8–12 miles | 12+ miles | birding hotspots | children's delight | dog's paradise |
|---|---|---|---|---|---|---|---|---|---|
| **NEW YORK: WEST OF THE HUDSON RIVER** | | | | | | | | | |
| 16 | Bear Mountain Doodletown Circuit | 98 | | | S | | | | ✓ |
| 17 | Black Rock Forest Peaks to Ponds Trail | 104 | | | | SI | ✓ | | ✓ |
| 18 | Fitzgerald Falls to Little Dam Lake (Appalachian Trail) | 111 | | | SI | | | | |
| 19 | Harriman Highlands Trail | 117 | | | SI | | | | ✓ |
| 20 | Harriman Seven Hills Loop | 122 | | | S | | | ✓ | ✓ |
| 21 | Hook Mountain Heights | 128 | | S | | | | ✓ | |
| 22 | Schunemunk Mountain Ridge Loop | 133 | | | S | | | | |
| 23 | Storm King Summit Trail | 139 | S | | | | | | |
| 24 | Tors' Thunder Tour | 145 | | M | | | | | ✓ |
| **NEW YORK: LONG ISLAND AND STATEN ISLAND** | | | | | | | | | |
| 25 | Caleb Smith Full Circuit | 152 | E | | | | | ✓ | ✓ |
| 26 | Caumsett Neck Loop | 157 | | E | | | | ✓ | ✓ |
| 27 | Clay Pit Ponds Connector | 162 | E | | | | | | ✓ |
| 28 | Connetquot Continuum | 167 | | | E | | | ✓ | ✓ |
| 29 | David Weld Sanctuary Tour | 172 | E | | | | | | ✓ |
| 30 | Jamaica Bay West Pond Trail | 177 | E | | | | | ✓ | ✓ |
| 31 | Muttontown Mystery Trail | 181 | E | | | | | | ✓ |
| 32 | Sunken Meadow to Nissequogue River Trail | 186 | | M | | | | | ✓ |
| 33 | Walt Whitman Sampler | 191 | E | | | | | | |
| **NEW JERSEY: NORTH OF INTERSTATE 80** | | | | | | | | | |
| 34 | Abram Hewitt's Bearfort Ridge | 198 | | | S | | | | |
| 35 | Farny Highlands Hike | 204 | | | S | | | ✓ | ✓ |
| 36 | High Point Duet | 210 | | | S | | | | ✓ |
| 37 | Mahlon Dickerson Discovery Trail | 216 | | | M | | | | ✓ |
| 38 | Norvin Green's Heart and Soul | 222 | | | SI | | | | |
| 39 | Ramapo–Ringwood Rally | 230 | | | | SI | ✓ | | ✓ |
| 40 | Sterling Ridge Trail | 238 | | | | SI | | | |

| REGION<br>Hike Number/Hike Name | page number | 1–4 miles | 4–8 miles | 8–12 miles | 12+ miles | birding hotspots | children's delight | dog's paradise |
|---|---|---|---|---|---|---|---|---|
| **NEW JERSEY: NORTH OF INTERSTATE 80 *(continued)*** | | | | | | | | |
| 41 Stokes Select | 244 | | | S | | | | ✓ |
| 42 Turkey–Egypt Connection | 249 | | | S | | ✓ | ✓ | |
| 43 Wawayanda 1: Way Way Yonder | 256 | | M | | | ✓ | | ✓ |
| 44 Wawayanda 2: Terrace Pond | 262 | | M | | | ✓ | ✓ | |
| **NEW JERSEY: SOUTH OF INTERSTATE 80** | | | | | | | | |
| 45 Allamuchy Natural Area Amble | 268 | | | M | | ✓ | | |
| 46 Black River Trail | 273 | | M | | | ✓ | | ✓ |
| 47 Cheesequake Natural Area Trail | 279 | | E | | | ✓ | ✓ | |
| 48 Great Swamp Wilderness Trail | 285 | | E | | | ✓ | ✓ | |
| 49 Hartshorne Woods Grandest Tour | 289 | | M | | | | | ✓ |
| 50 Jenny Jump Ghost Lake Loop | 294 | | M | | | | | |
| 51 Jockey Hollow Run | 299 | | M | | | | | |
| 52 Lewis Morris Loop | 304 | | M | | | | | ✓ |
| 53 Sandy Hook Hiking Trail | 309 | | | M | | ✓ | | |
| 54 Sourland Mountain Track | 314 | | M | | | | ✓ | |
| 55 Watchung Sierra Sampler | 319 | | M | | | | | |
| **CONNECTICUT** | | | | | | | | |
| 56 Babcock Circumference Trail | 326 | | E | | | | ✓ | ✓ |
| 57 Bennett's Pond and Beyond | 330 | | | M | | ✓ | | ✓ |
| 58 Devil's Den Concourse | 337 | | M | | | | | |
| 59 Trout Brook Valley Circuit | 343 | | | M | | | | |
| 60 Weir Pond and Swamp Loops | 349 | E | | | | | | ✓ |

# 60 HIKES BY CATEGORY (CONT'D.)

| HIKE CATEGORIES | | |
|---|---|---|
| history (H) & ruins (R) | leaf-peeping ops | multiuse |
| mushrooms (M) & wildflowers (W) | rock scramble | scenic vistas |
| water destinations | scenic hikes | |

| REGION<br>Hike Number/Hike Name | page | history & ruins | leaf-peeping ops | multiuse | mushrooms & wildflowers | rock scramble | scenic vistas | water destinations |
|---|---|---|---|---|---|---|---|---|
| **NEW YORK: EAST OF THE HUDSON RIVER** | | | | | | | | |
| 1 Angle Fly Amble | 14 | H | | | MW | | | |
| 2 Anthony's Nose Ascent | 19 | | ✓ | | | ✓ | ✓ | |
| 3 Butler Outer Loop Trail | 24 | | | | M | | | |
| 4 Fahnestock Catfish Loop | 29 | | ✓ | | M | | | |
| 5 Fahnestock Greater Hidden Lake Tour | 34 | H | ✓ | | M | | ✓ | |
| 6 Fahnestock Wilderness Trail | 40 | R | ✓ | | MW | | ✓ | |
| 7 Fishkill Ridge Trail | 45 | | ✓ | | | ✓ | ✓ | |
| 8 Hudson Highlands Breakneck Ridge Loop | 51 | R | ✓ | | MW | ✓ | ✓ | |
| 9 Mianus River Gorge Trail | 58 | | | | W | | | ✓ |
| 10 Pelham Bay Islands Loop | 63 | | | | | | | ✓ |
| 11 Rockefeller Medley | 68 | H | ✓ | ✓ | W | | ✓ | ✓ |
| 12 Teatown Triple | 73 | | | | MW | | | ✓ |
| 13 Ward Pound Ridge Star Loop | 78 | | ✓ | ✓ | MW | | | |
| 14 Westchester Wilderness Walk | 83 | | | | MW | | | |
| 15 Westmoreland Grand Tour | 90 | | | | MW | | | |

| REGION<br>Hike Number/Hike Name | page | history & ruins | leaf-peeping ops | multiuse | mushrooms & wildflowers | rock scramble | scenic vistas | water destinations |
|---|---|---|---|---|---|---|---|---|
| **NEW YORK: WEST OF THE HUDSON RIVER** | | | | | | | | |
| 16 Bear Mountain Doodletown Circuit | 98 | HR | ✓ | | | ✓ | ✓ | |
| 17 Black Rock Forest Peaks to Ponds Trail | 104 | | ✓ | | MW | ✓ | ✓ | ✓ |
| 18 Fitzgerald Falls to Little Dam Lake (Appalachian Trail) | 111 | | ✓ | | | ✓ | ✓ | ✓ |
| 19 Harriman Highlands Trail | 117 | | ✓ | | M | ✓ | ✓ | |
| 20 Harriman Seven Hills Loop | 122 | R | | | | | ✓ | ✓ |
| 21 Hook Mountain Heights | 128 | | | | W | ✓ | ✓ | ✓ |
| 22 Schunemunk Mountain Ridge Loop | 133 | | ✓ | | | ✓ | ✓ | |
| 23 Storm King Summit Trail | 139 | | ✓ | | | ✓ | ✓ | |
| 24 Tors' Thunder Tour | 145 | | ✓ | | | ✓ | ✓ | |
| **NEW YORK: LONG ISLAND AND STATEN ISLAND** | | | | | | | | |
| 25 Caleb Smith Full Circuit | 152 | H | | | | | | |
| 26 Caumsett Neck Loop | 157 | H | | ✓ | W | | ✓ | ✓ |
| 27 Clay Pit Ponds Connector | 162 | H | | | | | | |
| 28 Connetquot Continuum | 167 | H | | ✓ | | | | |
| 29 David Weld Sanctuary Tour | 172 | | | | W | | | |
| 30 Jamaica Bay West Pond Trail | 177 | | | | | | | ✓ |
| 31 Muttontown Mystery Trail | 181 | R | | ✓ | W | | | |
| 32 Sunken Meadow to Nissequogue River Trail | 186 | H | | | | | | ✓ |
| 33 Walt Whitman Sampler | 191 | | | ✓ | | | | |
| **NEW JERSEY: NORTH OF INTERSTATE 80** | | | | | | | | |
| 34 Abram Hewitt's Bearfort Ridge | 198 | | | | W | ✓ | ✓ | ✓ |
| 35 Farny Highlands Hike | 204 | HR | | | | | | |
| 36 High Point Duet | 210 | | ✓ | ✓ | | | ✓ | |
| 37 Mahlon Dickerson Discovery Trail | 216 | | ✓ | ✓ | W | | ✓ | ✓ |
| 38 Norvin Green's Heart and Soul | 222 | H | ✓ | | MW | ✓ | ✓ | ✓ |
| 39 Ramapo–Ringwood Rally | 230 | R | ✓ | | MW | | ✓ | ✓ |
| 40 Sterling Ridge Trail | 238 | HR | ✓ | | MW | ✓ | ✓ | |
| 41 Stokes Select | 244 | | ✓ | ✓ | W | | ✓ | |

| REGION<br>Hike Number/Hike Name | page | history & ruins | leaf-peeping ops | multiuse | mushrooms & wildflowers | rock scramble | scenic vistas | water destinations |
|---|---|---|---|---|---|---|---|---|
| **NEW JERSEY: NORTH OF INTERSTATE 80 (continued)** | | | | | | | | |
| 42 Turkey–Egypt Connection | 249 | R | ✓ | | | | ✓ | |
| 43 Wawayanda 1: Way Way Yonder | 256 | HR | ✓ | | | | | ✓ |
| 44 Wawayanda 2: Terrace Pond | 262 | | ✓ | | | ✓ | ✓ | ✓ |
| **NEW JERSEY: SOUTH OF INTERSTATE 80** | | | | | | | | |
| 45 Allamuchy Natural Area Amble | 268 | | | ✓ | W | | | ✓ |
| 46 Black River Trail | 273 | H | | | W | | ✓ | ✓ |
| 47 Cheesequake Natural Area Trail | 279 | | | ✓ | | | | ✓ |
| 48 Great Swamp Wilderness Trail | 285 | | | | W | | | |
| 49 Hartshorne Woods Grandest Tour | 289 | HR | ✓ | | | | | |
| 50 Jenny Jump Ghost Lake Loop | 294 | | ✓ | | W | | ✓ | ✓ |
| 51 Jockey Hollow Run | 299 | H | | ✓ | W | | | |
| 52 Lewis Morris Loop | 304 | | | ✓ | | | | |
| 53 Sandy Hook Hiking Trail | 309 | HR | | ✓ | | | ✓ | ✓ |
| 54 Sourland Mountain Track | 314 | | | | MW | | | |
| 55 Watchung Sierra Sampler | 319 | HR | | ✓ | | | | ✓ |
| **CONNECTICUT** | | | | | | | | |
| 56 Babcock Circumference Trail | 326 | | | | | | | |
| 57 Bennett's Pond and Beyond | 330 | R | ✓ | | MW | | | ✓ |
| 58 Devil's Den Concourse | 337 | H | | | MW | | ✓ | |
| 59 Trout Brook Valley Circuit | 343 | | | ✓ | MW | | | |
| 60 Weir Pond and Swamp Loops | 349 | H | | | | | | ✓ |

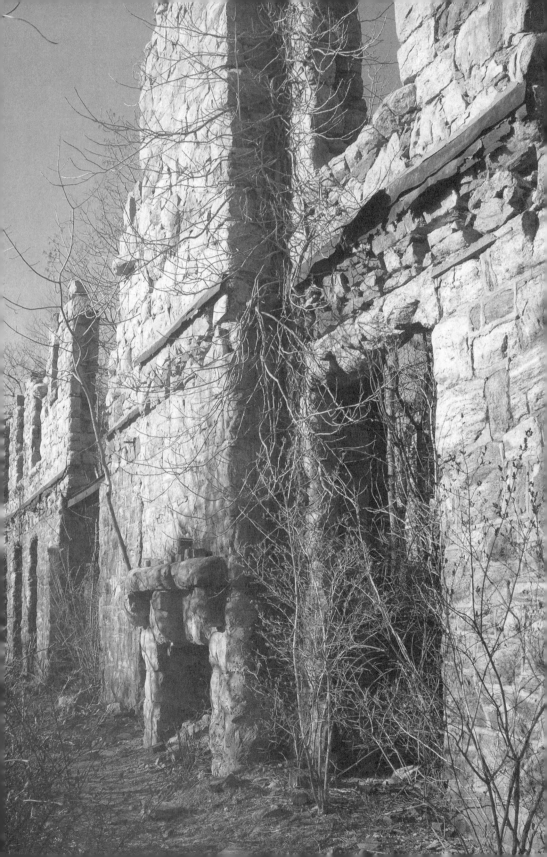

# INTRODUCTION

Welcome to *60 Hikes within 60 Miles: New York City*. If you're new to hiking or even if you're as seasoned a trail-hound as Bigfoot himself, take a few minutes to read the following introduction, which explains this book's organization and how to use it.

## HIKE PROFILES

Each hike contains eight key items: an In Brief description of the trail, a Key At-a-Glance Information box, directions to the trail, GPS coordinates, a trail map, an elevation profile, a trail description, and notes on things to see and do nearby. Combined, the maps and information provide a clear method to assess each trail from the comfort of your favorite reading chair.

### IN BRIEF

A "taste of the trail." Think of this section as a snapshot focused on the historical landmarks, beautiful vistas, and other sights you may encounter on the hike.

### KEY AT-A-GLANCE INFORMATION

This gives you a quick idea of the statistics and specifics of each hike:

**LENGTH** How long the trail is from start to finish. There may be options to shorten or extend the hikes, but the mileage corresponds to the described hike. Use the Description as a guide to customizing the hike for your ability or time constraints.

**ELEVATION GAIN** Indicates the cumulative increase in elevation, or all of the uphill stretches added together, you can expect from the start of the hike to its finish.

« Ramapo's Castle Point (Hike 39)

**CONFIGURATION** A description of what the trail might look like from overhead. Trails can be loops, out-and-backs (that is, trails on which one enters and leaves along the same path), figure-eights, balloons, or a combination of shapes.

**DIFFICULTY** The degree of effort an average hiker should expect on a given hike. For simplicity, difficulty is described as *easy, moderate,* or *strenuous.*

**SCENERY** A short summary of the hike's attractions and what to expect in terms of plant life, wildlife, natural wonders, and historic features.

**EXPOSURE** A quick check of how much sun you can expect on your shoulders during the hike. Descriptors used are self-explanatory and include terms such as *shady, exposed,* and *sunny.*

**TRAFFIC** Indicates how busy the trail might be on an average day, and if you might be able to find solitude out there. Trail traffic, of course, varies from day to day and season to season.

**TRAIL SURFACE** Indicates whether the path is paved, rocky, gravel, dirt, boardwalk, or a mixture of elements.

**HIKING TIME** How long it takes to hike the trail. A slow but steady hiker will average 2 to 3 miles an hour, depending on the terrain. Most of the estimates in this book reflect a speed of about 2 mph.

**DRIVING DISTANCE** One-way, measured from the George Washington Bridge.

**SEASON** Times of year and hours of the day when this trail is accessible. In most cases, the limiting factor is snow on the trail or the road to the trailhead, but in some cases trails are closed for reasons relating to wildlife habitat. When in doubt, call the information number to be sure you can hike it.

**ACCESS** Notes fees or permits needed to access the trail (if any), where wheelchair access is possible, and whether pets and other forms of trail use are permitted.

**MAPS** Which maps are the best, or easiest, for this hike (including U.S. Geological Survey topographic maps) and where to get them.

**FACILITIES** Includes restrooms, phones, water, picnic tables, and other basics at or near the trailhead.

**COMMENTS** These cover useful phone numbers and websites, advice, and tips.

## GPS COORDINATES

These may be used, in conjunction with the Directions to the Trail, below, to ascertain exactly where the trailhead is.

## DIRECTIONS TO THE TRAIL

Used with the GPS coordinates, these will help you locate each trailhead and its parking options.

## DESCRIPTION

The heart of each hike. Here, the authors provide a summary of the trail's essence and highlight any special traits the hike offers. The route is clearly outlined, including any landmarks, side trips, and possible alternate routes along the way. Ultimately, the Description will help you choose which hikes are best for you.

## NEARBY ACTIVITIES

Look here for information on appealing attractions in the vicinity of the trail— parks, historical sites, museums, restaurants, and the like.

# WEATHER

In an average year, the New York region receives 49 inches of rainfall and 26 inches of snow. And yet every month is well suited to hiking. Spring opens with a burst of wildflowers, songbirds, and cacophonous cascades. Even at its wettest, the unfolding forest canopies act as an umbrella, partially shielding hikers from precipitation. In summer, the woods become luminescent green; no matter how hot the days, there are always shady spots where you can mop the sweat from your brow and bathe your feet in the cool flow of clear-running streams. Autumn is leaf-peeping time, when hitting the trail allows you to enjoy the fall colors far from the crowds. Still fewer people venture out in winter, when a trip to a bald summit on a bright, crisp day can yield a spectacular view of the Manhattan skyline. And while snow may turn a path into a treacherous toboggan run, its glistening white carpet transforms the landscape into a different sort of paradise.

| AVERAGE DAILY TEMPERATURES BY MONTH: NEW YORK AND VICINITY | | | | | |
|---|---|---|---|---|---|
|  | JAN | FEB | MAR | APR | MAY | JUN |
| HIGH | 27°F | 29°F | 35°F | 45°F | 54°F | 64°F |
| LOW | 38°F | 42°F | 50°F | 61°F | 71°F | 79°F |
|  | JUL | AUG | SEP | OCT | NOV | DEC |
| HIGH | 69°F | 68°F | 61°F | 50°F | 42°F | 32°F |
| LOW | 84°F | 83°F | 75°F | 64°F | 54°F | 43°F |

# ALLOCATING TIME

On flat or lightly undulating terrain, the authors average 3 mph when hiking. That speed drops in direct proportion to the steepness of a path, and it does not reflect the many pauses and forays off trail in pursuit of yet another bird sighting, wildflower, or photograph. Give yourself plenty of time. Few people enjoy rushing through a hike, and fewer still take pleasure in bumping into trees after dark. Remember, too, that your pace naturally slackens over the back half of a long trek.

## MAPS

The maps in this book have been produced with great care and the assistance of a GPS unit. But as any experienced hiker knows, things can get tricky off the beaten path. When used with the route directions present in each chapter, the maps are sufficient to direct you to the trail and guide you on it. However, you will find superior detail and valuable information in the U.S. Geological Survey's 7.5-minute-series topographic maps.

Topo maps are available online in many locations. At **MyTopo.com**, for example, you can view and print topos of the entire United States free of charge. Online services such as **Trails.com** (a resource the authors recommend) charge annual fees for additional features such as shaded relief, which makes the topography stand out more. If you expect to print out many topo maps each year, it might be worth paying for such extras. The downside to USGS maps is that most are outdated, having been created 20 to 30 years ago; nevertheless, they provide excellent topographic detail. Of course, **Google Earth** (earth.google.com) does away with topo maps and their inaccuracies . . . replacing them with satellite imagery and its inaccuracies. Regardless, what one lacks, the other augments. Google Earth is an excellent tool whether you have difficulty with topos or not.

If you're new to hiking, you might be wondering, "What's a topographic map?" In short, a topo indicates not only linear distance but elevation as well, using contour lines. These lines spread across the map like dozens of intricate spiderwebs. Each line represents a particular elevation, and at the base of each topo a contour's interval designation is given. If the contour interval is 20 feet, then the distance between each contour line is 20 feet. Follow five contour lines up on the same map, and the elevation has increased by 100 feet.

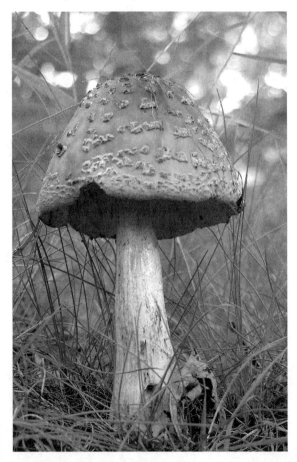

Blusher amanita

Let's assume that the 7.5-minute-series topo reads "contour interval 40 feet," that the short trail we'll be hiking is 2 inches in length on the map, and that it crosses five contour lines from beginning to end. What do we know? Well, because the linear scale of this series is 2,000 feet to the inch (roughly 2.75 inches representing 1 mile), we know that our trail is about 0.75 mile long (2 inches equals 4,000 feet). But we also know we'll be climbing or descending 200 vertical feet (five contour lines are 40 feet each) over that distance. And the elevation designations written on occasional contour lines will tell us if we're heading up or down.

In addition to the sources listed in Appendix B, you'll find topos at major universities and some public libraries. If you want your own and can't find them locally, visit **nationalmap.gov** or **store.usgs.gov.**

## TRAIL ETIQUETTE

Whether you're hiking in a city, county, state, or national park, always remember that great care and resources (from nature as well as from your tax dollars) have gone into creating these spaces. Treat the trail, wildlife, and fellow hikers with respect.

- **Hike on open trails only. Respect trail and road closures (ask if you're not sure), avoid possible trespassing on private land, and obtain all permits and authorization as required. Also, leave gates as you found them or as marked.**

- **Be sensitive to the ground beneath you. This also means staying on the existing trail and not blazing any new trails. Pack out what you pack in. No one likes to see the trash someone else has left behind.**

- **Never harass animals. An unannounced approach, a sudden movement, or a loud noise can startle them. A surprised snake or skunk can be dangerous to you, others, and itself. Give animals extra room and time to adjust to your presence.**

- **Plan ahead. Know your equipment, your ability, and the area in which you are hiking—and prepare accordingly. Be self-sufficient at all times; carry necessary supplies for changes in weather or other conditions. A well-executed trip is a satisfaction to you and to others.**

- **Be courteous to other hikers, bikers, skiers, or equestrians you meet on the trails.**

## WATER

"How much is enough? One bottle? Two? *Three?!*" Sure, carrying around all that extra weight can be a pain in the neck (or, more to the point, *back*), but taking off with an insufficient amount of water can ruin a hike—and possibly leave you vulnerable to heatstroke. One simple physiological fact should convince you to err on the side of excess when deciding how much water to pack: a hiker working hard in 80° heat needs approximately 2 gallons for a day's outing—that's 8 large water bottles or 16 small ones. In other words, pack along one or two bottles, even for short hikes.

For most people, the pleasures of hiking make the pain of carrying water a relatively minor nuisance, one that far outweighs the aggravation of going thirsty, or, worse yet, drinking "found water." No matter how clean that water appears, whether it is collected into a picturesque pond or flowing briskly down a river, there's a possibility it has been contaminated with giardia, a waterborne bug that attacks one's intestines. To be safe, plan to hydrate before setting off on your hike, carry (and drink) at least 6 ounces of water for every mile you intend to hike, and hydrate afterward.

## OTHER ITEMS TO STOW IN YOUR PACK

A typical outing may call for any of the following in addition to water:

**Ace bandages**

**Adhesive bandages (for treating blisters)**

**Aspirin or substitute**

**Flashlight (in case you unexpectedly stay out after dark)**

**Insect repellent**

**Matches or lighter**

**Pocketknife with tweezers (for removing ticks)**

**Rain poncho**

**Sunglasses**

**Sun hat**

**Sunscreen**

**Water-purification tablets or a water filter (on longer hikes)**

## HIKING WITH CHILDREN

No one is too young for a hike in the woods or through a city park. Be mindful, though, that flat, short trails are best with an infant. Toddlers who haven't quite mastered walking can still tag along, riding on an adult's back in a child carrier. Use common sense to judge a child's capacity to hike a particular trail, and always rely on the possibility that the child will tire quickly and need to be carried. Hikes suitable for children are noted in the chart on pages xx–xxii.

## SNAKES

Like bears and bobcats, snakes tend to appear when you least expect them. They like warm—but not hot—weather, and are active from midspring through midautumn. Most of the authors' encounters with such reptiles have involved

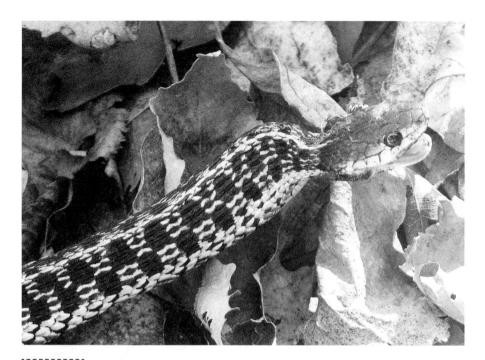

Garter snake

benign garter snakes (pictured above), rat snakes, ribbon snakes, and black racers. Venomous rattlesnakes and copperheads are also native to the New York area, but we have only rarely come across them. In general, their heads are more triangular than those of their nonvenomous cousins. You might spend a few minutes studying snakes before heading into the woods, but in any case, a good rule of thumb is to give whatever animal you encounter a wide berth and leave it alone.

## TICKS

Ticks tend to lurk in the brush, leaves, and grass that grow alongside trails. April through mid-July is the peak period for ticks in this area, but the authors have managed to pick up stray ticks in every month of the year. Of the two varieties that may hitch a ride on you while hiking—wood ticks and deer ticks—extensive research suggests that both need several hours of actual bloodsucking attachment before they can transmit any disease. Deer ticks, the primary vector for Lyme disease, are very small (often as tiny as a poppy seed), and you may not be aware of

Deer tick ready to dig in

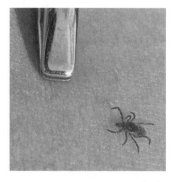

their presence until you feel the itchiness of their bite. The best avoidance strategy is to wear light-colored clothing (so that you can spot the ticks more easily); tuck the cuffs of your pants into your socks (sure, it looks geeky, but it helps); slather your ankles, wrists, and neck with a DEET-rich insect repellent; and remain on the beaten path. At the end of the hike, check yourself thoroughly before getting in the car; and later, when you take a posthike shower, do an even more thorough check of your entire body. Use tweezers to remove ticks that have bitten you, making sure to pull out the head.

## POISON IVY

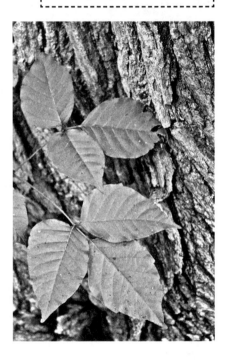

Poison ivy: "leaves of three, let it be"

Recognizing and avoiding contact with poison ivy are the most effective ways to prevent the painful, itchy rashes associated with it. In the Northeast, poison ivy occurs as a vine or ground cover. Its leaves, which are notched on one edge, are clustered in groups of three (hence the expression "leaves of three, let it be"). This is a chameleon plant, with its leaves—sometimes shiny, sometimes matte—assuming the tint and overall size of neighboring vegetation. The oil in its sap is responsible for the rash; thus, you may contract a case of poison ivy either through direct contact with the plant or by touching something—your clothing, boots, or pets—that has brushed against it. Within 12 to 24 hours of exposure, raised lines and/or blisters will appear, accompanied by a terrible itch. As with insect bites, scratching makes the situation worse, and bacteria under your fingernails may cause an infection. Wash and dry the rash thoroughly, applying calamine lotion or another desiccant to help dry out the rash. If the itching or blistering is severe, seek medical attention.

## BEARS

Many of the denser forests referred to in this book feature black bears as their largest and most fearsome residents. As they shake off their winter lethargy, typically in April, they start foraging for food, relying on their exceptional sense of smell to sniff out edible plants, nuts, and fruit, and fattening up for eight months before returning to their winter dens. While some truant bears have learned that campgrounds and suburban garbage cans hold easy pickings, these are, in general,

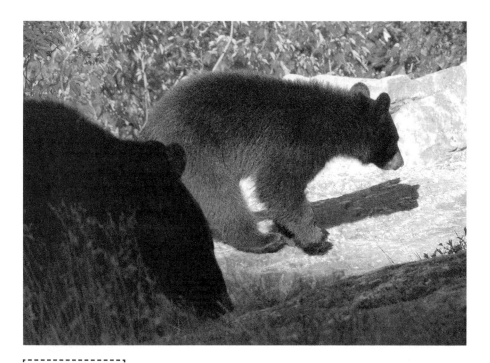

Mother bear and cub

shy animals. You are more likely to walk away a winner at three-card monte than encounter one on the trail. Should you be fortunate enough to come across an *Ursus americanus* waddling through the woods, give it plenty of space (getting off the path, if necessary), avoid direct eye contact, and don't offer it any food.

## A WORD ABOUT GLOBAL WARMING AND SEVERE-WEATHER IMPACT

Whether you're a confirmed skeptic or a true believer, there is no arguing that we are currently experiencing a period of what some have delicately described as "extreme weather events." The immediate effect of these storms is felt most deeply in the thousands of homes and businesses that are damaged, destroyed, or left without power. But there are ripples, too, out in the woods, where fallen trees and broken limbs force parks and preserves to close trails, or, in more severe circumstances, their gates. On going to press, some of the areas covered in this guide were still feeling the aftereffects of Hurricane Sandy, which battered the Northeast on October 10, 2012, just one year after Tropical Storm Irene did the same. But severe droughts can have an impact, too, by increasing the risk of wildfires, which in turn may lead park authorities to limit access to their domains. Thus, in every case (but in particular during and immediately after such extreme weather events), it would be wise to first call the park you intend to visit (or check its

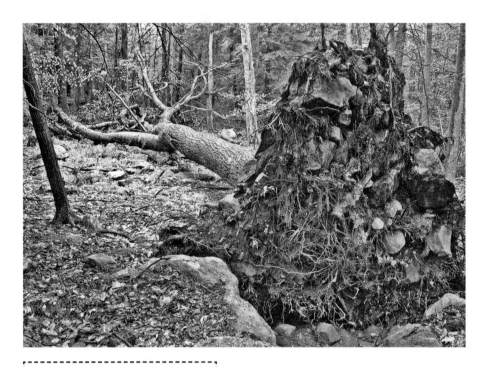

Windswept trees may require trail rerouting.

website) for an update on trails and any possible reroutings, pertinent river cross-ings, and bridge conditions. And if you are willing to acknowledge the possibility that global warming exists, and that it may be responsible for these catastrophic events, you might consider ways to reach the hike—for instance, carpooling or public transportation—that reduce your carbon footprint.

Black Rock Forest's boardwalks (Hike 17) »

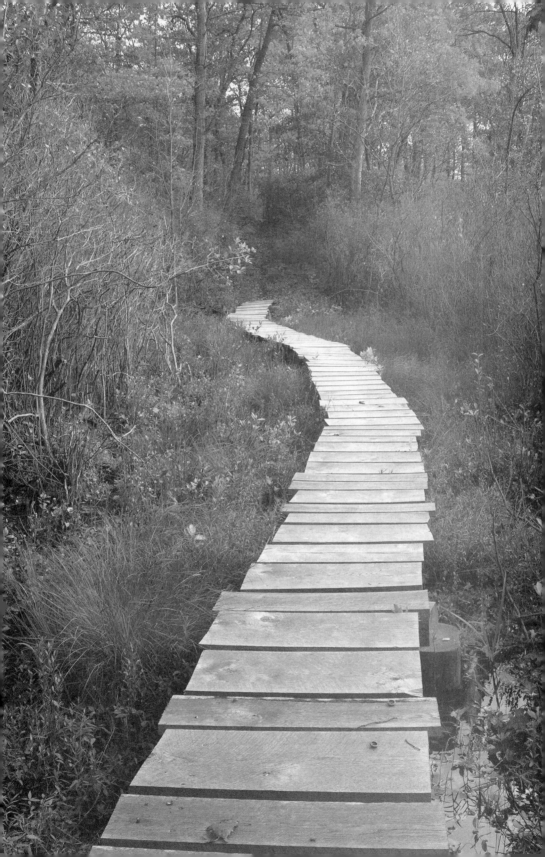

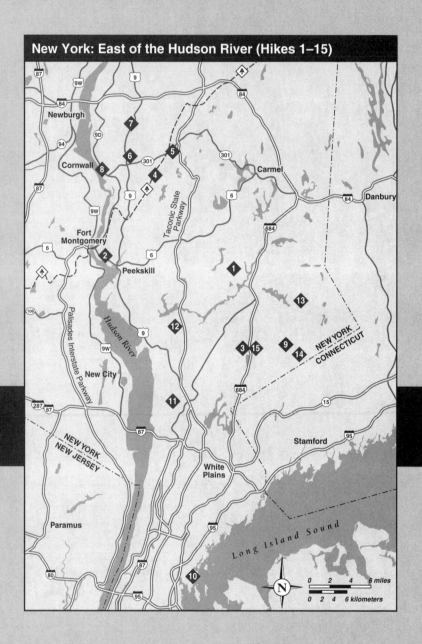

# New York: East of the Hudson River (Hikes 1–15)

# NEW YORK:
## EAST OF THE HUDSON RIVER

# 1  ANGLE FLY AMBLE

## KEY AT-A-GLANCE INFORMATION

**LENGTH:** 5.4 miles

**ELEVATION GAIN:** 1,045 feet

**CONFIGURATION:** 2 connected loops

**DIFFICULTY:** Easy to moderate

**SCENERY:** Rolling terrain, mixed forest, wetlands, and Angle Fly Brook, which bisects the preserve

**EXPOSURE:** Mostly shady

**TRAFFIC:** Mostly light

**TRAIL SURFACE:** Dirt, roots, rocks

**HIKING TIME:** 2.5 hours

**DRIVING DISTANCE:** 40 miles

**SEASON:** Year-round, sunrise–sunset

**ACCESS:** Free; no dogs

**MAPS:** Download from tinyurl.com /angleflymap

**FACILITIES:** Outhouse in parking lot

**COMMENTS:** This is a fairly new preserve and trails are still being developed. Beware of stumbling over small stumps. For details visit somerslandtrust.org.

## GPS COORDINATES

N41° 17.471'  W73° 43.155'

## IN BRIEF

Put away your fishing rod: the fun at Angle Fly has less to do with fly-fishing than with a lively jaunt along densely forested trails. The array of ecosystems highlighted here, from lowland swamps and bogs to upland meadows, from old-growth hardwoods to new-growth cedars and saplings, makes for a memorable hike. Toss in a few stream-hops and a historic ruin, and how can you go wrong?

## DESCRIPTION

Angle Fly Preserve owes its unusual name to the coursing stream, Angle Fly Brook, that bisects it. As for the preserve itself, if not for the concerted and determined efforts of the Westchester Land Trust, the state of New York, and the people of Somers, where it is situated, Angle Fly's 654 acres would have been whittled into a 104-unit townhouse development.

Long before bean-counting investors looked to carve up this land for profit, it was home to the Kitchawanks, an offshoot of the Mohegan tribe. Their word for the area, incidentally, was *Amapaugh,* which translates to "freshwater fish," an especially appropriate moniker given that Angle Fly Brook was once renowned as the Empire State's last source of naturally spawning brook trout. Traces of

## Directions

Drive north on the Henry Hudson Parkway to the Sawmill River Parkway North. Take Exit 6 and turn left on NY 35/Cross River Road. Proceed for 1.6 miles and go right (north) on NY 100/Somerstown Road. Continue 0.6 mile and turn left on NY 139/Primrose Street. Drive 1 mile and enter the preserve on the left. The parking lot is 0.4 mile down the road.

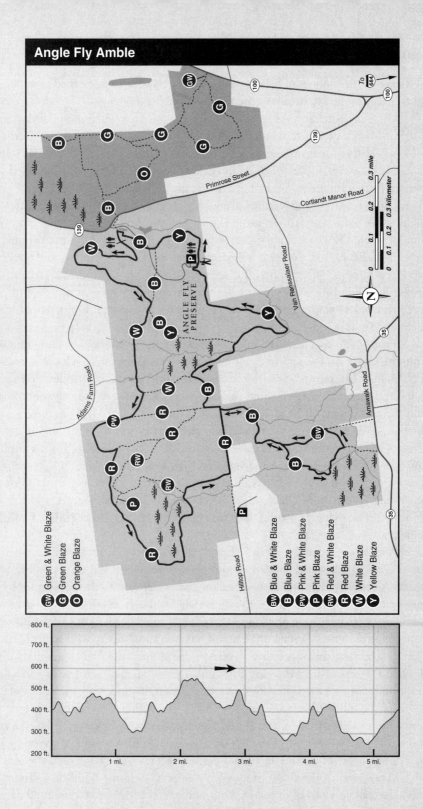

# Angle Fly Amble

**GW** Green & White Blaze
**G** Green Blaze
**O** Orange Blaze

**BW** Blue & White Blaze
**B** Blue Blaze
**PW** Pink & White Blaze
**P** Pink Blaze
**RW** Red & White Blaze
**R** Red Blaze
**W** White Blaze
**Y** Yellow Blaze

ANGLE FLY PRESERVE

To 684

100

139

Primrose Street

Cortlandt Manor Road

Van Rensselaer Road

35

Amawalk Road

35

Adams Farm Road

Hilltop Road

0.3 mile
0.3 kilometer
0.2
0.1
0.2
0.1
0

N

800 ft.
700 ft.
600 ft.
500 ft.
400 ft.
300 ft.
200 ft.

1 mi.    2 mi.    3 mi.    4 mi.    5 mi.

settlements, possibly used by the Kitchawanks, have been unearthed by archeologists along Angle Fly Brook to the north of the preserve.

Once the Kitchawanks were dispossessed, this area fell into one of the "great lots" of Cortlandt Manor that King George III granted to Stephanus Van Cortlandt in 1697. History does not record whether Stephanus enjoyed fly-fishing its waters, but it is known that part of the domain was kept open for pastureland and part was cultivated for crops. So productive was the land that during the Revolutionary War, British troops and various armed vagabonds took to raiding the area for plunder. A particular farmer–turned–local hero reportedly herded his cattle into one of Angle Fly's capacious swamps in order to hide them from the bandits.

In all likelihood, you won't find any cattle in Angle Fly today, and hopefully very few bandits. What you will discover is 654 acres of land that ranges from dense hardwood forests to open grassland, from old-growth woods to sprawling reed-rimmed swamps. There's even the ruin of an old mansion, parts of which date to 1803.

From the kiosk, start the hike by doing an about-face and heading due west into the forest, on the opposite side of the paved parking circle. This Yellow Loop (YL, yellow blazes) diverges in less than 10 yards, as the trail splits. Follow the left-hand path as it tapers behind the sage green outhouse at the edge of the parking lot and begins to head south among a mix of oaks, black birches, various maples, and sere cedars. After initially—and inauspiciously—brushing up against private property, the YL shifts east, then north-northeast, leading you downhill to an open swamp, where the morning sun can be quite striking. The path, now consisting of mowed grass, passes by cattail reeds and a variety of wildflowers, including Queen Anne's lace, ragged Robin, knapweed, goldenrod, and tick trefoil, before arriving at a three-way junction. Switch here to the Blue Trail (BT, blue blazes), bearing right.

Almost immediately, the BT slips through a gap in a stone wall, crosses the paved park road, and then starts steaming slightly uphill, still on a grass-surfaced track. A couple of minutes of easy walking will bring you to the parking lot by the preserve's entrance, just shy of the dilapidated old caretaker's cottage—if it's still standing. With pavement now underfoot, the BT breaks right, but you should swing left, following the old estate drive uphill, marked sporadically with white blazes.

Just as this maple-lined drive levels off, the White Trail (WT) darts to the right, leaving the macadam. Moseying back into the forest, the path passes beneath an enormous beech, a cultivated holdover from when this was domesticated land. The ruins of the old Mediterranean-style mansion are within view to the left, but your route lies straight ahead, or due north. Shortly after ascending a set of low concrete steps, the path steers toward the left through an area of successional scrub, circumnavigating the overgrown estate buildings. In perhaps half a mile, once the trail has arced back toward the south, it meets both the YL and the BT. Roll to the right, with the trail now blazed in yellow, blue, and white, and then—in about 70 paces—roll right again, sticking with the WT when it breaks off.

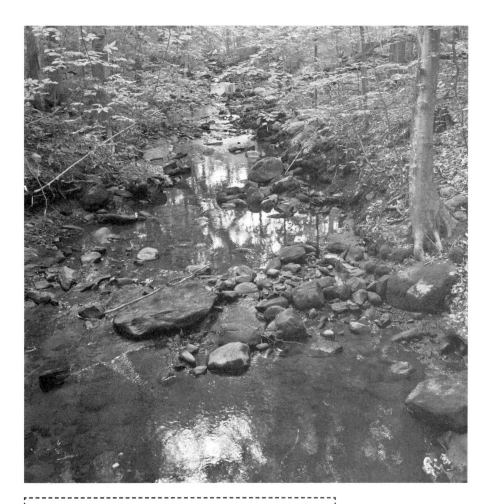

You'll need more than luck to fish Angle Fly Brook in the heat of summer.

In a handful of minutes the WT bends to the left, merging onto an old forest lane. After passing over a couple of streams, the white blazes then break right, departing the grass-surfaced road. When you come to a spur on the right that sports pink-on-white blazes, about 50 yards from the previous turnoff, take it. This shortcut to the Red Loop comes to a junction with another forest road in a couple of minutes, with pink-on-white heaving to the right, and a "Dark Red" trail (as distinct from the Red Loop) going left. Keep right, as the trail, now a little more enclosed by maples, oaks, shagbark hickories, and oversize tulip poplars, forges northward, only to lurch left off the forest road in a few additional strides.

Still strutting with the pink dots? Not for long, as this cutoff ends in a few minutes at a crossing with the Red Loop (RL, red blazes). Hang a right and stick with this route for the next half-hour or so, as it passes by both ends of a pink-blazed spur, neatly avoiding an expansive swamp. Along the way, the RL hops over a stream, joins—and then departs from—a grassy forest road, passes among an overgrowth of nettles and prickers (long pants advisable!), skips by a spur blazed with red crosses, and descends and climbs two steep hillocks. At the base of the second of these, the RL delivers you once again to the Blue Trail. Bear right, back on the BT.

In about a quarter-mile the BT meets a Blue Dot Trail. Keep to the right, still on the BT; you will return on the other path. In an otherwise-undermaintained area of the park, this stretch of trail shows welcome signs of improvement, having been cleared to a two-person width, with many of the pricker plants cut back or removed. There was even a spanking-new bridge evident late in 2012, succeeded by double-length duckboards, both of which aid in getting by the wettest stretches of an appealing swampland.

Veer left when you come to the other end of the Blue Dot Trail, and remain with it to that bit of the BT you traipsed along earlier. Go right there, on the BT, retracing your previous steps all the way back to the intersection with the RL, where you originally turned off. Swing right on that packed-dirt, pebble-strewn forest road and swing right again for about 2 minutes, still sticking with the blue blazes of the BT. A downhill stretch rapidly leads to the terminus of the WT, which you bypass, remaining instead with the BT. And approximately 5 minutes later, shortly after crossing Angle Fly Brook via a substantial bridge, Blue comes to a junction with the Yellow Loop.

In hoofing to the left, you have finally entered the home stretch of the hike. Your imminent arrival at the parking area is heralded by a series of informational signboards on such diverse topics as woodpeckers, red-tailed hawks, tree galls, and miscellaneous ferns.

## NEARBY ACTIVITIES

At **Muscoot Farm**, originally a gentleman's farm from the late 1800s, visitors can explore the original barns and commune with the resident animals. In addition to hiking trails it offers educational interpretive programs. Visit **muscootfarm.org** for more details.

# ANTHONY'S NOSE ASCENT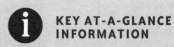

## IN BRIEF

It's not all uphill at Anthony's Nose—it only feels that way for much of the hike. The pay-off for this strenuous out-and-back's double ascent is an extended passage through an eye-fetching series of granite uplift and dramatic outcroppings, as well as one of the most striking vantage points along the entire Hudson River.

## DESCRIPTION

There are almost as many jokes relating to the name of this geological formation as there are explanations for how it came to be so dubbed. But once you get huffing and puffing up the steep and persistent slopes that define the first half of this outing, any smiles that you may have had about picking Anthony's Nose will likely be effaced. Try to keep in mind, however, that the stellar views from atop the crest, both of an impressively wide swath of the Hudson River and of the Bear Mountain Bridge, almost directly below the "nose," are worth every bit of the pain you endure during the grinding double ascent.

This southern tip of the Hudson Highlands has been known as Anthony's Nose since the 1600s, and it was registered as such on a

### KEY AT-A-GLANCE INFORMATION

**LENGTH:** 6.2 miles

**ELEVATION GAIN:** 2,358 feet

**CONFIGURATION:** Out-and-back

**DIFFICULTY:** Strenuous

**SCENERY:** Steeply sloping terrain in deciduous forest with some conifers and many granite outcroppings, leading to magnificent panoramic views

**EXPOSURE:** Some exposure along open ridges

**TRAFFIC:** Very popular

**TRAIL SURFACE:** Dirt, grassy patches, rocks and ledges

**HIKING TIME:** 3.5 hours

**DRIVING DISTANCE:** 39 miles

**SEASON:** Year-round, sunrise–sunset

**ACCESS:** Free; dogs on leash

**MAPS:** At Bear Mountain Bridge Toll House and at trailhead kiosk; USGS *Peekskill*

**FACILITIES:** Outhouse at trailhead

**COMMENTS:** Please yield the trail right-of-way when you encounter military personnel. The summit is a great raptor-observation point.

------------------------------------------

## *Directions* ⟶

**Drive north on the Henry Hudson Parkway to the Sawmill River Parkway North. Take Exit 25 and turn left on NY 9A. Proceed for 9.4 miles, then go left on US 9 North. Continue 8.5 miles and turn left on US 9 North/US 6 West/US 202 West. After 0.2 mile enter a roundabout and take the second exit for US 6 West/US 202 West. Drive 1 mile to the parking lot at the Bear Mountain Toll House, on the right.**

## GPS COORDINATES

N41° 18.088'  W73° 57.076'

# Anthony's Nose Ascent

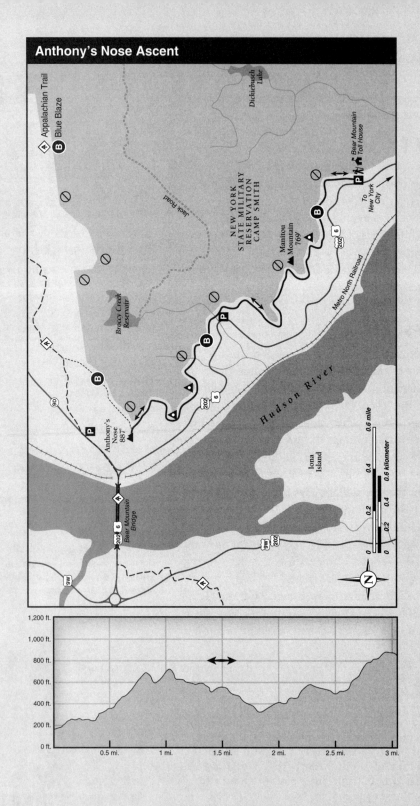

◈ Appalachian Trail
Ⓑ Blue Blaze

*Dickiebusch Lake*

*Jack Road*

NEW YORK STATE MILITARY RESERVATION CAMP SMITH

*Broccy Creek Reservoir*

Manitou Mountain 769'

Bear Mountain Toll House

To New York City

Metro North Railroad

202
6

Anthony's Nose 887'

90

202
6

*Hudson River*

Iona Island

0.6 mile
0.2    0.4
0.6 kilometer
0    0.2    0.4

202 6
Bear Mountain Bridge

9W

9W 202

N

1,200 ft.
1,000 ft.
800 ft.
600 ft.
400 ft.
200 ft.
0 ft.

0.5 mi.    1 mi.    1.5 mi.    2 mi.    2.5 mi.    3 mi.

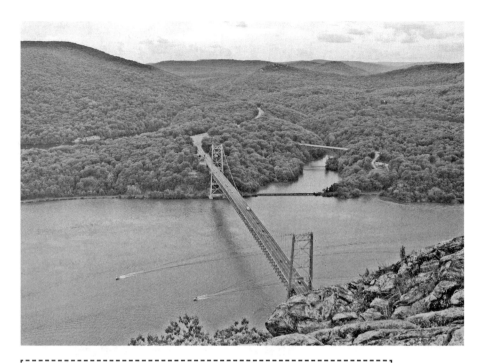

The Bear Mountain Bridge, at the foot of Anthony's Nose, carries the Appalachian Trail across the Hudson River.

grant patent in 1697. Pierre Van Cortlandt, who owned the land, claimed it was named for a Captain Anthony Hogan, whose Bergerackian nose was compared to the peak by one of his seamen when they sailed past it. Another account holds that the "nose" was a part of the Saint Anthony's Face formation of nearby Breakneck Ridge, a feature that was later destroyed by quarrying. And in his *History of New York,* Washington Irving puts forward the name of Antony Van Corlear as the likely origin of its name. Van Corlear, a trumpeter for New Amsterdam's garrison, was sent by Peter Stuyvesant up the river in 1642 to alert the Hudson Valley villagers of an imminent attack by the British, and he reportedly drowned while trying to swim across the river.

It is unlikely that you will face any such water hazards on your own march up the mountain, although a notice at the trailhead kiosk by the Bear Mountain Toll House does caution that the path is occasionally used by soldiers from neighboring Camp Smith, an outpost of New York's national guard. The bulletin reads, in part, "Do not be surprised to find military personnel using the trail, possibly carrying heavy packs and rifles. Please yield the right of way to them." Although we'd be willing to yield the right of way to armed *turtles*—let alone troops—we have yet to encounter either on the numerous occasions we've done this hike.

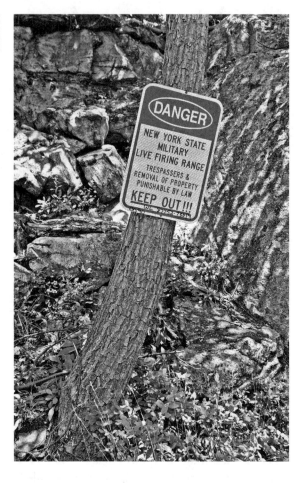

Don't cross this line unless you're ready to enlist.

When you embark from the Bear Mountain Toll House, you will actually have two peaks to look forward to summiting, with Manitou Mountain separating you from Anthony's Nose. With the road on your left side, head north from the kiosk, striking uphill on the blue-blazed Camp Smith Trail. The grass soon gives way to bare dirt, pocked with many loose and protruding stones, as the trail soars upward. The angular granite bedrock around you, colored in places by short-stemmed sassafras, blueberry shrubs, and other low-lying plants, is quite similar to the scenery elsewhere in the Hudson Highlands. What is unique to this stretch of trail is the yellow polypropylene rope that has been slung from oak to maple, one tree to the next, off to the right of the trail. This is a "do not cross" line that marks the park's border with Camp Smith, a prohibition that is spelled out more directly through the periodic placement of red and white warning signs.

The elevation gain comes rapidly once you are north of the trail register box (empty our last time through), in passing among a picturesque jumble of craggy rocks and massive erratics, rising high above the road. Yet, just as quickly, the path levels off and then, once by a seasonal streambed, descends. Of course, another steep climb ensues, this time aided by a set of crudely fashioned stone steps. The ascent through this lush, granite-studded landscape is interrupted by a break in the dense forest by a rocky shelf. Take a moment on this chunk of bedrock to catch your breath while soaking up the splendid view of the Hudson River, with Jones Point directly across the water. From here, the trail ascends through one of its more pleasing stretches, in which the glacial uplift achieves a level of high drama.

The climb grows less steep as the path threads through a copse of young birch trees, amid knee-high ferns and blueberry shrubs, ultimately rewarding you with yet another vista point, this one far broader than the previous. And then, shortly after this grand panorama, your descent from Manitou Mountain begins. There's a leveling off—briefly—amid a verdant pocket-meadow that is reminiscent of our favorite approach to Harriman State Park's Lemon Squeezer—followed by a resumption of the downhill traipse, all the way back to US 6 (albeit farther north than your starting point). Instead of dwelling on this disappointing development, bear right at the kiosk and get back in the saddle, slogging upward again with the blue blazes as your guide.

Although the trail surface borders at times on abominable, this second ascent is less strenuous than the first, with uphill stretches alternating with short spells of even ground. In about 15 minutes you should reach a protruding ledge that provides a great view of the Bear Mountain Bridge, and the marshes of Iona Island to its left. The subsequent shelf, a couple of minutes up-trail, also provides a Hudson view, albeit with more limited visibility through tree cover. From there, the path shoots inland across the granite, then indulges in some minor switchbacks to draw you higher still, meanwhile showcasing several impressive boulders. And then, just like that, you're standing on the angular, fractured dome atop Anthony's Nose, 880 feet above the river, with a number of scrub oaks all around you.

For the best views, stick with the Camp Smith Trail a few minutes longer. It drops off the dome on its north side (use care in winter, when it may be coated in ice) and almost immediately comes to a fork. Bear left, even as the blue blazes branch off to the right, and in a minute or two you will reach a broad granite outcropping, large enough to serve several hiking groups at once. From this Olympian outpost you can stare down at the bridge and the roiling waters of the Hudson, and wait for hawks, vultures, and the occasional eagle to fly by.

This is the turnaround point of the hike, though if time permits, you might consider exploring the other fork for a few hundred yards. More of a jeep road now than a forest trail, it initially cuts through some gorgeous scenery, rolling grassy turf well colored by various erratics, before meeting the Appalachian Trail in about half a mile.

## NEARBY ACTIVITIES

In addition to plenty of excellent hiking opportunities in the area, the following cultural gem is well worth visiting: the **Russel Wright Design Center**, in Garrison, just up NY 9D. Attractively landscaped Manitoga is the unique onetime home and studio of a leading U.S. designer. More information at **russelwrightcenter.org.**

# 3 BUTLER OUTER LOOP TRAIL

### KEY AT-A-GLANCE INFORMATION

**LENGTH:** 3.1 miles

**ELEVATION GAIN:** 675 feet

**CONFIGURATION:** Loop

**DIFFICULTY:** Easy

**SCENERY:** Lush deciduous forest with a few stands of conifers, swamps, streams, rock outcroppings, and a few steep hills

**EXPOSURE:** Shady

**TRAFFIC:** Light

**TRAIL SURFACE:** Dirt, rocks, and roots

**HIKING TIME:** 1.5 hours

**DRIVING DISTANCE:** 32 miles

**SEASON:** Year-round, sunrise–sunset

**ACCESS:** Free; no bicycles, dogs on leash; bridle trails

**MAPS:** At trailhead kiosk; download from tinyurl.com/butlersanctuary; USGS *Mount Kisco*

**FACILITIES:** None, but the Westmoreland Sanctuary, across the street, has restrooms and water.

**COMMENTS:** Bring binoculars and climb up to the bleachers of the Robert J. Hammerschlag Memorial Hawk Watch to observe raptors during their fall migration, mid-August–mid-November. For further information, call the Bedford Audubon Society at 914-666-6177 or visit tinyurl.com/arthurwbutler.

## GPS COORDINATES

N41° 10.934' W73° 41.196'

## IN BRIEF

*Boulders and bog crossings, hilltops and*
    *hemlocks,*
*Beech trees and pine groves, rock-hopping*
    *ravine romps,*
*Granite-strewn gorges and hawks flapping*
    *wings;*
*These are a few of our favorite things. . . .*

## DESCRIPTION

On lacing up your boots and heading into the Butler Sanctuary, a Nature Conservancy preserve, you will hardly be traveling to Timbuktu. It may seem that way, though, for while it's a scant half-mile from the Westmoreland Sanctuary, the bite-size Butler sees very few visitors—none at all on some of the days we've trekked through. Sure, at a mere 363 acres, it can feel hemmed in by suburbia on three sides and I-684 on its fourth. But once you set off into the woods, into its deep ravines and thriving marshlands, you'll hardly be aware of the outside world.

The roar of traffic racing along nearby I-684 is, unfortunately, omnipresent as soon as you step out of your vehicle. Don't despair, though, and by all means don't get back into your car and drive off. Once over the initial ridge, you can lose the earplugs, as the sounds of "civilization" recede, eclipsed by the rustle

----------------------------------------

## *Directions*

**Take the Hutchinson River Parkway North and keep left onto I-684 North. Drive to Exit 3N and merge onto NY 22 North. Continue for 3.4 miles and turn left onto Chestnut Ridge Road. Proceed for 1.5 miles, then hang a left across the bridge and park straight ahead.**

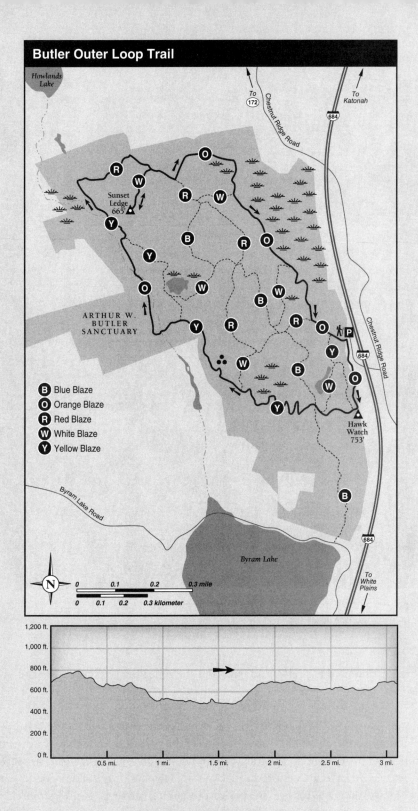

# Butler Outer Loop Trail

Howlands Lake

To (172)

Chestnut Ridge Road

To Katonah

684

**R** **W** **O** **R** **W** **O** **Y** Sunset Ledge 665' **O** **Y** **B** **R** **O** **W** **W** **B** **O** P Chestnut Ridge Road 684

ARTHUR W. BUTLER SANCTUARY

**Y** **R** **R** **O** **Y** **W** **B** **Y** **W** **O**

Hawk Watch 753'

**B** Blue Blaze
**O** Orange Blaze
**R** Red Blaze
**W** White Blaze
**Y** Yellow Blaze

Byram Lake Road

**B**

Byram Lake

684

To White Plains

N

0   0.1   0.2   0.3 mile
0   0.1   0.2   0.3 kilometer

1,200 ft.
1,000 ft.
800 ft.
600 ft.
400 ft.
200 ft.
0 ft.

0.5 mi.   1 mi.   1.5 mi.   2 mi.   2.5 mi.   3 mi.

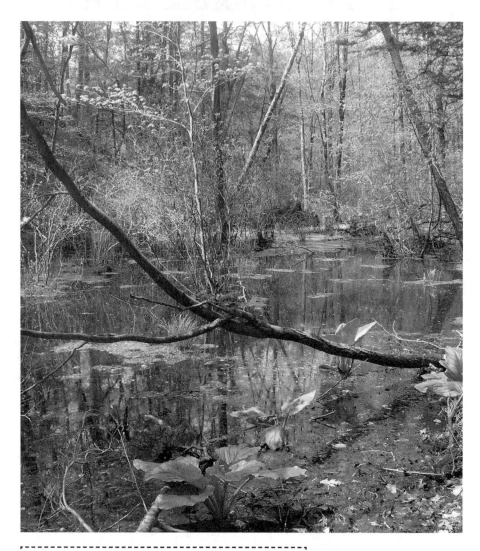

The trail hugs this lush jungle swamp at the heart of the sanctuary.

of breezes among the birches and oaks and the squealing cries of hawks and kestrels soaring high overhead.

To observe those raptors in flight during the autumn migration, a row of bleacher seats faces the open sky to the east. To reach that, and begin this hike, turn left, or south, at the dark-brown fence by the parking area and march directly uphill along the orange-blazed trail. Even if you fail to see a raptor (the migratory period runs from mid-August through mid-November), you should be able to spot the weathervane-topped steeple of the nature center at the Westmoreland Sanctuary across the highway. The trail, changing from orange to yellow blazes, veers inland here (to the right), passing among catbrier, sugar maples, oaks, beech trees, hemlocks, and a handful of pines.

The yellow-blazed trail begins to undulate, shifting first downhill past a white-tagged route to the right, succeeded shortly by an intersection with a path sporting blue swatches. Stick with yellow as it then rises through a gap in an old stone wall before descending steeply. This is an ankle-twisting stretch, where the trail narrows and involves a couple of rocky switchbacks, so be careful of your footing. A few well-placed stepping-stones by the fern-dappled marsh at the bottom are helpful in crossing the stream. Moving upward again, the track tops out by a series of granite boulders, offering a fine view over the swamp. With the hemlocks growing thicker here and animal trails adding to the confusion, you may have to be part bloodhound to sniff out the blazes. In a preserve this size, though, there is little chance of getting seriously lost.

As the trail briefly lingers on this higher ground, it swings slightly to the left and works along the saddle between two ridges before descending 25 feet or so into a small gully. Atop the next rise, where the ground is covered in sedge grass and granite and maples dominate, are a couple of old rock foundations, relics from the 1800s when this area was open farmland. Staying with the sparsely placed yellow blazes, edge gently to the left of the ruins, keeping to the left, or west, of the rocky knob. The terrain tapers downward from here, becoming rather steep before leveling off at an overgrown swamp. If you're feeling bogged down, watch for a white-blazed turnoff to the right that can be used as an early bailout back to the parking lot.

The yellow-tagged track wends onward between two rock walls and a marsh made all the greener by the presence of skunk cabbage and ferns. As you start to grind uphill again, keep a sharp eye out once more for yellow markings, though if you have a decent sense of direction, moseying off the path won't pose any risks. The undulating trace continues, but you should lilt left on the orange-blazed spur (just prior to a series of stones that are laid out like a narrow stretch of sidewalk to help ford a particularly moist patch of marshland). Remain with orange as it draws you first up a low, rocky bluff and then alongside a swampy, slowly moving stream, finally crossing the water at the base of an impressive bluff. Hang a left there, back on yellow, but before doing so consider reclining on one of the many lichen-crusted rocks and soaking up the wild, rough-hewn atmosphere of the ravine, where the low ground is littered with boulders.

This trail terminates at the far corner of the sanctuary, near a softly purling stream, its muddy banks festooned with oversized ferns. Roll right onto the red-blazed path and begin the steady climb uphill. Don't let the effort distract you, though, from the surroundings; we once spotted a herd of seven deer here snorting lustily through the oaks just below the ridge. The elevation gain over the course of 200 yards is perhaps 150 feet, though it may feel like more. Shortly after the crest, a poorly marked side trail to the right (GPS: N41° 11.337' W73° 41.831'), blazed white, leads to Sunset Ledge, about a quarter-mile away. The westward view from there is expansive, covering miles of hills, open sky, and a fair amount of new housing.

Back on the red trail, the walking remains relatively level and easy all the way to a left-hand turn onto the path marked with orange blazes. Long pants are a good buffer against the swarms of mosquitoes that thrive in Butler, and such garb is almost essential to get through the thicket of briar that encroaches on a lengthy part of this next stretch. That briar, incidentally, and the presence of blueberry bushes make this a popular area for foraging deer. (If you're here in summer, be on the lookout as well for such colorful wildflowers as wood lilies and butter-and-eggs.) As the trail descends, it parallels an old stone wall and a reed-rimmed swamp before coming to a vast network of rock walls that were once used for holding livestock.

Moving away from the swamp, you should see a white-blazed spur to the right, which runs back to the red-tagged track. Follow the orange markings and, in a fairly straightforward quarter-mile, a larger swamp appears left of you, with tulip trees thriving up the rocky slope to the right. The trail here threads over and around sundry stones and trees, requiring sharp eyes to find the elusive blazes. Drifting away from the marsh, the circuit showcases a few white pines and straggly cedars before rejoining, at the top of a small hill, the red-blazed route. You will notice as you go left that the roar of the highway has reasserted itself, and your hike is nearly at an end. With the parking lot only a couple of minutes ahead, just past the trail register kiosk, it is time to once more make use of those earplugs.

## NEARBY ACTIVITIES

When we're feeling energetic, we like to combine this hike with a longer spin through the **Westmoreland Sanctuary** (Hike 15), less than half a mile away. There's also the recently created **Angle Fly Preserve,** in nearby Somers (Hike 1).

History buffs should enjoy the **John Jay Homestead State Historic Site,** which is the farmhouse—maintained with period furnishings—where the first U.S. chief justice retired; it's on NY 22 in Katonah. For information, call 914-232-5651 or visit **johnjayhomestead.org.**

# FAHNESTOCK CATFISH LOOP

## IN BRIEF

These fun trails undulate so much you may be reminded of a roller-coaster ride. From moss-rimmed swamps to granite-struck ridges, this hike passes through an extraordinary clutch of boulders and includes a side trip to a hidden pond that appears to have been forgotten by time.

## DESCRIPTION

While Fahnestock State Park may lack the beautiful bald-dome qualities of Harriman State Park, or the rugged ascents and the almost cult-like appeal of the Hudson Highlands, it is most definitely the kind of park that grows on you. Sometimes, as we wander the trails deep in its boundless forests, it seems as though we've stumbled into a land that time forgot. From farmhouse ruins to intriguing remnants of 19th-century mining, from hidden lakes to secret pathways leading to a lonesome, abandoned reservoir, Fahnestock would appear to have all the essential ingredients of a gothic mystery. Add to that an abundance of wildlife and a natural setting that has been unsullied for generations, and you should find the hiking just as rewarding cerebrally as it is physically.

-------------------------------------------

*Directions* ———————————————→

**Drive north on the Henry Hudson Parkway to the Sawmill River Parkway North. Take Exit 25 and turn left on NY 9A. Proceed for 9.4 miles, then go left on US 9 North. Continue 8.5 miles and turn left on US 9 North/US 6 West/US 202 West. After 0.2 mile enter a roundabout and take the first exit onto US 9 North/Albany Post Road. Drive 10.3 miles, then go right on NY 301. After 2.6 miles turn right on Dennytown Road. The parking lot is 1.2 miles down the road, on the left.**

### KEY AT-A-GLANCE INFORMATION

**LENGTH:** 4.8 miles

**ELEVATION GAIN:** 745 feet

**CONFIGURATION:** Loop

**DIFFICULTY:** Easy

**SCENERY:** Dense deciduous forest, rocky ledges and boulder fields, lush wetlands, and a hidden lake, with a few steps along the Appalachian Trail

**EXPOSURE:** Thick, shady canopy in summer

**TRAFFIC:** Very light

**TRAIL SURFACE:** Very rocky with grassy stretches

**HIKING TIME:** 2.5 hours

**DRIVING DISTANCE:** 52 miles

**SEASON:** Year-round, sunrise–sunset

**ACCESS:** Free; pets on leash not exceeding 10 feet, no bikes, no motorized vehicles, no horses

**MAPS:** At park headquarters on north side of NY 301, 0.6 mile west of Taconic Parkway; download from tinyurl.com/fahnestockmspmap; USGS *Oscawana Lake*

**FACILITIES:** No restrooms or water on trails, but Canopus Beach, in the state park, has both and much more.

**COMMENTS:** Hunting is permitted in season; call 845-225-7207. For an overview of other activities, visit nysparks.com/parks/133/details.aspx.

## GPS COORDINATES

N41° 25.241'  W73° 52.122'

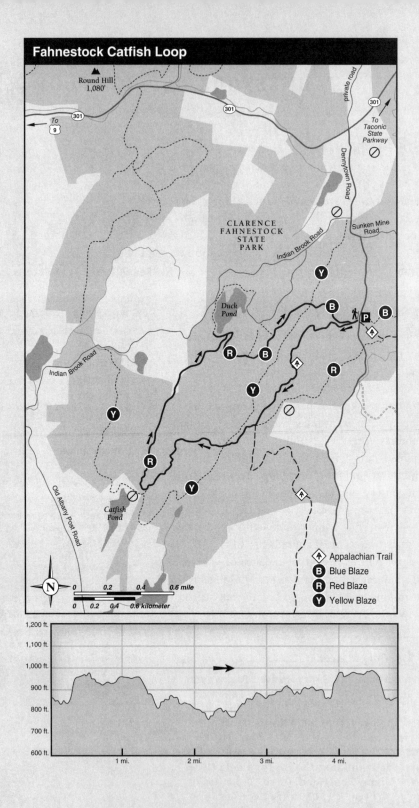

# Fahnestock Catfish Loop

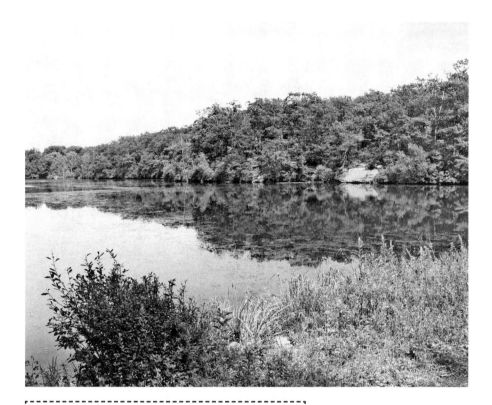

It takes some route-finding skills to discover peaceful Duck Pond.

Of the many possible hikes you might do in Fahnestock, the following serves as a great introduction to the area's wonderful allure. Although the Catfish Loop is relatively easy, at a hair under 5 miles and with a cumulative elevation gain of just 745 feet, it packs so much colorful scenery you'll probably return, like us, time and time again.

Be sure to pick up a park map at the kiosk before setting off from the gravel-and-dirt parking lot. Not only will it help guide you on this hike, you'll hopefully feel inspired to return at a later point to investigate some of Fahnestock's many other trails. With that folded slip of paper secure in your pocket, turn away from the kiosk (and the photogenic stone house ruin nearby) and cross the road. The trail, marked with both the blue blazes of the Three Lakes Trail (TLT) and the long white slash of the Appalachian Trail (AT), descends through a patch of poison ivy and wild grapes into the cover of a young forest of tulip poplars, birches, and oaks, with pricker bushes and lush ferns on either side of you. Almost immediately the TLT forks to the right; stick with the AT, straight onward. From dropping down through an old stone wall, the moss-limned path then starts climbing up a rock-strewn slope, with a couple of switchbacks making that effort akin to child's play. And so begins a delightful stretch of the AT atop a bedrock ridge well

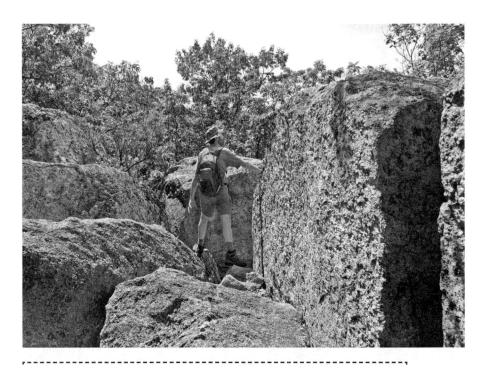

This secluded zone of giant lichen-speckled boulders makes a surprise appearance in the middle of the loop.

speckled with lichen and tufts of grass, with plenty of sunlight filtering through the surrounding laurels and birch trees.

Did we forget to mention boulders and extensive outcroppings? There are plenty of those, too, along this route, in addition to blueberry shrubs and lots of moss. All of which adds up to a subtle, almost subliminal, beauty that persists for much of the loop. You will leave the AT after 1.1 miles, turning right at the junction with the Catfish Loop trail (CL, red blazes), hard by an enormous segment of granite uplift. Fear not, the undulating attractiveness of the hike continues, even as the CL hops over a bridle trail (yellow blazes), troughs at a swampy stream (careful of the wobbly rock-crossing), and—now heading west— summits atop another narrow, sun-exposed rock ridge. From this brief glimpse through the trees of the western hills, the CL then pivots south, rapidly delivering you to one of this hike's true highlights, a clenched cataclysm of boulders, vaguely reminiscent of the megaliths at Schunemunk. If you packed a lunch or snack, this glacier-created clash of cyclopean rocks is the spot in which to enjoy it. Go ahead, climb on top of the tripe-crusted formation and soak up the views while you're enjoying a bite.

Back on the trail, 10 minutes of easy strolling will bring you to another swamp, where amid the ferns and moss the CL then heaves right, to the north-northwest, beginning the return stretch of the loop. Ignore the unblazed social trails in this area, and stay with the CL as it initially holds to the right side of a low ridge before finally ascending it. Note as you amble along how a few white pines and miscellaneous firs have appeared, further contributing to the primeval feeling of the forest. An aura that is additionally augmented, incidentally, by a trail so underused that it is overgrown in a couple of places, and occasionally poorly marked.

Although this hike does not lead to its namesake Catfish Pond, there *is* a connector trail to Duck Pond. The only problem is that spur is very difficult to spot. The easiest way to find it is by actually walking past it, to the point at which the CL reaches its northernmost point and begins to tack to the east. Just before that stage, shortly after you have passed over an extended bedrock plateau (and the highest elevation of the ridge), there is a narrow trace on the left (west) side of the trail, well hidden by undergrowth (GPS: N41° 25.174' W73° 53.033'). Look for it a step or two before the tree marked with staggered blazes, indicating the trail's shift to right, or do as we often do and backtrack to it from that arcing bend. Don't worry, tight as the spur is to start, it grows wider as you shuffle through the shrubbery, and in a couple of minutes you'll hit a nucleus of social trails. Keep going straight, as the path climbs some low rocks and ultimately reaches the southern foot of Duck Pond. Cross the stone dam, and after that a car bridge, and enjoy the solitude of this isolated setting, where such wildflowers as Deptford pink, Queen Anne's lace, and mullion grow abundantly. At the west end of this embankment, atop the stone uplift, are the white blazes of another trail, but save that exploration for another day, as this is your turnaround point.

If you succeeded in making your way out to Duck Pond (and back!), you should find the remainder of the return a snap. The CL, tailing from east to south, zigzags around various rocks and boulders, and then, eastbound again and losing ground, comes to an unceremonious end, its red blazes being replaced by the blue ones of the Three Lakes Trail. In something like six-tenths of a mile, the path jumps over the same bridle trail (yellow blazes) you crossed earlier and passes, along its route back to the closure of the loop, a couple of lush green swamps and no end of picturesque granite uplift. When the TLT rejoins the AT, you'll find the trailhead just a few strides farther on.

## NEARBY ACTIVITIES

From late March to late October, visitors can marvel at the horticultural creations of **Stonecrop Gardens,** in Cold Spring. For its bloom calendar and other programs, visit **stonecrop.org/index_cal_view.php.**

# 5  FAHNESTOCK GREATER HIDDEN LAKE TOUR

## IN BRIEF

Relatively smooth, wide pathways make this a foot-friendly environment, one in which you may see an array of avians at any of three ponds and their related wetlands. Glacial erratics, rocky uplift, ridgetop rambles, and a dynamic stream-crossing lend extra frisson to the shady terrain, while an elusive air of mystery emanates from the overgrown remnants of 19th-century iron-mining operations.

## DESCRIPTION

Don't be put off by the fact that Clarence Fahnestock State Park is smack in the middle of densely populated Putnam County. In combination with the Hubbard-Perkins Conservation Area, Fahnestock measures 11,000 acres and is the largest preserve in the entire Taconic area. Admittedly, when most people think of this facility, its sandy-shored Canopus Lake comes to mind. Others, hooked on angling, view the park's many other lakes and ponds as prime line-casting waters for pickerel, perch, bass, and trout.

Which is not to suggest that hiking in Fahnestock has all the appeal of a plunge into the Harlem River on a frosty November night.

## KEY AT-A-GLANCE INFORMATION

**LENGTH:** 9.7 miles

**ELEVATION GAIN:** 1,410 feet

**CONFIGURATION:** 3 connected loops

**DIFFICULTY:** Moderate

**SCENERY:** Dense deciduous forest with laurel patches and conifers, talus slopes, rock outcroppings, lush wetlands, three bodies of water, iron mine pits, and a 0.75-mile piece of the Appalachian Trail

**EXPOSURE:** Thick, shady canopy in summer, minimal exposure

**TRAFFIC:** Popular on weekends, otherwise light

**TRAIL SURFACE:** Mostly dirt with rocky and sandy stretches

**HIKING TIME:** 4.5 hours

**DRIVING DISTANCE:** 54.3 miles

**SEASON:** Year-round, sunrise–sunset

**ACCESS:** Free; pets on leash not exceeding 10 feet, no bikes, no motorized vehicles, no horses

**MAPS:** At park headquarters on north side of NY 301, 0.6 mile west of Taconic Parkway; download from tinyurl.com/fahnestockmspmap; USGS *Oscawana Lake*

**FACILITIES:** Canopus Beach, in the state park, has restrooms, water, and more.

**COMMENTS:** Hunting is permitted in season; call 845-225-7207. For other activities, visit nysparks.com /parks/133/details.aspx.

## GPS COORDINATES

N41° 27.170'  W73° 50.194'

*Directions* ————————————→

**Drive north on the Henry Hudson Parkway to the Sawmill River Parkway North. Take Exit 25 and turn left on NY 9A. Proceed for 9.4 miles, then go left on US 9 North. Continue 8.5 miles and turn left on US 9 North/US 6 West/US 202 West. After 0.2 mile enter a roundabout and take the first exit onto US 9 North/Albany Post Road. Drive 10.3 miles, then go right on NY 301. Proceed for 4.7 miles to the parking area by the lake, but both sides of the road have options.**

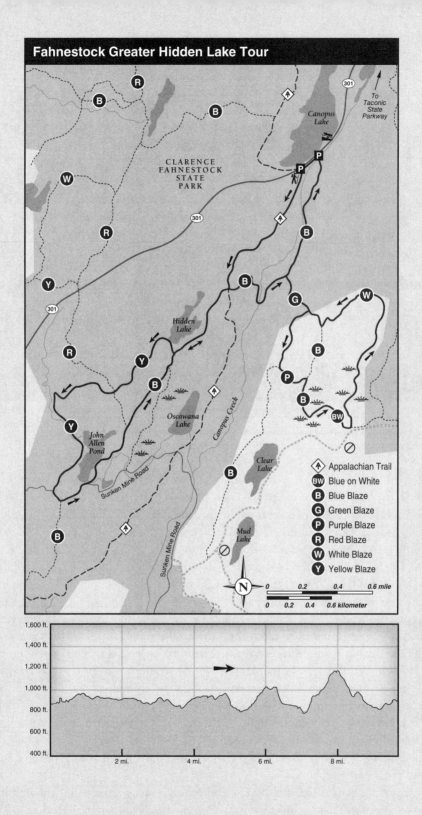

# Fahnestock Greater Hidden Lake Tour

CLARENCE
FAHNESTOCK
STATE
PARK

Canopus
Lake

301

To
Taconic
State
Parkway

Hidden
Lake

Oscawana
Lake

John
Allen
Pond

Sunken Mine Road

Canopus Creek

Clear
Lake

Mud
Lake

Sunken Mine Road

301

### Legend

- Appalachian Trail
- BW Blue on White
- B Blue Blaze
- G Green Blaze
- P Purple Blaze
- R Red Blaze
- W White Blaze
- Y Yellow Blaze

0    0.2    0.4    0.6 mile

0    0.2    0.4    0.6 kilometer

N

1,600 ft.
1,400 ft.
1,200 ft.
1,000 ft.
800 ft.
600 ft.
400 ft.

2 mi.    4 mi.    6 mi.    8 mi.

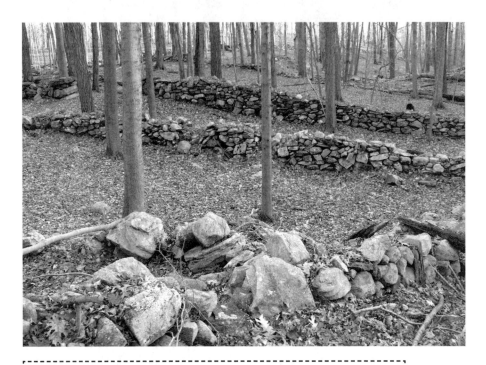

Field of dreams? These long rows of stone walls mark the borders of bygone pasture land.

On the contrary, most of the park's many miles of trails, including a portion of the Appalachian Trail (AT), run through dense, undertrafficked forestland. What the setting may lack in the dramatic peaks and views of the nearby Hudson Highlands, it more than compensates for in seclusion, tranquility, and a sublime sort of beauty.

The 9.7-mile Hidden Lake Tour is so secluded, in fact, you may have trouble finding its trailhead. From your parking spot just west of Canopus Lake, on the south side of the road, drop down off the shoulder by the end of the guardrail and pick up the white blazes of the AT. Keep right along the wide, well-trammeled track, where ferns decorate the rising ridge to the right, a stream courses noisily below to the left, and glacial erratics and hemlocks are scattered all around.

As the AT flows from the dense cover of conifers to a more open array of oak, maple, and beech trees, you will find that it is unusually well graded and slightly elevated from the forest floor—the curious effects of having been laid out over a defunct narrow-gauge rail line that was used in the 19th century to transport locally mined iron ore. Walking along this higher ground gives you an advantage in spotting wildlife, with wild turkeys among the more abundant of those that roam these parts.

In about half a mile, mountain laurel begins to crowd the path, making for a pretty pink floral display in early June. Follow the turnoff soon thereafter to the left, a rerouting due either to habitat restoration or flooded ground from work on the dam, according to a pair of contradictory signs posted there. This short side spur covers rocky land, where the occasional downed tree adds to the obstacle course, before depositing you on the other side of the loop. Turn right there, leaving the AT as it drifts onward (the left branch brings you back to the trailhead), with blue blazes guiding the way.

This is a scenic stretch, enhanced by a partial view of the not-so-well-hidden Hidden Lake to the right. Within 10 minutes, though, you'll be venturing off it to the right, onto a yellow-blazed spur. Although short, this yellow track has the virtue of heading directly to the southwest side of Hidden Lake, among knee-high sedge grass and wild grapes, where tall reeds fringe the shore and lilies dot its jade-green surface. When the water level is high, you'll need to rock-hop by the lakeside and possibly even wrestle with tall weeds to get through. When it is low, the entire lake may indeed be hidden—by mud. Stay to the left at the next junction, back on the trail from which you were diverted earlier, with yellow blazes now marking the trees.

Moving toward the third cut-through, which you ignore, there is an impressively large boulder with two black birches rising up against its side, as if they alone had checked it from tumbling farther down the hill. John Allen Pond comes into view just beyond the intersection. Perhaps 500 yards later, the grassy track bends to the right of a marshy gully and bends back again, and then the yellow blazes veer left off the smooth railroad grade. Follow them into the thicket of mountain laurel. With that shift, a more wild forest unfolds, as large stones poke through the surface of the path, which zigzags left and right past one large block of granite after another.

This leg connects momentarily to a second railroad bed, then spins by a couple of boggy spots and a series of slag heaps and mining holes. Some stepping-stones simplify a sticky stream crossing, but beware of that slippery moss. At the southwest side of the pond, where its overgrown edge is out of reach through a thicket, the trail jumps abruptly to the right, climbs over a moss-covered shelf of rocks and lichen-speckled talus, then swings toward the pond again. A couple of stone walls precede the next junction, where you stick to the left. The yellow-blazed trail ends in a few dozen yards, once by another group of slag heaps. Take a left onto the dirt-and-gravel road, and in roughly half a furlong you'll see a blue-blazed path join this route from the right. Continue straight and do the same at the next fork, in maybe 100 yards. The jeep road circles around toward the pond, and 50 feet from a walk-down access point to the water, the blue blazes lead you left, back into the forest.

From this overgrown, undertrafficked locale, the trail creeps below the concrete dam of the pond, where a few well-positioned stepping-stones ease the way across a stream that can be quite challenging after a heavy rain. For a brief spell, you'll walk on top of a narrow leg of the dam before returning to the darkness of the forest. Bear to the right of the enormous oak, which measures 5 feet in diameter, and as you encounter a second phragmites marsh, take a good look around.

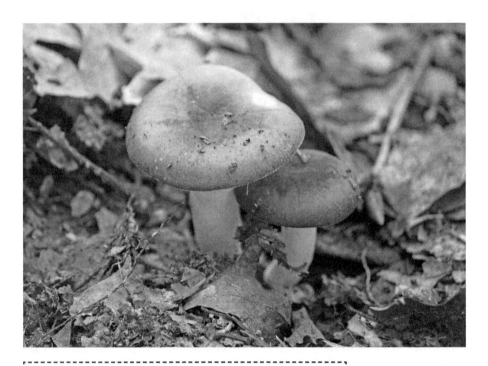

This snug duo is a member of the large and mostly inedible *Russula* family.

This area of aged oaks was formerly a hive of mining activity, its once-scarred ground now covered with grass and near a full recovery. If you're not in a hurry, you might wander off to the right once the path widens to explore other such remnants of ore mining. Otherwise, steer left to continue the tour.

For a time, you will be treading over rolling turf, passing from a setting of rugged, glacial erratics to an environment of fairly open, grassy swaths, punctuated by a healthy sprinkling of oaks, birches, and beeches. You should soon recognize the area you detoured through earlier, between the yellow-blazed option to the left and the intersection with the AT. Remain with Blue through the latter, as further undulations ensue, with the narrow path corralled by prickers and blueberry bushes.

After descending into an appealingly antediluvian concentration of hemlocks, the trail meets yet another stream, this one swelling up to 10 feet wide during periods of wet weather. Rock-hop across and then enjoy the view of that flowing water as you parallel it, heading east-northeast, for the next few minutes. On reaching the moss-covered forest road, Blue breaks to the left; if you're ready to call it quits, follow those markings all the way back to the road, reducing the hike by 3.5 miles. Otherwise, swing right on the green-blazed route to the right.

This mini-loop showcases a less-trammeled area of the park, rising to a series of isolated ridges and descending to a lowland swamp, while bringing a couple of impressive escarpments into high relief. Bear right with the blue blazes, about 15 yards after you see a large white sign, and march up to higher ground, where mountain laurel, scrub oak, and catbrier festoon the rocky surroundings. This modest elevation gain will be lost once you lunge left on the Purple Trail (GPS: N41° 26.250' W73° 50.330'), which speedily descends and dead-ends at a forest road. Step through the gap in the wall and trot to the right, again pursuing blue blazes, then dog it to the left when the forest road meets a junction with a similarly wide track, now sticking with blue dot on white markings. Proceed straight at the termination of the blue dots, as the swatches on the trees become all-white, and in 20 yards, in an area honeycombed with old farm walls, shift with those markings off the forest road. The ensuing ascent is the most prolonged of the day, encompassing three crests, with glimpses of Wiccopee Reservoir possible from two of them—when the trees are bare of leaves.

Remain with the haphazardly applied white blazes as the path circles north, then west, and drops off the rocky bluff, finally rolling right on Blue upon your return to the forest road (GPS: N41° 26.441' W73° 50.051'). In less than 5 minutes, the road delivers you to the spot where Blue earlier broke free from Green; keep to the right on the latter and retrace your steps back to the main trail, where you turn right, following blue blazes. Hang with this path past additional slag heaps, as the circuit dives deep within the hemlock canopy, before returning you to the road. Take a left on the unmarked frontage path there, and you should find your car directly ahead.

## NEARBY ACTIVITIES

**Canopus Beach** is the place to relax after a hot hike, with boating, swimming, fishing, picnicking, and even showering among its amenities. The park is open in winter for ice fishing and snow activities.

While in the area, plan to visit one of the grand mansions in the Hudson Valley area. Federal-style **Boscobel** dates from 1804 and is located on NY 9D near Cold Spring, overlooking the Hudson Valley. For information, call 845-265-3638 or visit **boscobel.org.**

# 6  FAHNESTOCK WILDERNESS TRAIL

## KEY AT-A-GLANCE INFORMATION

**LENGTH:** 13.5 miles

**ELEVATION GAIN:** 2,580 feet

**CONFIGURATION:** Enormous balloon

**DIFFICULTY:** Strenuous

**SCENERY:** Dense deciduous forest with laurel patches and some cedars, rock outcroppings, lush wetlands, two bodies of water

**EXPOSURE:** Thick, shady canopy in summer

**TRAFFIC:** Very light to virtually nil

**TRAIL SURFACE:** Mostly dirt, with stretches of pebbles, stones, and moss

**HIKING TIME:** 6.5 hours

**SEASON:** Year-round, sunrise–sunset, but winter is especially rewarding.

**DRIVING DISTANCE:** 49 miles

**ACCESS:** Free; pets on leash not exceeding 10 feet, no bicycles, no motorized vehicles, no horses

**MAPS:** At park headquarters on north side of NY 301, 0.6 mile west of Taconic Parkway; download from tinyurl.com/fahnestockmspmap; USGS *West Point*

**FACILITIES:** No restrooms or water on trails, but Canopus Beach, in the state park, has both and much more.

**COMMENTS:** Hunting is permitted in season; call 845-225-7207. For an overview of other activities, visit nysparks.com/parks/133/details.aspx.

## GPS COORDINATES

N41° 26.673'  W73° 54.900'

## IN BRIEF

This is not one of those blow-your-boots-off sorts of sorties, with killer views, phenomenal waterfalls, or anything else of a superlative sort. Its appeal is of a far more subliminal, cerebral nature, in which a rolling up-and-down terrain draws the hiker far into an unpopulated wilderness, a place in which the squealing of hawks overhead is more common than the squawking of other people, and mushrooms on the trail are a more frequent sight than hikers' litter.

## DESCRIPTION

Back when we were kids, the word *boondocks* was a pejorative used to describe being off in the sticks, without anything much to do. Now that we're a little older, and hopefully somewhat wiser, getting out into the boondocks, if only for a few hours, is one of our highest forms of pleasure. And while we hesitate to describe Fahnestock Memorial State Park's Hubbard-Perkins Conservation Area as a boondocks kind of place, few preserves can compete with it for that feeling of being far removed from so-called civilization. One thing

-------------------------------------------

## *Directions* ──────────→

Drive north on the Henry Hudson Parkway to the Sawmill River Parkway North. Take Exit 25 to NY 9A and turn left on NY 9A. Proceed for 9.4 miles, then go left on US 9 North. Continue 8.5 miles and turn left on US 9 North/US 6 West/US 202 West. After 0.2 mile enter a roundabout and take the first exit onto US 9 North/Albany Post Road. Drive 10.3 miles to the intersection with NY 301, continue for 0.2 mile, then turn right by the brown sign for Hubbard Lodge. Make a quick left on the deteriorating spur road, and in 0.3 mile park by the lodge.

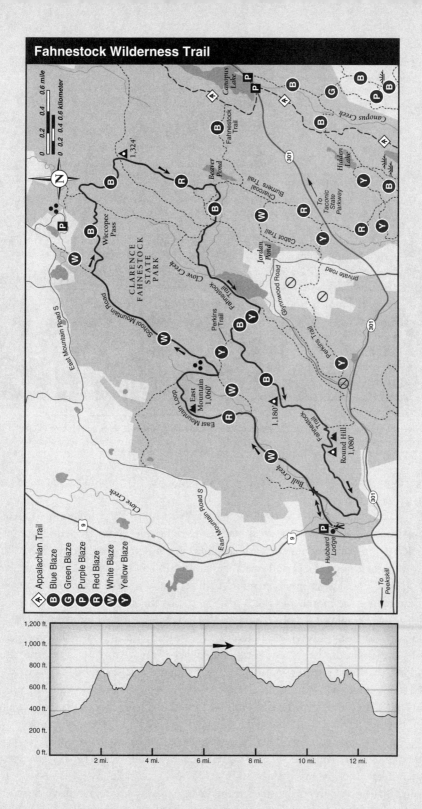

# Fahnestock Wilderness Trail

**Legend**

<table>
<tr><td>Appalachian Trail</td></tr>
<tr><td>B</td><td>Blue Blaze</td></tr>
<tr><td>G</td><td>Green Blaze</td></tr>
<tr><td>P</td><td>Purple Blaze</td></tr>
<tr><td>R</td><td>Red Blaze</td></tr>
<tr><td>W</td><td>White Blaze</td></tr>
<tr><td>Y</td><td>Yellow Blaze</td></tr>
</table>

Canopus Lake

Canopus Creek

Fahnestock Trail

Beaver Pond

Charcoal Burners Trail

Hidden Lake

301

To Taconic State Parkway

Cabot Trail

Jordan Pond

Glynnwood Road

private road

CLARENCE FAHNESTOCK STATE PARK

Clove Creek

Wiccopee Pass

School Mountain Road

Fahnestock Trail

Perkins Trail

Perkins Trail

East Mountain 1,060'

East Mountain Loop

1,180'

Round Hill 1,080'

Fahnestock Trail

Bull Creek

1,324'

East Mountain Road S

East Mountain Road S

Clove Creek

9

9

301

Hubbard Lodge

To Peekskill

1,200 ft.
1,000 ft.
800 ft.
600 ft.
400 ft.
200 ft.
0 ft.

2 mi.    4 mi.    6 mi.    8 mi.    10 mi.    12 mi.

0   0.2   0.4   0.6 mile
0   0.2   0.4   0.6 kilometer

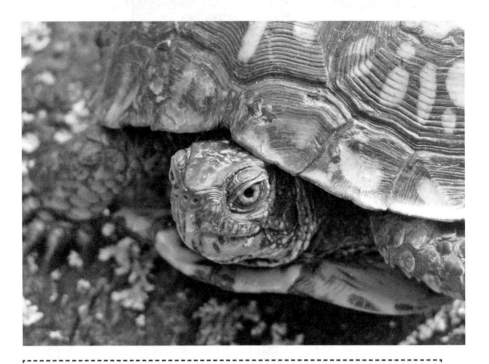

Eastern box turtles may be shy, but they devour almost anything—from slugs to mushrooms to our sandwich—if we're not careful.

is certain: if you treasure the aura of unsullied nature, you won't be at a loss for things to do there.

Pick up the trail to the right of the Hubbard Lodge, and follow the mowed-grass walkway down the gentle slope by the right side of the fenced-in butterfly garden. (If it's summertime or early autumn, you might browse in the latter for a few minutes among the coneflowers, bergamot, Indian blanket, blue vervain, and cinquefoil, looking for great spangled fritillaries and monarch butterflies, as well as hummers—the moths *and* the birds.) Step past the scraggly cedars and hang a left onto the unpaved School Mountain Road (SMR), marked by white blazes. As you proceed along this wide, relatively level (for now) route, note the emergence from the right of the blue-blazed Fahnestock Trail (FT), just after the third bridge—that's the return conduit you'll be making use of several hours from now. And just before that span, on the left, are the stone-and-concrete gateway pillars marking the entrance to the old Hubbard estate, which is about all that remains of it beyond a few nondescript pits and cavities here and there in the soil.

Continue straight ahead with the white blazes, breaking left through the grass after the fourth span onto the red-tagged East Mountain Loop (EML), just as the wider main track bends slightly right (GPS: N41° 27.264' W73° 53.656'). The bridge that once marked the start of the EML is badly disintegrated, with only its support logs remaining, so unless your sense of balance is great, you may have to cross the stream via a few rocks on the right. Here begins one of the steepest climbs of the hike, as the EML rises steadily, meandering by miscellaneous oaks and numerous black birch trees. In less than 15 minutes you should reach the summit, among a clutch of cedars, with filtered views west of Fishkill and Scofield Ridges your reward. Then, predictably, the path descends, gradually at first over a rocky shelf, followed by a jump over a stone-filled streambed, before swerving to the right along a grooved track. Near the base of this slope you'll encounter some stone foundations, and moments after that a colossal wall, with the wreckage of an old house appearing to the left roughly 10 minutes later. That hollow shell marks your return to the wide SMR (white blazes), where you lunge left on what has become a pebble-strewn, steady upgrade. This is perhaps the most tedious stretch of trail on the entire circuit, but in 1.7 miles you'll be done with it, rolling right onto blue-tagged Wiccopee Pass (GPS: N41° 28.552' W73° 52.159'). (If you're here in summer, this segment may be enlivened by the presence of exotic stinkhorn mushrooms, which we've seen growing in the vicinity.)

Wiccopee Pass (WP) is, to our thinking, great fun, with the moss-covered path bobbing up and down as it maneuvers over the corrugated texture of the ridge. On emerging by another wide woods road, the blue blazes dart left, and so should you. Three or four minutes later they steer you to the right, back onto a narrow forest path. (If you proceed straight on the woods road, now blazed yellow, you'll quickly come to the ruins of an old farmhouse.) The WP holds to a mostly eastbound track, leaping from one low, wrinkly hilltop to another, until it finally bends to the south and meets an unblazed spur on the right. The continuation of the loop is straight onward, as the blue blazes end and the red ones of the Charcoal Burners Trail (CBT) begin. The now-level terrain, hemmed in by blueberry bushes, persists for several minutes, until the path drops off the ridge and meets another wide woods road. The CBT breaks to the left there, while you switch to the right onto the Fahnestock Trail (FT, blue blazes), which you will follow for 5.4 miles (all the way back to the SMR). Before completing that turn, however, remain with the CBT for another 2 minutes (blue markings now running concurrently with red ones) for waterside access to Beaver Pond, a scenic spot where people sometimes ice-skate in winter.

Having retraced your steps to the previous intersection, hew to the left on the FT and tack left again in an additional 3 minutes when the blue blazes lead you off the wide, grass-covered road onto a single-file path. Moments later the FT rejoins a woods road, descends gracefully to a Y-junction, and rumbles right, only to lurch left at the subsequent intersection, which is heralded by stones piled into a cairn. Go left once more at the T, where a smattering of beech saplings lends a silvery sheen to the forest, and cross the remnants of the concrete car bridge, a welcome span over the stream feeding the north end of Jordan Pond. (If you're here in summer, look left among the rocks for the brilliant red of cardinal flowers.) As the FT arcs toward the southwest, it flanks the pond, providing a pleasant view of the water, a small island, and a cluster of white birches on the opposite shore. Just as the path begins to pull away from the pond, you'll have to bound to the right with the FT onto a side trail, as its blue blazes are overlapped by yellow ones. (The yellow markings also go straight ahead.)

In about 10 minutes of climbing you reach the top of the low rise, at which point the two colors diverge. Cruise left, with the blue blazes, as the final leg of the hike is now at hand. (If you've had enough of this roller-coaster romp, you can skip the last two peaks by bolting to the right, with the yellow markings, and hang a left, when that spur ends, onto the SMR, thereby sparing yourself 1.5 miles.) There are a couple of tricky spots to be alert to as you gradually make your way back to the SMR along the blue-blazed path, the first coming after a prolonged stroll along the ridge. When you finally descend from that, in roughly 30 minutes, you'll be heading directly toward the base of Round Hill (partridges often lurk among the understory on this west-facing slope). Just as the FT bends toward the right, on entering a narrow gully, it then hops left out of the ditch (GPS: N41° 26.654' W73° 53.860')—an obscure switch that's quite easy to over-look—and begins forging up the hill. The second challenge arises after you leave the sun-dappled summit, an idyllic spot crowned with cedars, oaks, and knee-high grass the color of ripe wheat. The route, which here and there resembles little more than a worn trace, begins to descend off the south side of the hill, reaching, shortly, a rock-shelf overlook of US 9. At that stage it appears to disappear alto-gether, but if you scan the ground carefully you'll observe that it actually slips off the rocks on the left side. When you've given up the last bit of elevation, the FT will draw close to a swamp stream, where an unblazed woods road materializes from the left. Motor to the right, still with blue blazes and paralleling the swamp stream, and in 5 more minutes the FT arcs left and slams into the white-tagged SMR. Turn left there, carefully crossing the collapsed bridge, and retrace your earlier steps back to the trailhead.

## NEARBY ACTIVITIES

If you enjoy a hearty beer after a hearty hike, think about visiting Fahnestock from Tuesday through Saturday. Why? Because those are the days when **Captain Lawrence Brewing Company,** just north of I-287, between the Sawmill River and Sprain Brook Parkways in Elmsford, holds open tastings. Brewer Scott Vaccaro, who honed his skills at the Sierra Nevada brewery in California, keeps a number of flavors flowing, including Liquid Gold, a spicy Belgian-style ale; the hoppy, citric Freshchester Pale Ale; Smoked Porter, rich with chocolate and caramel malts; and Captain's Reserve Imperial IPA, a big-bodied, highly hopped ale. For hours and directions, call 914-741-2337 or visit **captainlawrencebrewing.com,** and consider buying a six-pack to go, just so you have something to sip after your *next* hike.

# FISHKILL RIDGE TRAIL

## IN BRIEF

When Walt Whitman penned "a leaf of grass is no less than the journeywork of the stars," he might have been thinking of Fishkill. There is indeed a celestial atmosphere to its extended ridge, a sedge-sprinkled granite plateau of unsurpassed beauty and calm. The various Hudson River vistas along the way are a breathtaking bonus.

## DESCRIPTION

We hesitate to mention Fishkill Ridge in the same breath as the Hudson Highlands. The former, after all, at just over 1,000 acres, is but one-quarter the size of the latter. And while the Highlands, a state park, is fine hiking terrain most any time, Fishkill, operated as a conservation area, allows hunting in late autumn, when hikers who value their health had best stay away—or color themselves like oversize pumpkins.

That Fishkill Ridge is often associated with the Hudson Highlands is certainly no coincidence, given its position at the north end of that range. Naturally, such geographic

- - - - - - - - - - - - - - - - - - - - - - - - - - - - -

### *Directions* ———————→

Take US 9 North to the junction with I-84 West. Follow I-84 West briefly to Exit 12 for NY 52. Turn left on Main Street/NY 52/ NY 52 BR. Proceed for 0.3 mile and go left on Old Glenham Road. Continue for 0.9 mile and swing left on Maple Street. After 0.1 mile make a slight right on Washington Avenue, and after another 0.1 mile turn left on Old Town Road. Drive 0.4 mile and go right on Sunnyside Road. Follow it to the end, then bear left on an unpaved gated road and go 0.1 mile to the grassy parking lot where the trailhead is located.

---

### KEY AT-A-GLANCE INFORMATION

**LENGTH: 8 miles**

**ELEVATION GAIN: 2,937 feet**

**CONFIGURATION: Balloon**

**DIFFICULTY: Strenuous**

**SCENERY: Rugged, steep trail ascends through hardwood forest to panoramic views of Fahnestock State Park, Hudson River, Manhattan skyline, and quarry.**

**EXPOSURE: Pretty shady all the way, with exception of highest ridges**

**TRAFFIC: Very light**

**TRAIL SURFACE: Mix of packed dirt, rocks, roots, ledges and a couple of grassy patches; quite uneven at times**

**HIKING TIME: 4 hours**

**DRIVING DISTANCE: 59 miles**

**SEASON: Year-round, sunrise–sunset**

**ACCESS: Free, but donations accepted; dogs on leash**

**MAPS: USGS *West Point***

**FACILITIES: No restrooms or water on trails**

**COMMENTS: Stellar viewpoints for leaf-peeping in autumn, great raptor-observation spots. For further information, call 845-473-4440 or visit scenichudson.org/parks /fishkillridge.**

## GPS COORDINATES

N41° 30.474'  W73° 55.707'

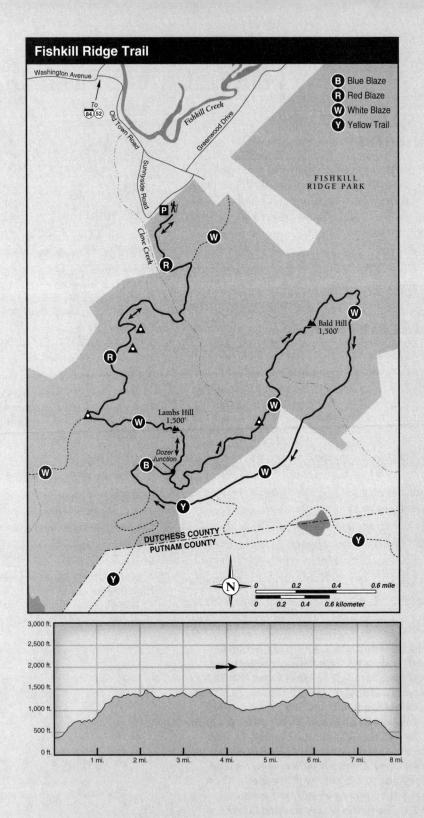

kinship blesses Fishkill with many of the same attributes that make its neighbor such a happy hiking ground, including rugged climbs to rocky ridges and craggy domes, awe-inspiring views of the Hudson River and surrounding hills, and a massive gain in elevation.

This last characteristic should not be underestimated. From the trailhead by Sunnyside Road to the highest point of the ridge, plan on climbing more than 1,200 feet. But whereas in previous editions of this book the initial part of the route involved a grueling, stamina-draining ascent up a grooved track, the trail we now recommend is more meandering and scenic, and much less fatiguing.

The hike begins at the far end of the unpaved parking lot, where you pick up the red-circle blazes of the Overlook Trail (OT). Swing left around the wooden barrier, moving toward the kiosk (maps usually available), then, in about 10 paces, pivot to the right, following the blazes uphill into the forest. After initially climbing and circling around and above the parking area, the dirt-packed track levels off, for a time, passing among maples, oaks, and an occasional telephone pole. The ascent resumes shortly, however, over well-eroded, root-and-shale-filled turf, zigzagging by miscellaneous hardwood trees and reaching, in 5 minutes of huffing and puffing, a turnoff to Malouf's Camp, a private campground. Bypass that acute left turn, sticking instead with the rising track, and in another 2 minutes the trail reaches a deeply eroded hole in the hill, as if a colossal mudslide sucked the trees and topsoil off the ground. The moss-sided path cuts around that rending and for a brief spell descends, then evens out and crosses a pour-off of Clove Creek, where asters and goldenrods thrive and the cascading water in spring can make for a challenging rock-hop.

Subsequent to that fun stretch, the OT snakes higher over increasingly moss-and-shale-studded ground, with mountain laurels gradually creeping into the forested mix. As you begin gaining serious elevation, most of the river views will be limited by tree cover, especially when leaves hang from their limbs. But in due course, as you ascend to a bald patch of granite, a magnificent panorama unfolds, with Beacon looming below and the Hudson River stretching across the horizon beyond.

Further vistas ensue as you climb higher, even as the upward angle of the OT begins to moderate. After a few minutes, a stellar view of the Newburgh Bridge is added to rewards of this splendid piece of trail, where pitch pines and scrub oaks, having largely supplanted the maples and birches of earlier, add to its subliminal beauty.

Following a short additional rise, the red-blazed route finally hits flat ground, now traveling west through a maple grove. From paralleling an old stone wall, it soon shifts left through a gap in the rocks, then wobbles between west and south. The climbing then resumes, over rocks and packed dirt, with knee-high grass and occasional ferns coloring the trailside, ultimately yielding additional views of the Hudson (and Breakneck Ridge to the south) from the granite-based side of the mountain. Persisting along this rocky shelf, one of the figurative high points of the hike, you will have to look sharply to find the

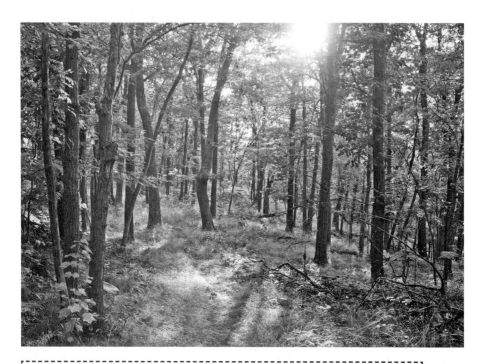

The lush deciduous forest of the lower elevations stands in stark contrast to the stunted shrub growth atop the ridge.

continuation of the OT: a hard left about 20 feet shy of the end of the bedrock, slipping between a couple of pitch pines.

The Overlook Trail comes to an end as you emerge from the tree cover, with the prosaically named White Trail (WT, marked with—you guessed it!—white blazes) succeeding it. Take the left fork (right leads to the Mount Beacon trailhead). From fairly full exposure to the sun on an open patch of rock, the WT dips back into a shady mix of maples and oaks, heading due north to northeast. Ignore the social trails and overgrown forest tracks that you may see among the high grass and sundry mushrooms, sticking with the WT as it hops left over a tumbledown stone wall and spears over an impressively craggy bluff.

Once atop that outcropping, the WT meanders over bedrock on its way to the crest of Lambs Hill (at 1,500 feet), ultimately delivering the payoff of a fabulous 180-degree vista toward the west, with Breakneck Ridge looming to your left and the Hudson River occupying center stage. The peaks of Storm King may bring you closer to the river, but we know of few other viewpoints that showcase its majestic, never-ending length so dramatically. This is the place for a memorable picnic or to sip a solitary brew while savoring the approach of a colorful sunset.

You may want to save that brew for later, however, as there is still plenty of trail left to hike. Continuing along the circuitous WT, in about 10 minutes—and a drop of about 150 feet—you will arrive at Dozer Junction. Named for the rust-crusted earthmover permanently parked down the Blue Trail to the right, this bulldozer is a vivid reminder of the threat of "development" that hangs over many a similar woodland. Save the study of that rusty relic for now, though, and instead of going right, head directly across the wide forest road, remaining with the white blazes as they draw you over a chunky track up to a sun-struck stone terrace, a peaceful nook blessed with expansive views arcing from the northeast to southeast. A short descent over talus debris leads to a similar ledge, with a bird's-eye position over a quarry pond and a pocket of the Hudson River; the trail creeps from there in a northerly direction toward the twin Bald Hills. Much of this appealing plateau is decked with knee-high wild grass and fragrant blueberry bushes, while scrub oaks, shagbark hickories, a few tulip trees, and a fistful of cedars round out its rough-cut beauty. The Hudson is a little more visible from atop the next ridge, and the crest beyond yields an equivocal view of an active quarry and industrial site, and, more happily, a glimpse of the Manhattan skyline. (There was a rustic rocking chair left behind by someone the last time we passed this way, and we were all too happy to avail ourselves of its comfort for a few moments' rest.) You may have difficulty locating the blazes along this section of the route, for most are painted on rocks and are easily confused with the many guano splotches deposited by birds. Similarly, don't be lured off-track by the numerous animal trails that crisscross the grass up here. Simply remember that the path hews largely to the eastern fringe of the summit as it heads north, pressing onward first downhill, then up, through an unmarked intersection on the approach to the first Bald Hill.

With so many rocky, denuded peaks peppering one ridge, you may wonder how you'll identify the Bald Hills. Relax: the U.S. Geological Survey has rendered that child's play by implanting markers in the middle of their diminutive crowns. Immediately before the first, though, is a grass-covered access road. The white blazes cross that wide, flat surface at the lull between ridge nodes and climbs steadily from there, still chugging northward. Both Bald ones top out at 1,500 feet of altitude, though with oak trees encircling the peaks like tonsured heads, the vistas are limited and thus a bit anticlimactic.

The descent that succeeds the second Bald Hill is surprisingly painless. True, you pass from tall, golden grass to hard, rock-impregnated earth, and from immovable boulders to a brief patch of ever-shifting scree. But it is seldom the tooth-grinding test of the lower joints that the march up might have led you to expect. The path bends right at a faint T onto the lower ridge, and after 20 to 25 minutes of ease along this spacious lane, the WT ends, with a yellow-blazed trail emerging from the left.

To return to Dozer Junction, continue marching straight ahead, with the wide path now bearing yellow markings. Eventually, it will arc to the right, slipping through a notch between two promontories via some towering granite outcroppings and a scree-covered slope, where boneset blooms in late summer. Ignore the unmarked spur to the right, steering right on the blue-blazed route instead in

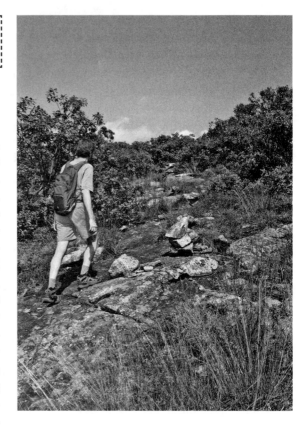

Climbing to the summit of Lambs Hill requires an almost continuous ascent of more than 1,000 feet.

another 100 yards, when the yellow markings shift sharply through a rock wall on the left. Remain with blue, to the right, at the wide intersection that immediately follows, as it carries you into a disheveled upheaval of rocks and trees, past the flattened remnants of a shack and some rusty remains of farm implements. Several minutes later of slogging uphill, and you will find yourself standing beside the bulldozer of earlier. To return to the trailhead, turn left onto the WT (about 150 feet up-trail from the rusty relic), and retrace your previous steps.

## NEARBY ACTIVITIES

The historic **Van Wyck Homestead** is an important showpiece of the Fishkill Historical Society. The museum displays artifacts that evoke Hudson Valley colonial life, with a special emphasis on the American Revolution. For information, call 845-896-8755 or visit **fishkillhistoricalsociety.org.**

If you are inclined to take a more cultural stroll, **Dia:Beacon** will entice you with its magnificent art collection—encompassing the 1960s to the present—in a breathtaking environment. For details call 845-440-0100 or visit **diaart.org.**

# HUDSON HIGHLANDS BREAKNECK RIDGE LOOP

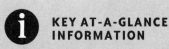

## IN BRIEF

Stupendous views, rock-scrambling, and strenuous climbs are a good part of what this thrilling jaunt is about, with a special accent on *strenuous*. This is one of the more memorable hikes in the Highlands, with a colorful finish by the remnants of an old estate and dairy farm—ruins far more extensive than the average ghost town. For many, this is the Holy Grail of highland trails, but don't try it without sturdy hiking boots and plenty of water.

## DESCRIPTION

Many hikes are so mild in nature, so undemanding of one's physical strength and capacity for endurance, that we think of them as woodland walks or streamside strolls, nothing to break a sweat over. Then there are the hugely challenging calorie-burners, the ones where the elevation gain is measured in four digits, not two or three; rocks are to be summited, not sidestepped; and no matter how much water we've brought along, it never seems enough. Hudson Highlands, a relatively undeveloped park of 4,000 acres, features just such a monster hike, a strenuous haul in which you are less likely to finish up with a spring to your step than a stumble down the slope. And if you're at all like us, you'll love every minute of it.

---

## Directions →

**Take US 9 North to the junction with NY 403 (Garrison Road). Turn left and drive 2.2 miles to the junction with NY 9D, where you head north (right). Proceed for 4.9 miles through the village of Cold Spring and turn right into a small parking lot. There is additional parking across the street, at Little Stony Point Bridge.**

## KEY AT-A-GLANCE INFORMATION

**LENGTH: 8.8 miles**

**ELEVATION GAIN: 2,968 feet**

**CONFIGURATION: Figure-eight**

**DIFFICULTY: Strenuous**

**SCENERY: Rugged trail crosses two elevated ridges, yielding stunning views of Hudson River and mountains, and passes extensive dairy farm ruins.**

**EXPOSURE: Partial tree canopy; many open sun-exposed areas**

**TRAFFIC: So popular (on weekends) the trails can seem like a near-continuous conga line.**

**TRAIL SURFACE: Mostly dirt and rocks, some rock-scrambling, 0.5 mile of pavement at finish**

**HIKING TIME: 6 hours**

**DRIVING DISTANCE: 50 miles**

**SEASON: Year-round, sunrise–sunset**

**ACCESS: Free; dogs on leash not exceeding 10 feet**

**MAPS: USGS *West Point***

**FACILITIES: No restrooms or water**

**COMMENTS: Best views are from late fall through early spring, but snow and ice in winter can make trail surface treacherous. Hunting is permitted in season. For information, call 845-225-7207 or visit nysparks.com /parks/9/details.aspx.**

## GPS COORDINATES

N41° 25.597'  W73° 57.931'

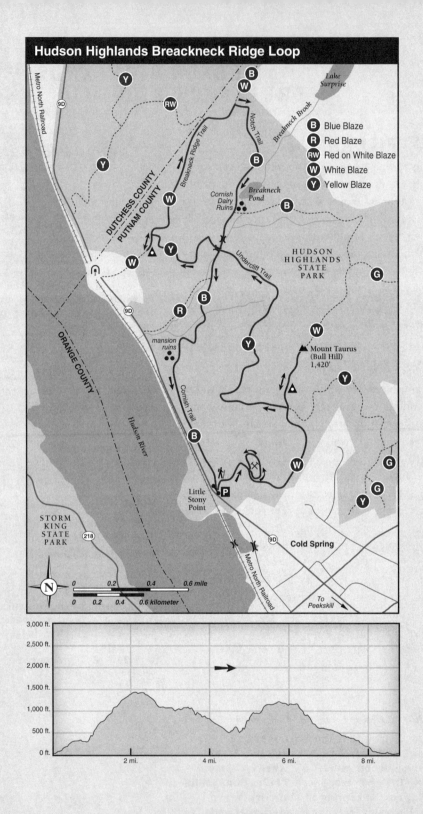

# Hudson Highlands Breackneck Ridge Loop

**B** Blue Blaze
**R** Red Blaze
**RW** Red on White Blaze
**W** White Blaze
**Y** Yellow Blaze

Lake Surprise

Breakneck Brook

Notch Trail

Breakneck Ridge Trail

DUTCHESS COUNTY
PUTNAM COUNTY

Cornish Dairy Ruins

Breakneck Pond

HUDSON HIGHLANDS STATE PARK

Undercliff Trail

mansion ruins

Mount Taurus (Bull Hill) 1,420'

Cornish Trail

ORANGE COUNTY

Hudson River

Little Stony Point

STORM KING STATE PARK

Cold Spring

Metro North Railroad

9D

218

To Peekskill

N

| 0 | 0.2 | 0.4 | 0.6 mile |
| 0 | 0.2 | 0.4 | 0.6 kilometer |

3,000 ft.
2,500 ft.
2,000 ft.
1,500 ft.
1,000 ft.
500 ft.
0 ft.

2 mi.    4 mi.    6 mi.    8 mi.

On leaving the diminutive parking area, proceed around the gate that bars the quarry road and keep right, following the white blazes up the sandy slope. Even with vegetation growing thickly around the trail and a number of dogwoods, oaks, and shagbark hickory trees in the vicinity, the sun exposure is intense and a hat should be considered mandatory summer apparel. The climb is steady for the first 10 minutes, brushing by slag heaps from bygone quarrying, before arriving at the quarry itself. The path continues by the crater's right rim, but take a moment to tour the hollowed-out core—and catch your breath!—while observing a recovery in progress, as sumac, cottonwoods, oaks, and cedars now thrive among the knee-high grass that covers this damaged ground.

The going gets steeper on resuming the trail, but with the elevation gain comes a series of false summits where you can rest and enjoy striking views of the town of Cold Spring below, the Hudson River beyond, and the rising rocky profile of Storm King across the water. If it's a warm day, you may share that panorama with plenty of lizards sunning themselves on the pale slabs of stone littering the area. Indeed, the higher you get, the greater the quantity of rubble, with the climax being a scramble over rocks to a plateau that rests about 650 feet above the trailhead.

On rising another 250 feet through blueberry bushes and sassafras, the path forks, with yellow blazes launching leftward and white blazes pointing to the right (GPS: N41° 25.964' W73° 57.552'). Don't be put off by the low-swooping turkey vultures: opt for the right leg, which leads to the crown of Mount Taurus. For a brief spell, the way doesn't seem so strenuous, hopping over shelves of buff-colored granite, darting between black birch trees and scrub oaks, even descending a bit. Then, all too soon, the bill comes due and it's back up the mountain, leapfrogging over melon-size chunks of stone from one false summit to another (with limitless views at each), more scrambling over a slanted rock face, before finally reaching the top, at 1,420 feet of elevation. The laurel-and-oak-sprinkled setting of Taurus, also known as Bull Hill, is an ideal spot in which to swap some real whoppers with your companions.

For vistas that are no less enchanting and to get on with the hike, return to the Undercliff Trail (UT) at the aforementioned yellow-blazed turnoff. Although it is a couple hundred feet lower, the UT offers several stellar vantage points, including a spectacular view from a rocky knob outpost, a towering perspective of NY 9D and the tunnel to the north, Storm King over the river, and of course the Hudson itself. The verdant plateau beyond is Breakneck Ridge, beautifully tree-covered and looking deceptively easy to reach. Shuffling onward, the stone-studded path finally enters a touch of shade cast by oaks that loom larger and taller.

In less than half an hour, the UT starts a seriously steep descent down a talus slope, switchbacking through maples and laurels, creeping in the general direction of Breakneck Ridge. Stone steps in strategic places help make this drop more foot-friendly than you might otherwise expect, before hitting a grass-topped carriage lane with a surface smooth enough to push a baby carriage. As you proceed

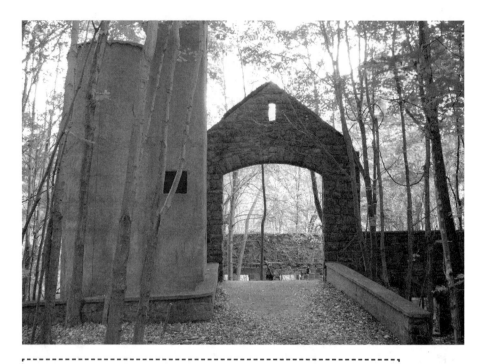

Don't be cowed: exploring the eerie ruins of the Cornish dairy farm is all part of the fun.

downward at a more gradual angle, listen for the *rat-a-tat-tat* of pileated wood-peckers, which can often be heard drilling into the beeches and birches coloring this part of the park.

Cross the seasonal streambed, near a small grove of hemlocks, swing left on a larger carriage road, blazed red, and then roll right and ford the wooden foot-bridge. You've lost 925 feet since descending from Mount Taurus—no bull!—and are about to regain a good portion of that. Did you enjoy that strenuous stretch to the last peak? Let's hope so; some hikers maintain that this next yellow-blazed bit is even tougher, an assertion we're not inclined to argue with. All we know is if it were any steeper, you'd probably need rappelling ropes to make your way up. Switchbacks help, wending their way through the moraine field, and when a series of boulders appears to block further progress, the makeshift trail somehow snakes to its left, sparing you—for now—the need to scramble. Another 40 yards and you'll be facing the vertical side of a large knob, with a fine glimpse of Taurus behind your back.

On moving forward under the limbs of wild dogwoods, another angular escarpment surfaces. It is possible to climb over the rocks here (beware of rattle-snakes sunning themselves on the upper reaches!) to the pitch pine–dotted ledge above for a moment of off-trail solitude in a rough-hewn, wildly beautiful spot. There are even faded orange blazes that lead up there and beyond. Ultimately, though, it is the yellow markings to the left of this grand protrusion to which you want to adhere, avoiding the oblong blocks of granite and sharp-edged rocks as the path zigzags downward through another moraine patch. Having dodged a couple of oversize boulders, you'll begin to climb again, surmounting a steep talus slope and threading through a few more switchbacks. At the base of the next bluff—a dramatic protrusion of dark-gray rocks—below a hanging garden of ferns and weeds, are the remains of a crude rock shelter.

The yellow blazes expire abruptly just north of that, once you've passed through a rocky notch. This is the start of the Breakneck Ridge Trail (white blazes); stay to the right as the strenuous, rocky climb grinds on. (For yet another thrilling view of the Hudson, however, first take a brief detour to the left, up to the top of the rocky knob.) Yet one more igneous crag follows near the crest, with a fun hand-over-hand scaling of stones required to reach its dome. The worst—or best, depending on your outlook—of the ascent is finished, so rest a moment and enjoy the sublime views and serenity of the setting. The wrinkled promontory directly across the wide, rollicking Hudson is Storm King Mountain, with the extended ridge of Schunemunk Mountain looming beyond it. That spot of land near the east shore of the river is Pollepel Island, where the largely intact ruin of a five-story castle, built in Scottish baronial style early in the 20th century, still stands. And of the many possible birds overhead, you may be fortunate enough, in warm weather, to observe osprey flying by.

From this stage onward, Breakneck is just a name (rather than an actual hiking risk) as it flows from one rising knuckle to the next along the spine of this ridge, with low, grassy saddles in between. The highest point, at the third pinnacle, tops out at 1,150 feet. Once the fourth rise is behind you, the inevitable descent begins, dropping 60 feet over rock fill in a matter of seconds.

Not so fast, though, for from that minor gully there is another peak. Ignore the spur to the left and remain on Breakneck as the ridge, almost level for a change, draws gradually to this last summit, one that yields a splendid 360-degree panorama, with Lake Surprise beaming brightly to the northeast. Shifting downhill, hew to the right in about 150 yards, at a junction with the Notch Trail (blue blazes) (GPS: N41° 27.348' W73° 57.774').

The Notch heads lower immediately, at first over rocky ground, but soon giving way to an easier, packed-earth surface. The forest is denser here, and the use of blazes not too generous, so some hard squinting may be in order to find the blue discs. In a little less than a mile—and a loss of 500 feet—the path hits a T with a carriage road, Breakneck Pond lying just beyond. Veer right onto the pebbly road, which leads in a few minutes to the impressively large ruins of the Cornish Dairy, consisting of a number of stone-block and concrete structures scattered on both sides of the lane. This is a fun area to explore, but as always in such locales, be cautious about entering ruined buildings.

The blue blazes make a sharp left up another carriage lane (circling back eventually to Mount Taurus), but you should saunter straight ahead as the road trends downward, serenaded for a spell by the pleasant tinkling of Breakneck

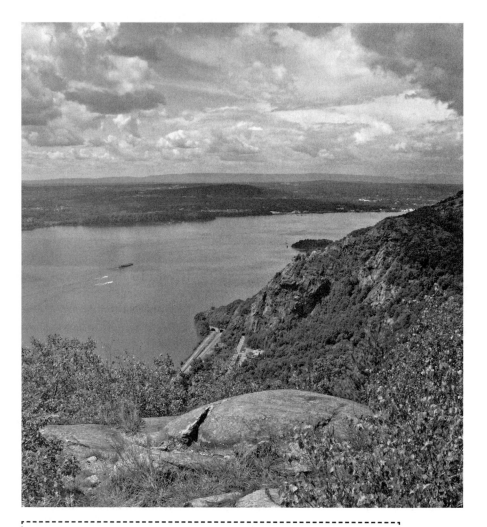

The New York Water Gap: the Hudson River cuts through the mountain ridge, separating mighty Storm King from challenging Breakneck Ridge.

Brook. Eventually, after crossing the brook on a narrow bridge, you'll walk by the Undercliff Trail (both right and left) and the bridge (to the right) you used earlier on the way up to Breakneck Ridge. When the trail diverges, perhaps 100 yards beyond a derelict pump house, stay to the left on the blue-blazed route.

From there onward, an enticing network of grassy lanes cuts through the forest. Simply adhere to the main drag, which imminently turns to asphalt, and you'll be fine. Though this section of the park lacks the views and raw beauty of the higher elevations, its upside in spring and early summer is so rich an explosion of wildflowers that paisley looks drab by comparison. Because of the lush vegetation, white-tailed deer often graze the area. We once saw a black racer snake, too, curled up on the path, in no hurry, apparently, to race anywhere. Shortly after you

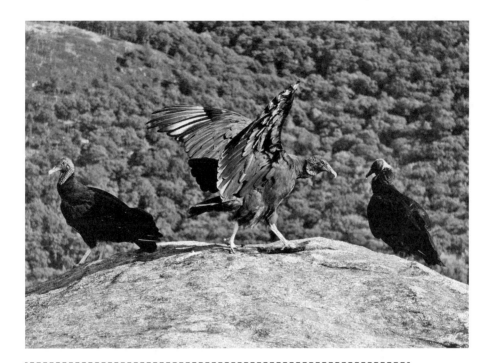

Black vultures—like hikers—favor the high elevation ledges as superior vantage points.

encounter the round foundation of an old cistern, the ruins of the estate's green-house appear cloaked among the bushes to the right. Several yards beyond that is the prize, the remains of the stone mansion itself, partially overgrown by a tangle of rhododendrons (GPS: N41° 26.255' W73° 58.189'). When the paved lane reaches the pillared gate by NY 9D, slice left on the trail leading into the over-growth. You'll arrive at the trailhead in 5 minutes.

## NEARBY ACTIVITIES

This hike is plenty for one day, but experiencing a sunset on **Little Stony Point** by the Hudson River, just across the road, will jump-start your revival.

Did the glimpse of **Bannerman Castle** on Pollepel Island pique your interest in this state-owned land? Kayak and boat tours there run on weekends from mid-June through October. For details, call the Bannerman Castle Trust at 845-831-6346 or visit **bannermancastle.org**.

# 9   MIANUS RIVER GORGE TRAIL

## IN BRIEF

A great gorge and reservoir vistas, old-growth hemlocks, an intricate network of 19th-century farmstead walls, glacial erratics, and granite outcroppings highlight one of the better short treks in the region. Mianus is at its best in springtime, when the streams and cascades are most watery—but its cool, well-shaded paths also offer a respite from the heat of summer.

## DESCRIPTION

Hold the snickering, please. Contrary to what some wits might suggest, Mianus River Gorge owes its peculiar sobriquet to Sachem Myanos, leader of a local band of Mahican Indians that reportedly summered on the sandy shores of Long Island Sound in the late 1600s, using the gorge as their happy hunting grounds during colder months. That white-tailed deer still roam these woods (along with the occasional red and gray fox, raccoons, and, every so often, a polecat) owes less to the dietary discretion showed by the Mahicans and their white supplanters than to the ongoing success The Nature Conservancy and the Mianus River Gorge Preserve have enjoyed in jointly managing the domain.

Though Mianus, at 738 acres, is hardly a mighty oak, it has grown quite a bit from the

### KEY AT-A-GLANCE INFORMATION

**LENGTH:** 4.5 miles

**ELEVATION GAIN:** 868 feet

**CONFIGURATION:** Out-and-back

**DIFFICULTY:** Easy

**SCENERY:** Undulating trail winds through old-growth and successional forests, along cool slopes of a gorge, past cascades and lush quarry.

**EXPOSURE:** Very shady canopy throughout

**TRAFFIC:** Popular but seldom crowded

**TRAIL SURFACE:** Packed dirt, some rocky and rooty stretches

**HIKING TIME:** 2 hours

**DRIVING DISTANCE:** 37 miles

**SEASON:** April–November, 8:30 a.m.–5 p.m.

**ACCESS:** Donations encouraged; no pets, no bicycles

**MAPS:** At entrance kiosk; download from tinyurl.com/mianusmap; USGS *Pound Ridge*

**FACILITIES:** Water and vault toilet near entrance

**COMMENTS:** To learn about special events and for other information, call 914-234-3455 or visit mianus.org.

## GPS COORDINATES

N41° 11.153'  W73° 37.289'

### *Directions* ⟶

Follow I-684 North to Exit 4. Go right on NY 172/South Bedford Road. Drive 1.6 miles and stay left on NY 172/NY 22/Old Post Road. Continue 1.9 miles and make a right on Long Ridge Road. Proceed 0.7 mile and turn right onto Millers Mill Road, then left, after the bridge, on unpaved Mianus River Road. The parking lot is 0.5 mile ahead, on the left.

# Mianus River Gorge Trail

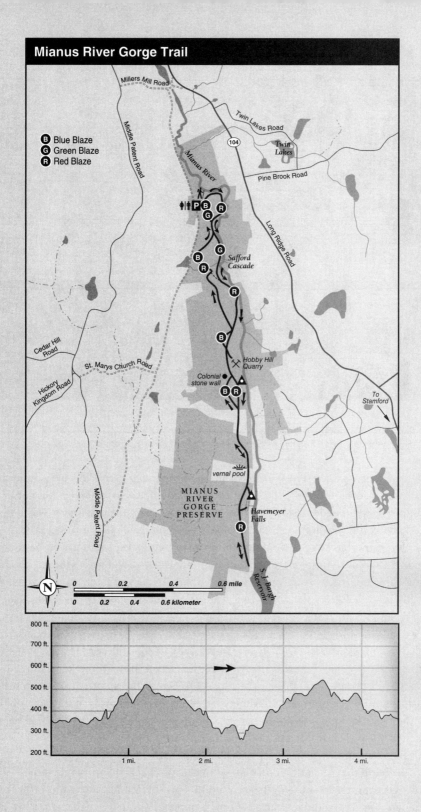

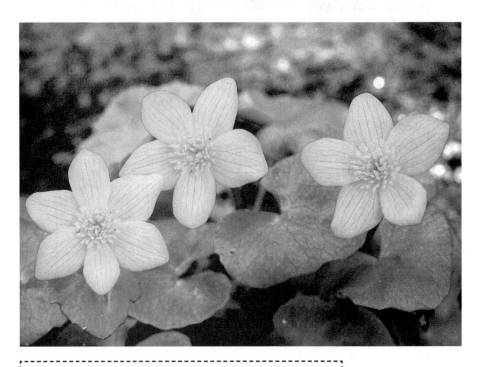

Spectacular marsh marigolds help brighten the darkest recesses of a forest.

littlest of acorns, when The Nature Conservancy created it in 1955 with an initial purchase of just 60 acres. Before a decade elapsed, this woodland habitat was recognized by the federal government to be of such significance that it was designated the country's first National Natural Landmark. That status stems in part from a remarkable concentration of old-growth hemlocks, some dating back 350 years, clustered along some of the steeper slopes of the gorge. More-accessible features include rocky outcroppings jutting high above the river, superb views of the S. J. Bargh Reservoir, a seasonal waterfall, an 18th-century mica-and-quartz quarry, and an intricate series of solid stone walls.

Trails fall into three color groups—Red, Blue, and Green—that overlap over the course of a relatively easy out-and-back hike of 4.5 miles. Maps are available at the kiosk, though you are unlikely to get lost if you bear to the left throughout the walk. Take a moment prior to setting off to peruse the picture display on stone walls, a useful backgrounder on Mianus's many mortarless walls that run throughout the woods. These are relics from the 19th century, when most of the trees in this area were cleared for farming and pastureland and farmers lined their fields with the many stones unearthed by their plows.

Begin on the Red Trail to the left of the kiosk. It and the subsequent paths are very well maintained, ranging from a wood-chip surface initially to hard-packed earth later on. Protruding rocks pose only a minimal hazard, one that is fairly typical of this sort of rolling, up-and-down, glacier-wracked terrain.

Once past a couple of aged cedars and a few sugar maples, you come directly to a shade-sheltered bench by an appealing overlook of the Mianus River, some 40 feet distant. For the first half-mile or so of the hike, the trail meanders past beech trees, hemlocks, and an occasional oak, sticking fairly close to the river. Roughly halfway along that distance, after a slight ascent, is a grassy patch to the right; it's a piece of pasture in succession, slowly being swallowed by the resurgent forest.

Yet another reminder of this area's bygone agricultural era follows, as you descend again toward the water. Look for a tree with a "4" mounted on it, by a stepping-stone bridge that fords a seasonal tributary. That marks the spot where farmers routinely rode their wagons across the river, with the old lane they used still faintly discernible uphill on the right.

A short series of ascents and descents ensues, culminating at yet another great view into the gorge. Then, on turning left onto the Green spur, the trail drifts steadily lower past numerous hemlocks until it meets a rather still section of the river. Though buggy in the spring, this is a peaceful glade, with skunk cabbage and ferns coloring the mossy bank, and a large stone wall running through the woods on the opposite side of the water. We once came upon a pileated woodpecker here, noisily knocking its beak into a fallen beech.

The Safford Cascade, to the right in roughly 100 yards, is generally active only from springtime through early summer, when a stream of water crackles photogenically down the rocky hillside, and dragonflies flit about in the moist spray. (Even when the cascade is dry, though, the moss-covered stepping-stones can be surprisingly slick.) A few paces beyond is a fork, with the right option retreating to the trailhead, and left, or straight ahead, joining the Red Trail for the continuation of the hike.

This begins one of the few sustained uphill stretches in the preserve, with the path threading toward the Hemlock Cathedral, home to most of the old-growth conifers and yielding one more overlook of the river. Predictably, it descends from there, reaching in a couple of minutes the Rock Wall Breach, the narrowest point in the gorge, where glacial ice sculpted this sharp bend in the river more than 15,000 years ago.

The trail now meanders upward, passing in the process several fine specimens of mature beech trees and a growing number of granite boulders, many mottled green with lichen. Keep to the left at each of the succeeding two intersections, as an increasing amount of mica specks glitter on the humus-laden path—a sure sign that you are approaching the Hobby Hill Quarry. A well-marked spur to the left ends, in perhaps a furlong, at the quarry, where ferns and lianas protrude like a hanging garden from the carved-out rock wall.

Back on the main trail, proceed on Red as the undulating route brushes by a series of well-preserved stone walls. On heading through a rather open stretch of such hardwoods as maple, oak, and black birch, the path veers toward the gorge, dropping down a few feet in elevation to Vernal Pool, a boggy spot marked by a "10." Throughout Mianus, such wetlands are rife in spring with trillium, trout lily, mayapple, and marsh marigold, and in early summer you may find frogs, horned toads, snapping turtles, and Eastern ribbon snakes in the vicinity.

A spur to the left appears a few minutes later, once you've climbed a bit, going out to a fair view of the reservoir. The laurel-fringed mound of granite there, shaded by oaks and hemlocks, is a choice place to rest or have lunch. A sign cautions that this is a DEER TICK RESEARCH AREA, a warning that would be no less applicable to much of the Northeast. It is probably a bluff meant to discourage bushwhacking down the embankment to the water, though the prevalence of poison ivy should prove a sufficient deterrent.

Goldfinches occasionally bathe in the small pool below Havemeyer Falls, which is just ahead via the next spur. The stream that makes up this scenic splasher is reputedly the healthiest tributary in Mianus's 37-square-mile watershed, though it is often dry by late summer. With a bit of rock-scrambling, you can easily reach the bank of the Bargh Reservoir. Not too many years ago, the falls marked the hike's turnaround point. Additional land acquisitions, however, have extended the route by nearly a quarter-mile, right to the rocky shore of the reservoir. The elevation there is just under 300 feet, lower than the trailhead by a mere 50. Post 15, nearly halfway back, is the highest point, where the elevation tops 550 feet. The return along the Blue Trail follows much the same route as the Red, with a few side branches providing the illusion that you are on a loop rather than a straight track.

## NEARBY ACTIVITIES

Finished the 4.5 miles at Mianus and you're still hot to trot? The Bedford Audubon Society's **Henry Morgenthau Preserve** is in the vicinity, with a short trail to the pristine Blue Heron Lake. For further information, visit **henrymorgenthau preserve.com.**

You might add another mile or so to your trekking total with a stop at the **Bye Preserve,** another Nature Conservancy unit just north of the Connecticut state line, on the east side of NY 137. Beech, black birch, and a variety of oaks are the predominant trees along the small ravine at the heart of this peaceful pocket-park. For additional information and some more pretty preserves, visit **thesalmons.org/lynn/walks.**

# PELHAM BAY ISLANDS LOOP 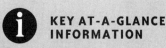 10

## IN BRIEF

Giant beech, birch, and tulip trees provide the gift of shade to this tranquil oasis, which is within a tennis ball lob of one of the area's more popular beaches and sports complexes. Close proximity to a lagoon, the bay, and a salt marsh make this a birding paradise, especially during the spring and fall migrations, so don't forget to bring your binoculars.

## DESCRIPTION

In the mood for a trivia question? Name the Big Apple's biggest park. Hint: it consists of land the city acquired in 1888 and now totals 2,766 acres, including 13 miles of shoreline. If you guessed Pelham Bay Park, you're one of the few, the proud, the informed, and you may just be ready for an appearance on *Jeopardy!*

Of the 28 estates that once lined Pelham Bay, only the Bartow-Pell Mansion (circa 1840) remains. Which is not to suggest that this coastal park is largely undeveloped. On the contrary, visitors with a penchant for play can indulge in a panoply of pursuits, including tennis, basketball, golf, sunbathing, even horseback riding. Oh, did we overlook hiking? There is that, too, with the excellent—if unchallenging—Hunter Island and Twin Island double-dip just off Orchard Beach.

### KEY AT-A-GLANCE INFORMATION

**LENGTH: 2.9 miles**

**ELEVATION GAIN: 116 feet**

**CONFIGURATION: 2 connected loops**

**DIFFICULTY: Very easy**

**SCENERY: Saltwater marshes alternate with views of Long Island Sound and tidal inlets along partially forested trails**

**EXPOSURE: Mostly shady trails; exposed when exploring shoreline**

**TRAFFIC: Moderate, although most people remain on the beach.**

**TRAIL SURFACE: Gravel and dirt, boardwalk and grass**

**HIKING TIME: 1.5 hours**

**DRIVING DISTANCE: 11 miles**

**SEASON: Year-round, sunrise–sunset**

**ACCESS: Parking fee is $6 weekdays and $8 weekends Memorial Day weekend–Labor Day; dogs on leash. Boardwalk is wheelchair-accessible.**

**MAPS: At Orchard Beach Nature Center during summer; online at tinyurl .com/pelhambaymap; USGS *Harlem***

**FACILITIES: Restrooms along beach boardwalk, summer concession stands, picnic areas, tennis, golf, playground**

**COMMENTS: Bring insect repellent May–September, when mosquitoes reign. For further information, call 212-NEW-YORK or 718-430-1890, or visit nycgovparks.org/park /pelhambaypark.**

### Directions

Take I-95 North to Exit 8B (Orchard Beach/ City Island) and follow the signs to Orchard Beach for about 2.5 miles until you reach a large paved parking lot on the right. Drive straight across the lot and park by the tennis courts. Orchard Beach lies directly beyond.

## GPS COORDINATES

N40° 52.196'  W73° 47.574'

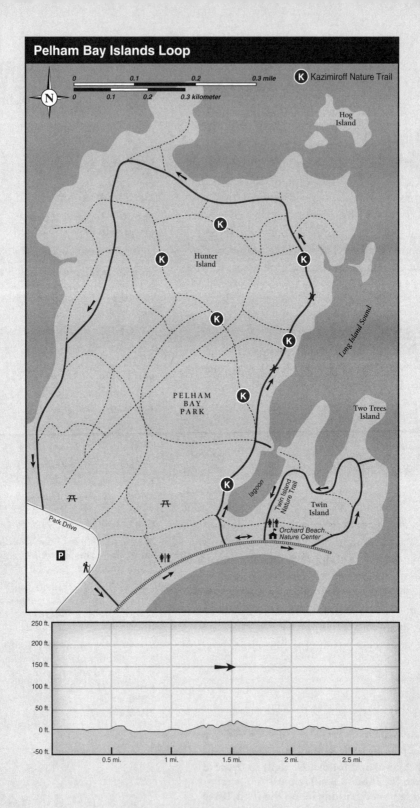

# Pelham Bay Islands Loop

**K** Kazimiroff Nature Trail

N

0    0.1    0.2    0.3 mile
0    0.1    0.2    0.3 kilometer

Hog Island

Hunter Island

Long Island Sound

PELHAM BAY PARK

Two Trees Island

lagoon

Twin Island Nature Trail

Twin Island

Orchard Beach Nature Center

Park Drive

P

250 ft.
200 ft.
150 ft.
100 ft.
50 ft.
0 ft.
-50 ft.

0.5 mi.    1 mi.    1.5 mi.    2 mi.    2.5 mi.

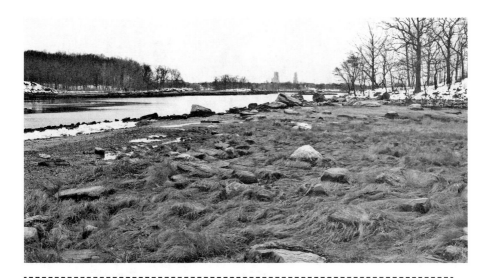

Except for some hearty waterfowl and a few hungry squirrels, Twin Island is mostly deserted in winter.

Start at the northeast end of the parking lot and stroll toward the water. No, this is not going to be a sandy beach walk; when you hit the concrete boardwalk, turn left and go to the Orchard Beach Nature Center, at section two of the beach, where you can pick up an interpretive brochure. Continuing along the boardwalk, hang a left at the next break in the inland side of the railing and take the middle trail, the widest of your three options, rapidly entering into the shade of oaks, birch, black locust, and shagbark hickory trees, with beggar squirrels scrambling around by your feet. This is Twin Island, which, as you may have observed, is not actually an island at all. It *was* until 1947, when the New York City parks commission filled the water between it and the mainland with rocks, effectively extending the peninsula. (A similar stunt was pulled on nearby Hunter Island, 13 years earlier.) Nonetheless, the contrast between the calm of this peaceful retreat and the rollicking sounds of the picnic parties and beach bathers beyond is sharp enough to feed the illusion of being on a distant speck of land.

Ignore the social trails that have been worn into the soft, loamy soil, sticking instead with the main track as it passes by a patch of phragmites and wild blackberries before arriving at a spur, on the right, that leads to the rocky, glacier-scoured shore. Go ahead and explore this scenic spot, which is attractive despite a plethora of plastic and other flotsam, then return to the path, which soon begins to arc toward the west, or left, passing, meanwhile, additional access points to the photogenic waterside. Within a minute or three, as the trail curves southward, you are delivered onto the sandy beach, with a tidal inlet—look for herons and egrets—to the right. Keep moving south until you reach the crotch of the inlet, where the path breaks left, straight, and to the right (GPS: N40° 52.277' W73° 47.097'):

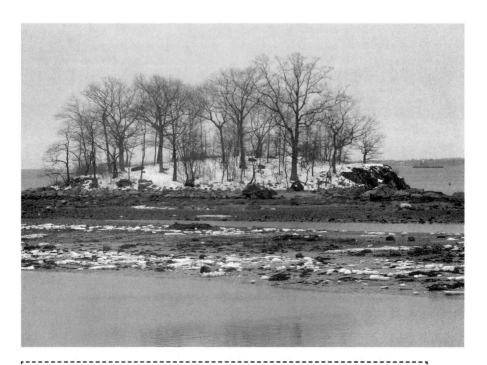

Several spits of land, frequented by marine and winged creatures and the occasional kayaker, surround Hunter Island.

take the last option and, now heading west, use the rocks to hop over the stream where a tidal pool seeps into the inlet. Leap left at the next intersection, by the interpretive sign about shorebirds, joining a wide trail, and stay with this as it emerges by the nature center.

The ensuing stage of this convoluted course lies to the right, about 100 yards along the boardwalk. March inland directly opposite the sign for section three of the beach, by another gap in the barrier (GPS: N40° 52.213' W73° 47.306'), and move toward the woods, steering to the right of the picnic area. In a jiffy you'll be standing under a dense canopy of mature shade trees, on the first leg of the Kazimiroff Nature Trail, where the numbered posts are pegged to the brochure you picked up at the nature center. Don't get too carried away with the reading, though, or you may miss the great white egrets and other waterfowl that fish and nest in the weeds and shallows of the surrounding marshes. Actually, there is little chance of that, as the abundance of spurs to water and marsh viewpoints makes bird sightings almost as common as the swarms of mosquitoes that hover over hikers like cumulus clouds.

Toward the center of Hunter Island, a tangle of sassafras, silver-barked beech, and black birch—many aged and goitered—lend an air of seclusion to this part of the park. Feel free to dart inland and explore the rat's maze of interlacing trails; with water on three sides of the peninsula, you'll have to work hard to get lost.

For the easiest water access, though, hang around the perimeter, sticking to the right at almost every major junction. Head through the first such intersection, which occurs just as you encounter a cluster of mature tulip trees. Bear right at the next fork, brushing by a massive oak and over a pair of long wooden bridges. At the four-way crossing, continue straight, as the path descends perhaps 12 feet over a large stelelike stone, then bends left, yielding glimpses of a salt marsh and the north end of the bay.

Edge onward through the intersection that appears right after a superannuated tulip tree; the left leg returns to the Kazimiroff, while the trace to the right leads to water access and a picnic table amid the sandy marsh. The trail circles to the left, then parallels the lagoon and begins a great stretch for watching birds and boats—have your binoculars handy. Remain walking southward, by majestic oaks and a few mature cottonwoods, while keeping the cordgrass and water to your right. The odd popping sound of tennis balls indicates the trail's imminent end, by a cluster of white birch trees and picnic tables at the north side of the parking lot.

## NEARBY ACTIVITIES

The **Bartow-Pell Mansion Museum,** on Shore Road within the park, showcases upper-crust country living of the 1800s. The 9-acre estate includes plush period furniture, art collections, and a carriage house. For information, call 718-885-1461 or visit **bartowpellmansionmuseum.org.**

If you feel like donning a tourist's hat, plan to explore **City Island.** All sorts of art galleries, antiques, and craft shops, as well as many popular seafood restaurants, are wrapped up in the picturesque atmosphere of this quaint fishing town. More at **cityisland.com.**

# 11  ROCKEFELLER MEDLEY

## KEY AT-A-GLANCE INFORMATION

**LENGTH: 9.6 miles**

**ELEVATION GAIN: 1,147 feet**

**CONFIGURATION: 2 connected loops**

**DIFFICULTY: Easy to moderate**

**SCENERY: Dense network of carriage roads circling a lake and threading through deciduous forests and open fields traversed by streams, many spanned by rustic bridges**

**EXPOSURE: Balanced between shady forests and open meadows**

**TRAFFIC: On weekends, people flock to most corners of the preserve.**

**TRAIL SURFACE: Gravel-and-dirt or cinder-surfaced carriage roads; only a half-mile of dirt-grass trail at end**

**HIKING TIME: 4 hours**

**DRIVING DISTANCE: 23 miles**

**SEASON: Year-round, sunrise–sunset**

**ACCESS: $6 vehicle-entry fee April–October and on weekends year-round, or Empire Passport ($65) for year-round use. No bicycles, pets on leash, horses allowed.**

**MAPS: At visitor center; download from tinyurl.com/rockefellerspmap**

**FACILITIES: Restrooms, water, and public phone at visitor center**

**COMMENTS: Access via Sleepy Hollow Road is free. For further information, call 914-631-1470 or visit nysparks.com/parks/59/details.aspx.**

## GPS COORDINATES

N41° 6.619'  W73° 50.028'

## IN BRIEF

This walk travels largely over an extensive network of wide, smooth carriage lanes, but don't be fooled. Rockefeller's scenery runs the gamut, from the serenity of a small lake to the backwoods beauty of rock-studded beech forests, from photogenic bridges and stream crossings to lush meadows. With many, many miles of trails, this is a great spot for short strolls or all-day outings. Visit early or late in the day to improve your chances of seeing deer.

## DESCRIPTION

The distance between Rockefeller Center and Rockefeller State Park is only 23 miles. It might as well be 23 *light-years*, though, for all the similarity they bear to each other. The immensely popular 1,000-acre park boasts a broad mix of habitats, including woodlands, wetlands, grassy meadows, and a 24-acre lake, with hikers rubbing up against joggers and equestrians on its 20 miles of carriage lanes. As for Rockefeller Center, well, you already know about that.

Originally, the preserve was a part of the Rockefeller family's Pocantico Hills estate, before being deeded to New York in 1983. Unlike other land the Rockefellers have given to the public, such as that in Acadia National Park and Grand Teton National Park, this realm won't require you to don hiking boots

- - - - - - - - - - - - - - - - - - - - - - - - - - - - - - - - -

## *Directions* ────────────→

**Follow I-87 North to Exit 9 and turn left on NY 119/White Plains Road. Continue 0.3 mile and turn right on US 9/South Broadway. Drive 3.3 miles and merge right onto NY 117 East. Proceed 1.5 miles to the park entrance on the right. Parking is 0.2 mile ahead.**

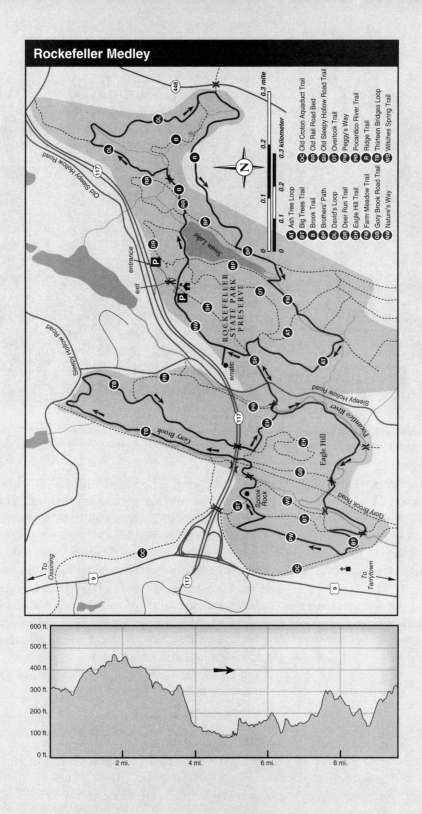

# Rockefeller Medley

**Legend:**

- **AT** Ash Tree Loop
- **BT** Big Trees Trail
- **B** Brook Trail
- **BP** Brothers' Path
- **DL** David's Loop
- **DR** Deer Run Trail
- **EH** Eagle Hill Trail
- **FM** Farm Meadow Trail
- **GB** Gory Brook Road Trail
- **NW** Nature's Way
- **OC** Old Croton Aquaduct Trail
- **RB** Old Rail Road Bed
- **SH** Old Sleepy Hollow Road Trail
- **OT** Overlook Trail
- **PW** Peggy's Way
- **PR** Pocantico River Trail
- **R** Ridge Trail
- **TB** Thirteen Bridges Loop
- **WS** Witches Spring Trail

ROCKEFELLER STATE PARK PRESERVE

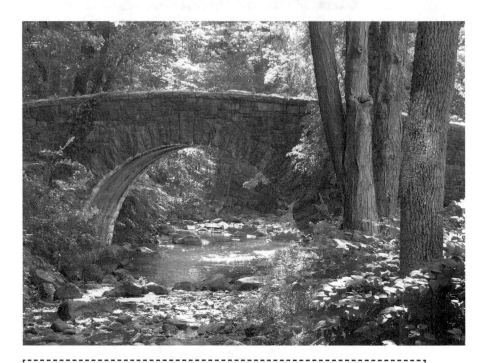

A bridge too far? Not if you're in reasonable hiking shape, and it beats wading across the river.

to survey it. Almost all the trails are graded carriage lanes, and thus the most challenging obstacles you are likely to contend with are pebbles on the path. That said, this is one dazzling domain, laced with more than enough loops to put in a long, enjoyable workout.

Stop by the modern visitor center, uphill from the parking area, and pick up a map. Trails are extremely well signposted, but a map is necessary to get the most out of this sprawling park. Continue onward to the pastoral Swan Lake, where lilies dot the water and oaks thrive by its cattail-lined shore, and you'll probably see more people jogging, strolling, and sunning themselves than over the remainder of this 9.6-mile jaunt. Follow the left side of the lake, and just after fording its grass-covered dam, hang a left onto Old RR Bed. You may be relieved to observe that the well-groomed look of the lake area, with the lawn snipped just so, does not carry over to the undulating forestland beyond the water. In fact, as you move right onto the Brook Trail, wildflowers, ferns, and sassafras begin to vie for space with the strip of grass that flanks the gravel-and-sand-surfaced track.

Your next turn is to the left, loping uphill on David's Loop among dogwoods, birch, beech, and tulip trees. Hilly and nearly a mile long, this is one of the park's more secluded—and prettier—pieces of trail. It ends back on Brook, where you jump left, only to swing right directly after that on the Ridge Trail. Also about a mile in length, the Ridge runs by fairly open grasslands that evoke the times when farms still operated in these parts. For a while it is also within earshot, alas, of NY 448, picking up a disturbing amount of traffic noise before wending away to the right.

Eventually, the Ridge dead-ends back at Swan Lake; bear left on the Brothers' Path, then right at the subsequent four-way crossing in perhaps 125 yards. Keep right at the ensuing junction, where a conduit flows off the lake, then pivot sharply left, leaving Brothers' Path for the Farm Meadow Trail. This parallels a small creek for a bit as you proceed straight at the first turnoff for Ash Tree Loop, heaving right only at the second option for the latter. Swing left at the bottom of the hill, onto the Overlook Trail, and tack left again when Overlook meets the Old Sleepy Hollow Road Trail. Stay with Sleepy Hollow across the pavement (look out for cars!) and over the bridge, until it slams into the Pocantico River Trail. Lunge left there.

This 0.75-mile stretch by the scenic, meandering river is especially enjoyable in spring, when the water level is high. A modest cascade, maybe 100 yards below the bridge, has a number of viewing spots atop the retaining wall from which to gaze at the purling water. You might also choose to leave the path and sit on a rock by the river, sandwich or sketchpad in hand. At the finely wrought Romanesque bridge—one of several such structures in the preserve—canter to the right and persevere along Pocantico until it eventually hits the Gory Brook Road Trail. Veer left at the span, then hang an immediate right and stride straight through the intersection with the abandoned road. At the next junction, hew to the left, just before the bridge, marching onward for an eighth of a mile, eventually crossing Gory Brook via one of the more impressive bridges in the preserve, this one supported by three arches. Go left at the ensuing turn, now trending more steeply upward, with a thick grove of pines off to the side. Shift right at the subsequent intersection, shortly after a partly hidden cemetery, onto the secluded Peggy's Way. Remain with this for three-eighths of a mile, at which point hang a right on Big Tree Trail, where you may see, as we have, a red-tailed hawk perched among the giant poplars. Your next turn, in an eighth of a mile, is a left; then bear right at the ensuing junction of trails. Continue downhill and circle to the right, keeping an eye out on that side of the path for Spook Rock, a gray, oblong erratic streaked with black varnish. Whether this sarcophagus-like stone resembles a ghost that's gone to sleep, an ogre lying on his back, or whatever, depends upon the light, your imagination—and, just possibly, the sounds emanating from the forest at that particular moment.

Ambling onward down the hill, step left at the first fork, and ditto at the base of the triangle. You should now be in the boggy area of Witches Spring Trail, passing over a bridge and then swinging left onto Gory Brook (once more) at the top of the rise. Stagger straight ahead on Thirteen Bridges Trail at the ensuing intersection, which appears a few seconds later. (Or, to save 2 miles, turn right and go on to Eagle Hill—see next paragraph.) This route passes directly under NY 117 and quickly puts the roar of traffic behind you. As to whether there are actually 13 bridges along this mini-loop, well, go ahead and count: we've tried to do so many times, but, frankly, the subtle pulchritude of this section of the park, its extended cluster of hemlocks, the rising ridge of granite, even its aura of isolation, all combine to distract us from our census. Ignore the side spurs to the left as you head north, gradually gaining modest elevation, and do likewise on your return, as the path gently meanders southward.

Once you've passed back under NY 117, launch left on Eagle Hill. When it hits Pocantico, go left briefly, then right, recross the bridge at the end of Old Sleepy Hollow Road Trail, and then hop over Sleepy Hollow Road itself. This is familiar ground—a retracing of your earlier steps until you meet the somewhat overgrown Nature's Way on the left.

Nature's Way is the one trail in Rockefeller that is restricted solely to hikers. While it's a pity that only a half-mile is so designated in a park this large, and that it runs *ear*-fully close to busy NY 117, Nature's Way does have its pretty points. It arcs by locust trees, hemlocks, and Tarzan vines that hang invitingly from broad-limbed white pines. A granite outcropping just off the trail adds to the rustic charm of this path, as did the three white-tailed stags and a brood of wild turkeys we encountered on different visits. About a third of the way along this narrow stretch, a spur to the left has been carved into the undergrowth. It dead-ends, in less than a quarter-mile, by an odd, enormous erratic, just to the side of a partly overgrown remnant of a large stone bridge. The hike ends at the overflow parking area, with the main lot just ahead.

## NEARBY ACTIVITIES

This area is quite rich in Rockefeller-themed cultural attractions. **Kykuit: The Rockefeller Estate,** in Pocantico Hills, features a magnificent art collection, antique carriages, and automobiles, as well as terraced gardens overlooking the Hudson River. Call 914-631-8200 for information.

**Philipsburg Manor,** in Sleepy Hollow (on US 9), is a Dutch-style estate with 18th-century furnishings, a barn, and a working gristmill. Call 914-631-8200 for information.

The **Union Church,** on Bedford Road (NY 448), is open to the public and contains stained-glass windows by Chagall and Matisse. For tours, call 914-332-6659.

For more details on all attractions above, visit **hudsonvalley.org.**

Highlights of the **Lyndhurst** estate, in Tarrytown (also on US 9), include oil paintings, Tiffany glass, silk rugs, and trompe l'oeil ceilings and walls. Call 914-631-4481 or visit **lyndhurst.org** for details.

# TEATOWN TRIPLE  12

## IN BRIEF

A lake with an island devoted to wildflowers, a couple of streams, and a number of boardwalks and bridges make this a can't-miss for family outings. The wild-at-heart should beat a path to the forested hillsides, too, where granite outcroppings, bogs, and meadows round out this diverse park. Teatown is crosscut by numerous paths, including a stretch of the Briarcliff–Peekskill Trail, so you can create as long or short a hike as fits your time or energy.

## DESCRIPTION

Some people feel that a hike is not complete without at least one animal sighting. A lone deer grazing on spruce needles, a fuzzy-tailed squirrel gathering acorns, even a swarm of bloodsucking mosquitoes in some intangible way validates the experience of being outdoors for a few hours. No hike comes with a guarantee, of course, that a focus on things feral will come to fruition. But Teatown Lake does the next best thing: it offers up a fail-safe selection of animals within its half-timbered, cream-colored nature center.

Want to know what a corn snake looks like? The nature center has one, along with a black rat snake, a garter snake, green and gray tree frogs, a bearded dragon, a couple of cuddly ferrets, a bobcat, coyote, barn owl, and

### KEY AT-A-GLANCE INFORMATION

**LENGTH:** 5 miles

**ELEVATION GAIN:** 1,037 feet

**CONFIGURATION:** 3 connected loops

**DIFFICULTY:** Easy to moderate

**SCENERY:** Gently rolling trails meander through shady forest, around a lake, and among a few swamps.

**EXPOSURE:** Dense, protective canopy and only one open meadow

**TRAFFIC:** Light across Blinn Road, but Lakeside Trail is quite popular on summer weekends.

**TRAIL SURFACE:** Dirt with occasional rocks and roots, and boardwalks

**HIKING TIME:** 2.5 hours

**DRIVING DISTANCE:** 30 miles

**SEASON:** Year-round, sunrise–sunset

**ACCESS:** Free, but donations welcome; pets on leash, no bicycles

**MAPS:** At nature center; download from tinyurl.com/teatownmap; USGS *Ossining*

**FACILITIES:** Water and restrooms at nature center; picnic area and public phone

**COMMENTS:** The 2-acre Wildflower Island sanctuary is open mid-April–September. To preregister for a guided tour or for further details, call 914-762-2912, ext. 110, or visit teatown.org.

## *Directions* ⟶

Follow the Taconic State Parkway North to the NY 134 exit toward Ossining. Turn left on NY 134/Kitchawan Road and after 0.2 mile turn right on Grants Lane. Continue for 0.2 mile and go right on Spring Valley Road. Proceed 0.6 mile and make a right on Blinn Road. The Lakeside parking lot is 0.1 mile ahead, on the left.

## GPS COORDINATES

N41° 12.816' W73° 49.596'

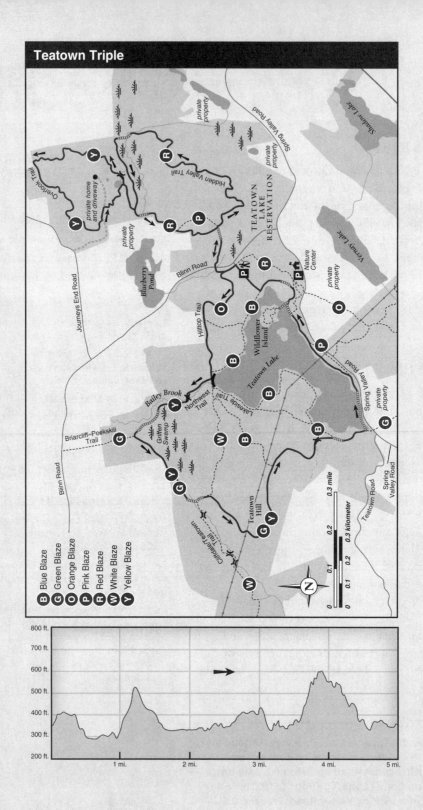

# Teatown Triple

moose. Well, okay, the last four are stuffed, but you get the idea: this is very much a family-friendly operation. Managed by a nonprofit corporation, Teatown was established in 1963 with just 190 acres. It has since grown to 759 acres, which consist of a large lake and wildflower island and several scenic loops showcasing swampland, meadows, hardwood and conifer forests, and a craggy gorge.

Most of these features may be seen over three loops that amount to 5 miles of fairly easy walking. (These circuits may, of course, be tackled separately for shorter excursions.) Two of these routes start near the road on the right side of the parking lot, and yes, there is indeed a good chance of encountering wildlife along the way. The trail forks as you leave the lot, with the orange-blazed Hilltop heading left and the red-slashed Hidden Valley cutting across the road. Keep to the left for now (careful of the poison ivy); you'll return to the Hidden Valley Trail in about an hour and a half. Initially the fairly open dirt track parallels the parking lot, followed in a few minutes by private dwellings to the right, in addition to a number of weather-stained erratics. The path brushes by maples, shagbark hickories, hemlocks, and a handful of withered cedars, then shifts downhill through a shady patch of pines.

It arrives near the base of that slope at the north end of Teatown Lake, with the latter's shimmering green surface lit up by lily pads. Cross the concrete edge of the dam and then, after a short wooden walkway, hang a right onto the Northwest Trail (yellow tags). This gravel-lined track hugs Bailey Brook (more rocks than water much of the year) for perhaps 200 yards before crossing a bridge and continuing to the right, away from the lake. Diverging slowly from the brook, this northwest passage threads precariously through the moist, mucky Griffen Swamp (look for red cardinal flowers among the slippery rocks), with grass and ferns at ankle level and maple, beech, and tulip trees towering above.

On the far side of a wooden span is a fork; stick with the yellow (now paired with green) blazes to the left. From there, the meandering begins in earnest, and like a magician dazzling his audience with a succession of tricks, there will be fleeting glimpses of a high, rocky ridge rising dramatically to the right, more swampy conditions along a couple of boardwalks, another boulder-filled bluff, maybe a red-tailed hawk soaring low over the birch trees, and then a series of intersections. Stride straight through the first junction (by the boardwalk), and bear right—still on yellow—at the next. Ten minutes of marching uphill should put you among laurels, hemlocks, and a mound of jagged granite.

Savor this setting, for in a few more steps the scenery takes a definite—though momentary—turn for the worse, as you emerge on an open hillside under a nucleus of power lines. The climb continues in the shadow of those cables and their colossal support stanchions, with blueberry bushes, sassafras, Queen Anne's lace, and wild grapes thriving beneath the sun's strong glare. Stay to the left at the ensuing four-way intersection, and keep stomping up the steep, rock-filled slope. Finally at the top, canter left and descend on the other side of the power lines through knee- to waist-high grass and winged sumac. The yellow-green blazes veer off to the right at

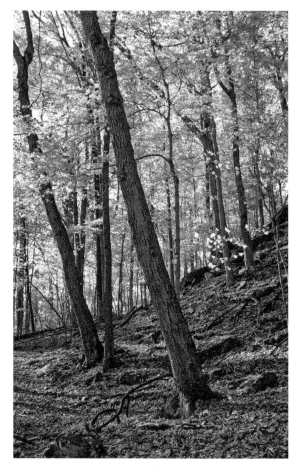

The Overlook Trail may not offer a view, but in autumn its golden maples are the attraction.

the base of one stanchion, bending at last away from those eyesores and back under a mantle of maples and oaks, among a range of rocky ridgelines.

The trail shifts left by a stone wall, near a boggy patch, yielding in the process a pretty fair view of Teatown Lake. From there, it's downward by an imposing series of boulders, seemingly frozen in place as they were cascading down the hill. Roll right on the 20-foot-long boardwalk at the junction with the blue-blazed Lakeside Trail and, as soon as you've hit the west side of the lake, shift left (just prior to the road) onto a pontoon boardwalk that runs directly over a section of the water. This segment of the hike rewards your decision to bring field specs, as the birding is typically excellent and it's easy to whittle time off the clock counting mallards, swans, and Canada geese (and occasionally something more exotic).

In due time, press onward through the shady nook by the shore, over the next span, and into a second maple-graced recess. Note the spruce grove near the small access pavilion to Wildflower Island; the farmers who tilled the earth here planted it as a windbreak more than a century ago. Moving east by the water, lope left at the wooden stairs to the nature center and pass over the boardwalk. Stroll by the enormous tulip tree, go straight across the trail junction (left leads down a boardwalk to a view of Wildflower Island through a bird blind), then hop off blue to the right and return to the parking area.

Once more at the trailhead by the road, this time follow the red blazes of the Hidden Valley Trail (HV) across the asphalt for an entirely different look at the park. Proceed through the rock wall and over the boardwalk into a grassy, fern-speckled meadow, with an apple orchard on one side, black walnut trees on the other, and a handful of dogwoods, maples, and sycamores tossed in for good measure. Shuffle right at the four-way junction and remain with the red blazes throughout the entire 1.6-mile loop, seeing along the way thick clusters of pines and hemlocks, and several dramatic escarpments with rocks spilling down their angular sides. There is even another boardwalk by an extended marsh.

The yellow-blazed spur of the Overlook Trail (OT) appears a couple of minutes past an impressively high granite formation (GPS: N41° 13.055' W73° 49.439'). If your soles still have good spring, consider adding this 1.1-mile mini-loop to the tour: it leads to one of the park's more untamed areas, where the rough-cut beauty is highly appealing and the flush of wildflowers in the spring and summer adds to its allure. From the short series of stone steps that lead away from the HV, the path ascends to a small reed-rimmed pond, its muddy banks blooming with lobelia in summer. Continue to the right, over additional steps, making use of the guide rope as you climb uphill. Take a moment to catch your breath, enjoying meanwhile, in the break of the rock formations to the right, the great view of the swamp you passed through earlier, and the tree-lined hills beyond; the trail snakes higher still, but the vistas won't get any better. The next set of steps heralds the summit, and the highest point of the hike, at 584 feet of elevation. The wild look to the woods here, with lichen-speckled rocks scattered among miscellaneous maples, oaks, birches, and mountain laurels, suggests a deeply forested wilderness—even though there's a house tucked just out of sight below the crest. That illusion dissipates rapidly as the OT descends to a paved driveway, where a couple of monster homes are visible to the right. Swing left on the asphalt and in 50 paces head right, returning to the shelter of the trees. Back at the pond, retrace your steps to the turnoff from the HV, and veer right, once more following the red blazes. Stay with those markings all the way to the meadow, and from there to the parking lot.

## NEARBY ACTIVITIES

Nearby Ossining offers—in addition to quaint eating and drinking spots—attractions such as the **Ossining Heritage Center**. Its exhibits focus on historic town buildings, the Old Croton Aqueduct, and such Sing Sing–related themes as weapons made by prisoners, replicas of cells, and an electric chair. Free admission; for information, call 914-941-3189 or visit **hudsonriver.com/hudson-river-ossining**.

# 13  WARD POUND RIDGE STAR LOOP

## KEY AT-A-GLANCE INFORMATION

**LENGTH:** 6.6 miles

**ELEVATION GAIN:** 1,053 feet

**CONFIGURATION:** Loop

**DIFFICULTY:** Easy to moderate

**SCENERY:** Swamps, hemlock, laurel, and hardwood forests, rock outcroppings, scenic overlook of a reservoir, and historic cave

**EXPOSURE:** Shady canopy cover in summer, few exposed spots

**TRAFFIC:** Heavy summers and most weekends; seldom crowded

**TRAIL SURFACE:** Dirt, rocks, roots

**HIKING TIME:** 3 hours

**DRIVING DISTANCE:** 42 miles

**SEASON:** Year-round, 8 a.m.–sunset

**ACCESS:** $5 with Westchester County Parks Pass ($60 for county residents), $10 without pass; pets on leash, no bicycles, no swimming

**MAPS:** At entrance booth; posted at trailhead; USGS *Pound Ridge;* download from tinyurl.com/wprmap

**FACILITIES:** Restrooms and water at park office and some picnic areas; telephone at park office

**COMMENTS:** Fishing is possible in the Cross River. For other activities and further information, call 914-864-7317 or visit parks.westchestergov .com/ward-pound-ridge-reservation.

## GPS COORDINATES

N41° 14.876'  W73° 35.657'

## IN BRIEF

You could easily while away a day or two on the trails here and still not see the entire park. Its sublime scenery is a marvelous medley of hardwood forests, glacial ridges, lowland bogs, granite outcroppings, and high-rising bluffs, with a couple of ravines, a river, and a far-reaching viewpoint as added attractions. The main trails are wide and very popular with family groups, while many narrower routes provide a more rugged experience.

## DESCRIPTION

Ward Pound Ridge Reservation—or simply Pound Ridge—is the largest preserve in the Westchester County Parks system, with 35 miles of trails slicing seamlessly, almost artistically, through its 4,700 acres. It is also the most beautiful of the county's parks, where litter on the ground is as rare as candy in a dentist's office, and the camping shelters (stone lean-tos constructed by the Civilian Conservation Corps more than 65 years ago are raked clean by park personnel.

A nucleus of 32 abutting farms was purchased back in 1924 to create the reservation. Extensive tracts have since been added, and with almost every step you take, Pound Ridge's

-------------------------------------------

### *Directions* ⟶

**Follow the Hutchinson River Parkway North and keep left onto I-684 North. Drive to Exit 6 and merge onto the Saw Mill River Parkway North. Take Exit 6 onto NY 35 East/Cross River Road and drive 4 miles, then turn right (south) at the junction with NY 121. The reservation entrance is immediately to the left. Continue for 0.5 mile to the entrance booth. About 0.2 mile beyond, steer right onto Michigan Road and proceed for 0.7 mile to the parking lot.**

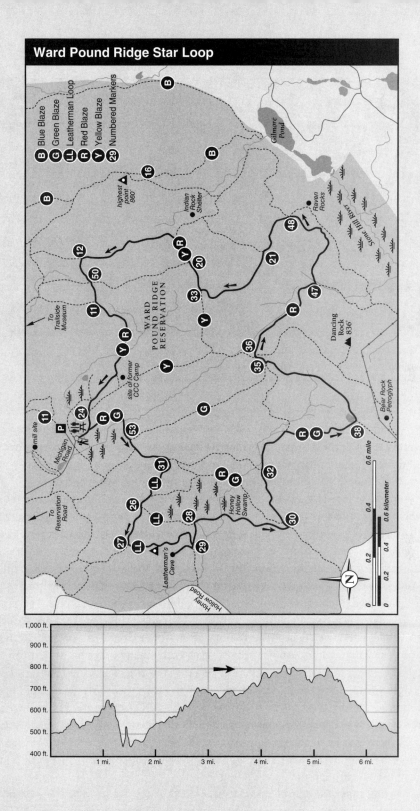

# Ward Pound Ridge Star Loop

**B** Blue Blaze
**G** Green Blaze
**LL** Leatherman Loop
**R** Red Blaze
**Y** Yellow Blaze
**29** Numbered Markers

highest point 860

Indian Rock Shelter

Raven Rocks

Stone Hill River

Gilmore Pond

WARD POUND RIDGE RESERVATION

To Trailside Museum

site of former CCC Camp

Dancing Rock 836'

Bear Rock Petroglyph

mill site

Michigan Road

To Reservation Road

Honey Hollow Swamp

Leatherman's Cave

Honey Hollow Road

0.6 mile
0.4
0.6 kilometer
0.4
0.2
0
0

N

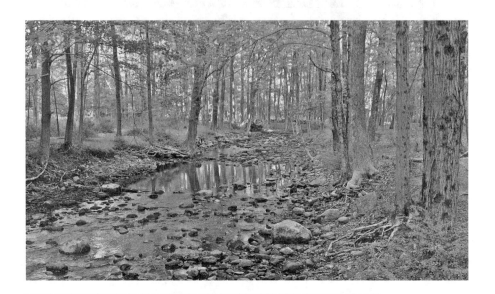

You know it's been a hot, dry summer when you can rock-hop over the Cross River.

agricultural antecedents are evident in the form of the rock walls running from the upland forests through the lowland swamps. A Trailside Nature Museum recounts some of this history, plus that of the indigenous people who earlier occupied the land, and it also has exhibits on native wildlife.

Regarding that wildlife, black bears have reportedly returned to these woods, yet you are far more likely to encounter white-tailed deer. Commonplace as those herbivores are nowadays, it remains a thrill to see them dart through the hemlock and beech groves, bound over granite ridges, or spring past the park's rippling streams. But if the most one can boast of is having witnessed a turkey vulture fly overhead, or heard a chipmunk yelping its squeaky alarm from within the chinks of an ancient wall—well, spending a few hours in such a wild, uncorrupted setting, without a house in view or car horn audible, is reward enough.

It's hard to go wrong with any of Pound Ridge's trails, but for a good overview of the park, we suggest the red-blazed 5.7-mile circuit. It is a wide, lilting loop, clearly marked and easy to follow, crossed by many other paths that can be used to create a longer or shorter hike. Begin at the Michigan Road trailhead, to the right of the picnic area. Almost immediately, there is a fork in the trail, near a couple of cedar trees; keep to the right. The red-blazed route (RT) runs first through a low swamp, highlighted by stands of hickory and black birch; then, after a quarter-mile, it starts edging up a pebbly slope. Bear left at the next intersection, as the upward slant gives way to a more rolling terrain, with dark boulders scattered through the surrounding woods.

During one of the level stretches that ensue, look for a slight trace branching off to the left, indicated by the number "25" mounted on a tree (GPS:

N41° 14.561' W73° 35.751'). That leads through Wildcat Hollow, a more challenging, highly appealing ravine trek of nearly a mile in length. This secluded detour is haphazardly marked with faded pink blazes, which zigzag from one side of the creek to the other, departing the ravine at its southeast end. On emerging from the hollow, the pink spur meets the Green Trail (GT), a main conduit, and you can return to the parking lot by taking it to the left, or resume the longer loop by going right and in 5 minutes veering left, back onto the RT.

If, on the other hand, you forgo the Wildcat Hollow side trip, the well-marked trail to the Leatherman's Cave lies just ahead, on your right. This, too, is a wonderful patch of the preserve, not so much for its namesake cave (which is really more of an indentation at the base of a rocky bluff), but for the splendid views from atop that bluff, and the varied topography you pass along the way. Stick with the spur's white blazes, which are overlain with double Ls (for "Leatherman Loop"), as they lead you into a forest that is initially dominated by silvery-barked beech, later giving way to maples and oaks. From this fairly open area, the grass-lined track moseys uphill away from the bog and passes, in about 6 minutes, a turnoff to the left by a tree tagged with a "26," before hitting a T at the base of a lichen-spotted granite rise. Steer left (the other way exits the park) and slog on to the top of the next rise. There are many traces worn into the mossy ground here, but straight ahead, beyond a few fallen limbs and rotting logs, is a bench that crowns an open viewpoint. This summit, at 665 feet, is nearly 200 feet lower than Pound Ridge's highest point, where a fire tower once stood. Nonetheless, the isolated aerie offers hands-down the finest, most far-reaching vistas in the park, with the Cross River Reservoir to the west assuming center stage.

From the bench the LL-blazed trail snakes south, over a slick of bedrock and by the mound of granite, hewing to an extension of the ridge. Keep right as the well-padded route descends from the bluff, passing by and under an angular overhang as it nears the bottom and approaches a stone wall. Just before you reach the signboard by that wall, turn right and march up the deeply eroded rut, the rubble of the bluff now to your right. In less than a minute you'll find the recess where "The Leatherman," Jules Bourglay, periodically sought shelter (GPS: N41° 14.490' W73° 36.185'). Seen by some to be a tramp, Bourglay was the ur-hiker, reportedly covering 365 miles in 30 days, a cycle he maintained for 30 years in peregrinations throughout western Connecticut and the Hudson Valley. To return to the loop, backtrack to the stone wall and jog left onto the wide track.

Skip the LL-blazed turnoff to the left that appears in roughly 2 minutes, by the tree marked with a "28," remaining instead on the broad path as it bends toward the south. For a few hundred yards you'll be treading through swamp country, this particular area going by the handle of Honey Hollow. The next intersection is a critical and rather convoluted one, a kind of triangle in which the straight option leaves the preserve. Head to the left and, in 15 strides, when you arrive at a four-way junction, continue directly ahead in a resumption of the RT.

In approximately 20 minutes, the GT, which has run concurrently with the RT thus far, diverges to the left. (You may pick up the far end of the previously described Wildcat Hollow Trail by walking 5 minutes down the GT and turning left on the vague trace by a tree with the number "34" on it.) The RT, meanwhile, forges onward, branching right at a Y in another 5 minutes. The hard-packed track alternately gains and loses ground after that turn, while heading first toward the southeast, before swooping around toward the north. Once it begins to tack to the left, now northwest, you will come to a "21," which marks a descending path to Indian Rock Shelter, a picturesque jumble of grass-topped boulders set among an overgrown, laurel-filled wetland. (A continuation of the spur, blazed white, leads to Pound Ridge's highest point.) In another 10 minutes, the RT hits a T, where it is joined by a yellow-blazed route (YT), and shifts to the right. The return leg from the Indian Rock Shelter appears on the right at the following major fork, while the red and yellow blazes swerve to the left.

Now heading north, you come, after 15 minutes of brisk walking, to a further series of turns, with the first and third rights leading to the Pell Hill picnic area and the Trailside Nature Museum (1 mile away), respectively. Keep with the clearly marked blazes as they head west, with the RT finally branching off to the right away from the YT through an open parcel of grassland. They merge once more in nearly a thousand feet, just before the trailhead. As you amble by the kiosk with the marsh nearby, you may catch sight of the glistening black domes of turtles among the tufts of grass, while being serenaded by peepers and bullfrogs.

## NEARBY ACTIVITIES

If you didn't spot a single specimen of wildlife, perhaps a visit to the **Wolf Conservation Center,** in South Salem, is in order. For more information, call 914-763-2373 or visit **nywolf.org.**

# WESTCHESTER WILDERNESS WALK

## IN BRIEF

Some trails naturally overlap animal paths or ancient forest roads, while others are created from scratch to showcase the wilds with a minimum impact. This hike takes a third approach, playfully, artistically, and circuitously winding around old walls and glacial erratics, through an attractive blend of hardwood highlands (complete with craggy bluffs) and soggy lowlands, where stepping-stone staircases draw visitors into the middle of streams and cascades.

## DESCRIPTION

Like most hikers, we have our favorite stomping grounds, little-known secluded spots where one is more likely to see wildlife than an ambling ambassador of civilization. The Westchester Wilderness Walk (WWW) is one such oasis. Although the preserve has been open for more than a dozen years now, it remains a fairly well-kept secret, and on most days you will probably see more hawks flying overhead than people on the trails. WWW, which is also known as the Zofnass Family Preserve, consists of a little more than 150 acres tucked into the heart of suburban Pound Ridge, just over the Connecticut state line. While that acreage may seem meager for anything bearing the word *wilderness* in its sobriquet, consider that creative—at times, *rococo*—trail construction has

---

### *Directions* ⟶

**Follow the Hutchinson River Parkway North to the Merritt Parkway/CT 15. Take Exit 34 onto Long Ridge Road/CT 104, and drive north on it for 5.5 miles to Upper Shad Road. Turn right on it and continue for 0.3 mile to a tiny parking lot on the left, opposite a small pond.**

---

### ⓘ KEY AT-A-GLANCE INFORMATION

**LENGTH:** 5.9 miles total; Southern Loop is a 2.7-mile self-guided nature hike.

**ELEVATION GAIN:** 932 feet

**CONFIGURATION:** 3 connected loops

**DIFFICULTY:** Easy to moderate

**SCENERY:** Mixed hardwood forest with upland rocky ridges, lowland swamps, and lots of stepping-stones

**EXPOSURE:** Only in winter, when dense canopy is absent

**TRAFFIC:** Pleasantly light

**TRAIL SURFACE:** Mostly dirt and rocks, with occasional streambed rock-hopping

**HIKING TIME:** 2.5 hours

**DRIVING DISTANCE:** 39 miles

**SEASON:** Year-round, sunrise–sunset

**ACCESS:** Free; pets on leash, no bicycles

**MAPS:** At trailhead; USGS *Pound Ridge;* download from westchester landtrust.org/wilderness-walk-map

**FACILITIES:** None

**COMMENTS:** This preserve is very attractive in spring, after snowmelt has filled the creeks; rock-hopping over streambeds is a fun challenge. For further information, call 914-241-6346 or visit westchesterlandtrust.org /westchester-wildnerness-walk.

## GPS COORDINATES

N41° 10.547'  W73° 35.963'

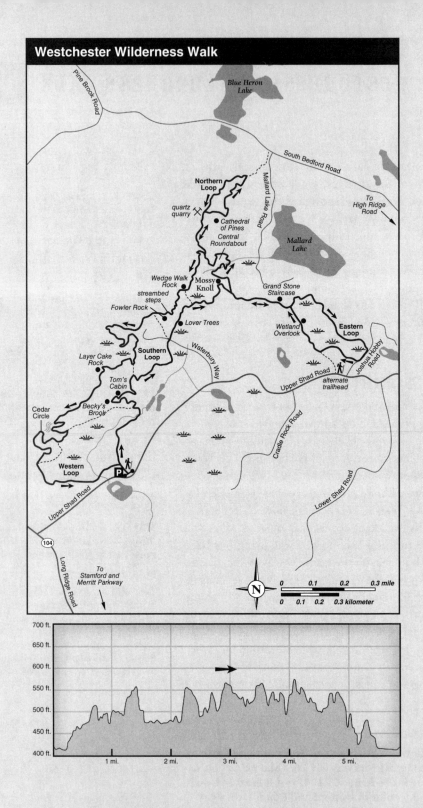

# Westchester Wilderness Walk

Blue Heron Lake

Pine Brook Road

South Bedford Road

To High Ridge Road

**Northern Loop**

quartz quarry

Cathedral of Pines

Central Roundabout

Mallard Lake Road

Mallard Lake

Wedge Walk Rock

Mossy Knoll

Grand Stone Staircase

streambed steps

Fowler Rock

Lover Trees

Wetland Overlook

**Eastern Loop**

**Southern Loop**

Layer Cake Rock

Waterbury Way

Upper Shad Road

alternate trailhead

Joshua Hobby Road

Tom's Cabin

Cedar Circle

Becky's Brook

**Western Loop**

P

Upper Shad Road

Cradle Rock Road

Lower Shad Road

104

Long Ridge Road

To Stamford and Merritt Parkway

N

| 0 | 0.1 | 0.2 | 0.3 mile |
| 0 | 0.1 | 0.2 | 0.3 kilometer |

700 ft.
650 ft.
600 ft.
550 ft.
500 ft.
450 ft.
400 ft.

1 mi.    2 mi.    3 mi.    4 mi.    5 mi.

resulted in four interconnected loops, amounting to 5.9 miles of densely forested pathways that wind circuitously through skunk cabbage–filled bogs, over seasonal streams, and by high-rising granite bluffs.

From the trailhead parking area (four- to five-vehicle capacity), slip through the rail fence and pick up a map at the wooden kiosk. Proceed north on the forest road, skipping the left-hand spur of the West Loop that appears in 100 yards— that's your return route. In a few minutes, the carriageway narrows to single-file and brushes up against a swamp—minor rock-hopping required—before hitting a low stone wall by post 5. Jump up on the wall and head left along the railing, thus avoiding the murky, meandering creek that covers the ground on either side of you. The trail resumes at the end of this span, shifting to the left before meeting a fork. Bear right, gaining a bit of elevation as you leave the lush wetland habitat behind—for now—and enter into a hardwood forest. Gneiss and schist, metamorphic rock outcroppings deposited by the Wisconsin Glacier when it withdrew from the area 12,000 to 15,000 years ago, lend an air of drama to the understory here.

In a moment or three, the path plunges through a gap in a wall and arrives at Becky's Brook, a small cascade tumbling over an array of rocks. A well-worn trace just before that leads to the right up a low embankment, but it's more fun to simply walk up the stream itself. That's correct, *up* the stream. In a whimsical bit of trail construction that recurs later in the hike, a crude stone stairway has been set directly into the flow, providing an over-the-top view of the water as it rolls and spills downhill. The main route, near the top of the cascade, presses onward along the upper lip of a granite fin.

From this colorful spot, the green-blazed track doglegs right, then left, shuffling through the ruins of an old cabin. Although it is referred to locally as Tom's Cabin, no one really knows who lived here. The site, much overgrown by hemlocks and beech trees, was left to squirrels and raccoons decades ago—and not much remains beyond its fireplace and foundation stones. The trail loops by a jumble of gray boulders, then swings left and ascends that mound via an improvised stair of stones. Stroll by post 11, which commemorates the decline of the American chestnut (due to a fungus accidentally introduced from overseas a century ago), and vault right in 25 yards at the junction with the South Loop cutoff.

The trail holds largely to the well-treed high ground for the next tenth of a mile, zigzagging between oaks, maples, and miscellaneous chunks of granite. On descending by a network of old mortarless walls toward a swamp on the right, it crosses a private drive and continues into an extension of the wetland (the track to the left is a shortcut to Fowler Outlook on the other side of the loop). A staggered line of oversize stone steps, fringed appealingly with large-leaf skunk cabbage, aids in fording a particularly wet portion of this bayou before the path once again starts to ascend. A couple of minutes' steady striding brings you to an intersection, with the hike proceeding to the right on a loop dubbed the Central Roundabout (CR).

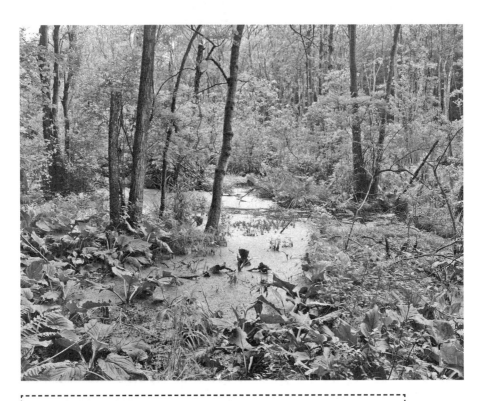

The Eastern Loop circles a large swamp teeming with all kinds of swimmers, but we don't recommend that you join them.

As the leaf-strewn track rises gently, a stone bench appears in a little more than a tenth of a mile, providing a splendid overlook of a serpentine stream coursing through the bog below. (From this vantage point, we were once thrilled to see a red-tailed hawk soaring aloft with a squirrel gripped in its talons.) This is listed as Mossy Knoll on the map, with the turnoff to the East Loop (EL) a few paces distant to the right. Shift onto that latter spur, as the EL surges through an open half-acre of grassy meadow, gradually being overgrown, before reaching a craggy bluff. Take the right fork to descend the series of steps (the left option is your return trail), officially dubbed the Grand Stone Staircase. This impressive display of amateur masonry delivers hikers to the lower terrain, where you should hang with the path as it tapers downhill in an easterly direction. In about a minute, take the hard left toward the north as the trail splits (you will return on the right spur). The ensuing area has a wild aura, with a boulder-littered bluff extending to your left and an expansive swamp simmering on the right. Within 5 minutes, the trace bends right, away from the rocky high ground, only to emerge at a paved road, where bit by bit houses are being built. Heave to the right there and remain on the right shoulder for the next 75 paces, slicing right by the large maple, next to a stone wall, as the blazes reenter the forest. Hew to the right at the subsequent juncture (the EL trailhead lies to the left) and persevere with the undulating loop as it reconnects, in 5 more minutes, with your earlier turnoff. Scoot left and proceed to the foot of the bluff, using the stone stairs on the right to reach its top. Backtrack from there to the CR, where you cruise right.

The CR earns its title of Roundabout during the succeeding quarter-mile, as it hugs the undulating terrain, darting to the right or left of various trees, loping around glacial debris, and cutting through ubiquitous bogs. Stay straight when you come to a left fork across a small stream by a hefty erratic, but remember that spur—you'll need to grab it on your return. This is the start of the North Loop, which rises initially before dipping toward a slightly lower elevation. In 5 minutes, as the Cathedral of Pines grove of conifers comes into view toward the east, the green blazes diverge, with your tour branching to the right.

Over the next 10 minutes, the trail approaches that large patch of pines, then lurches over some oblong stepping-stones, slips through gaps in a couple of stone walls, and drops toward a watery, fern-flecked swamp. You may require the steely vision of a French trapper here to spot the return spur to the left, as the natural flow of the trail appears to be straight onward, a rock-skipping route through the marsh. Don't worry if you miss the intersection (GPS: N41° 11.387' W73° 35.452'), because the South Bedford Road trailhead (no parking) is only a couple of minutes away, and you can easily double back from there.

The return from this shady, appealing swamp can be concluded in a fairly expeditious 5 minutes, after a brief climb and more stepping-stone marsh crossings. The mini-loop's end occurs just beyond the Quartz Quarry, where you transfer to the right and retrace your steps back to the earlier junction by the stream, beside the large, dark erratic. Before you hasten on, though, dawdle a moment to inspect this small, leaf-filled quarry site. Digging here ceased in the first half of the 19th century, and from then on the cavity was used as a garbage pit, with some of the trash, which consists largely of odd bottles and an occasional earthenware jug, reportedly dating back to the Civil War.

Having spun right at the fork by the stream, you are now traveling once more on the CR. The path gains a touch of elevation initially and then—predictably—loses it, meandering meanwhile around several sizable globs of granite and gliding over a handful of stone steps, with rock-hopping through a slow-moving creek preceding the CR's terminus. Tack right at the intersection and slip between the fractured rocks, listed on the map as Wedge Walk Rock, as the track gradually edges uphill. The minimal effort involved in this climb yields, in a moment or two, a fine overview of the surrounding swamp, and the chance, in spring, to observe bluebirds in flight. Then it's downward again, drifting beneath the bluff. On reaching a stream, the track veers left, only to cut suddenly to the right, where it ascends, as at Becky's Brook, over the very center of a trickling cascade. Well-positioned stones make this enjoyable stretch child's play, but as always when striding on wet rocks, be careful of your footing.

This improvised walkway arcs to the left away from the water in a couple of seconds, grinding up to a pair of erratics and a four-way intersection. Dead ahead

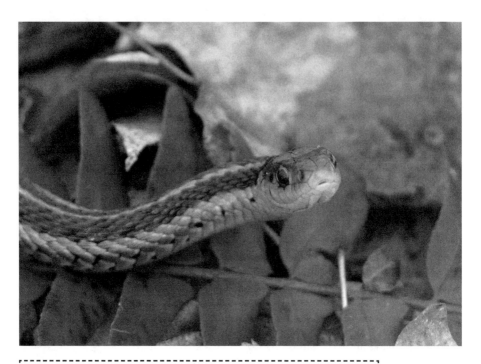

Don't tread on me: this little ribbon snake doesn't bite like a rattler, but it *may* know how to spit like a llama . . . .

is Fowler Outlook, a viewpoint from atop a large rock, with the hike continuing to the right on the faintly discernible trace. (Left is the aforementioned cutoff to the private road you crossed earlier.) A few spindly hemlocks leaven the hardwood mix of trees as you sputter upward by some fair-size boulders, and after an additional pair of lookout ledges, the green blazes guide you by a seasonal stream and alongside a broad bog. When you hit the T, bolt right.

The next portion of the hike is a resumption of the interpretive loop, with the numbered posts interspaced with such playfully named natural phenomenon as Pooh's Stump, Layer Cake Rock, and the World's Largest Poison Ivy Vine. That last curiosity, by the way, is at post 20, by a small, attractive cascade, where Dutchman's breeches flower in early spring. The trail hooks left there, descending over stone steps to the fairly level ground of a bog. Lurch right in about 100 yards, just shy of the large vine of fox grape roping across the main path. This is the new West Loop (WL), a short side trip through appealing swamp terrain.

On slipping through the gap in the wall, the WL swings right, keeping to the side of that wall. Turn right again at the subsequent T, as this fanciful, fern-flecked circuit hops over moss-covered rocks while showcasing some appealing craggy uplift, as well as colorful trillium and wild geranium in spring. Just as it appears that you're destined to revisit the cascade of earlier (the one abutting the giant vine of poison ivy), the trail hooks left and comes to a fork. Bear right, heading toward higher ground.

Shortly after circling by additional granite outcroppings and a collection of desiccated cedars, the WL breaks left, passing—as it begins to descend—a stone "fort," dubbed Mayo. (Though why is anyone's guess.) The trail bends sharply to the left just shy of this "fort" (more of a hook in the wall, really), as an avenue of cedars, maples, and black oaks unfolds around you. Veer right when you come to the other end of the spur you bypassed a few minutes earlier and hop through the gap in the wall directly in front of you.

The environment here is distinctly swampy, with knee- to waist-high ferns abundant and a string of stepping-stones helpfully provided to maneuver through the mud. As you work your way through the bayoulike conditions, be sure to stop occasionally to look for animal tracks in the ooze. You may not find those of alligators, but raccoons and other small critters are quite likely. Listen attentively, too, along this stretch of rococo routing through the dense undergrowth, and you should be able to hear the calls of various birds, including pileated woodpeckers and various warblers.

All too soon, the swampland rambling comes to an end at a junction with the main trail. On swinging right there, you'll see the kiosk straight ahead, and the parking area just beyond.

## NEARBY ACTIVITIES

Another short hike worth considering is a tour through the **Leon Levy Preserve,** a 386-acre parcel that was established in 2005 through a joint effort by the town of Lewisboro and the Westchester Land Trust. Several blazed trails have since been created that showcase much of the preserve's beauty, including a second-growth forest, swamplands, dramatic rock outcroppings, even a 25-foot-high ravine. The trailhead is just south of NY 35 on NY 123, in the town of Lewisboro, marked by a sign on the west side of the road. For further information, call 914-241-6346 or visit **westchesterlandtrust.org/leon-levy.**

The **Bartlett Arboretum,** in North Stamford, Connecticut, is of a more manicured nature. Swamps and ponds thrive next to woodlands and meadows, and the unique collection of champion trees makes this a special place. For more information, call 203-322-6971 or visit **bartlettarboretum.org.**

# 15   WESTMORELAND GRAND TOUR

## KEY AT-A-GLANCE INFORMATION

**LENGTH: 5.6 miles**

**ELEVATION GAIN: 1,117 feet**

**CONFIGURATION: Double loop**

**DIFFICULTY: Easy to moderate**

**SCENERY: Mixed forest houses rock cliffs and stone walls, lush swamps, cascading streams, and kettle-hole pond.**

**EXPOSURE: Mostly shady**

**TRAFFIC: Heavy on some weekends or when student programs take place, but usually light on Coles Kettle Trail**

**TRAIL SURFACE: Packed dirt, rocks, and roots**

**HIKING TIME: 2.5 hours**

**DRIVING DISTANCE: 35 miles**

**SEASON: Year-round, sunrise–sunset**

**ACCESS: Free; no pets, no bicycles**

**MAPS: At entrance kiosk; USGS *Mount Kisco;* online at tinyurl.com/westmore landsanctuary**

**FACILITIES: Restrooms and water inside Museum & Nature Center**

**COMMENTS: The sanctuary management offers a great range of public programs, such as an annual fall festival, maple sugaring, bird-watching, slide shows, and the like. To inquire about special activities and for further information, call 914-666-8448 or visit westmorelandsanctuary.org.**

## GPS COORDINATES

N41° 10.822'  W73° 41.066'

## IN BRIEF

With paths ranging from wide and smooth to narrow and rocky, family groups and hardened hikers alike can find the circuit that suits their interests—the common denominator being sensational scenery. Over the course of a handful of miles through rolling forestland, you will encounter impressive rock outcroppings, seasonal streams, and a few ponds where birds often flock. Deer sightings, too, are virtually guaranteed early and late in the day.

## DESCRIPTION

A bearded dragon is housed among the animals on exhibit in Westmoreland's nature center, but don't let that deter you from heading into the woods of this attractive sanctuary. This abandoned pet is native to Australia—not Westchester County—and was adopted by the resident naturalist. The most threatening animals you are likely to encounter along the 5.6 miles of trails that rope through Westmoreland's 625 acres are the snapping turtles that inhabit its three ponds.

Which is not to suggest that this is a buttoned-down suburban park with all the beauty of a backyard tomato garden. On the contrary, Westmoreland offers an opportunity for a good up-and-down workout along some of the area's more exciting granite bluffs, in addition to a striking kettle-hole pond dating

------------------------------------------

## *Directions* ———————————→

**Take the Hutchinson River Parkway North to I-684 North. Take Exit 4 and drive west on NY 172/South Bedford Road for 0.3 mile, then turn left onto Chestnut Ridge Road and proceed for 1.3 miles. The entrance and parking lot are on the left.**

# Westmoreland Grand Tour

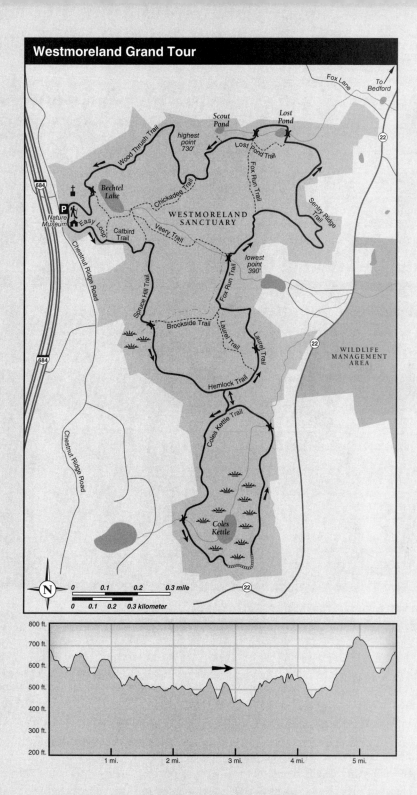

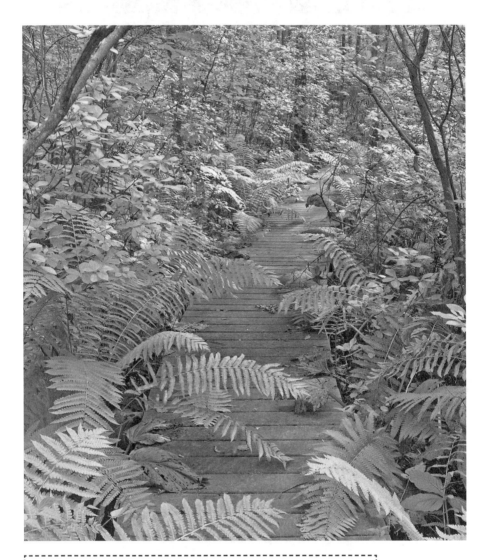

A secluded boardwalk traverses the lush swamp at the far end of the kettle hole.

to the last ice age. Deer herds teem through groves of oaks, beeches, and black birch trees, and the abundance of water, including numerous streams and minor seasonal cascades, draws a wide range of songbirds as well as downy, pileated, and red-bellied woodpeckers, turkey vultures, and red-tailed hawks. Bobcat tracks have also been observed within the domain, according to the naturalist.

This circumference of the park starts on the Easy Loop, by a wooden arch (where maps are usually available) to the right of the nature center. Stay with the red blazes as they trend downhill past a few maples and spruce trees, and continue straight in a tenth of a mile, through a break in the stone wall, onto the Catbird Trail (white markings). More stone walls and a couple of open fields ensue as you persist downward, and in 2 or 3 minutes, swing right at the junction with Spruce Hill Trail (SHT, yellow).

With pines hanging low over short stretches of the ascending path, this section of the sanctuary feels appealingly wild. After a 40-yard stretch, the SHT crests by an uplifted mound of glacial moraine, one of many dark, lichen-mottled ridges that run through Westmoreland. Spruce Hill then descends into a concentration of beech trees, where it meets Brookside and Hemlock Trails. Step right onto Hemlock and cross the wooden-plank bridge fording a marshy stream. Wild lilac grows nearby, and in July and August its sweet perfume fills the air, attracting swallowtail butterflies in search of nectar.

The trail, now blazed orange, moves uphill, past desiccated hemlocks and a few shagbark hickories. On leveling off in 150 to 200 yards, it enters a bog that can be very, very moist in winter and early spring. As you begin to descend once more, take a glance behind at a hitherto-hidden granite outcropping that rises an impressive 30 feet off the forest floor.

The right-hand turnoff to Coles Kettle Trail (yellow) (GPS: N41° 10.330' W73° 40.462'), a 1.5-mile mini-loop, is signposted, but that indicator faces the opposite direction. In any case, you are unlikely to miss so clear an intersection. The kettle hole, or pond, measuring about 100 yards wide by 170 yards long, is at the far end of the loop, but because it is ringed by greenbrier and a variety of hardwood trees, it's most visible in winter and early spring. That is also the time, alas, when the trail is likely to be soggy with snowmelt and a surfeit of water. No matter; this less-trafficked circuit, part of which runs along a boardwalk, is well worth the detour. Remain wide-eyed, not just for wild turkeys, of which we once spied a dozen here, but also for flowering pickerelweed at the north end of the pond.

On your return from Coles Kettle, roll right onto the eastern stretch of the Hemlock Trail. It presses forward another eighth of a mile, descending past a cluster of maple trees in advance of an intersection with the Laurel Trail. March right and pass over a couple of small bridges, with some hefty boulders and a massive moraine field on either side of the laurel-fringed path. The rugged rock outcroppings extend for a quarter-mile, at which point the track emerges at a slightly sloping, grassy meadow. Head directly across this birdhouse-festooned sward, keeping to its southern side until you hit the intersection with the Brookside Trail (white), where you veer right along the stone wall.

This trail is bordered by a wide stream (dry in summer) while tapering downward among beech, birch, maple, and (later on) hemlock trees. Ultimately, and just after a wooden bridge, Brookside bottoms out at 390 feet of elevation, which is the lowest point in the sanctuary, before—you guessed it!—beginning a gradual ascent. Step through a rock wall, and hew to the right on Fox Run (orange) at the trail junction.

Here starts one of the steeper stretches in Westmoreland, though it lasts only for something like 150 yards. A dramatic bluff looms to the left, extending outward as the trail levels off, culminating in a protrusion of boulders 50 feet above the ground. Roughly a quarter-mile up the path is your turn onto Sentry Ridge, but before hanging a right there, check out the solidly built stone wall that runs directly up the opposite hill, finishing in a nearly vertical position. This sturdy relic indirectly reveals how thoroughly this land was cultivated little more than a century ago.

As its name implies, Sentry Ridge (yellow) offers pretty fair views, although a good portion of those are of NY 22, well below and to the east. In addition to the chance to see more wildlife (we've spotted a score of wild turkeys here recently and, on other occasions, several herds of deer), this stretch features a series of uphill–downhill bursts past rocky knobs, through a congregation of maples, and around a ledge and granite ridge, before finally meeting the right-hand turnoff to Lost Pond (white). A bench at the northeast side of this man-made pond provides a fine spot to idle and look for frogs among the lilies. Your Walden-like reverie concluded, follow the trail away from the water as it threads through a bog, across a small bridge, and uphill to the next intersection, where you should point your paws to the right.

For the upcoming quarter-mile, the trail shifts steadily higher into a rocky landscape, skipping by Scout Pond—really more of a marshy flat—and its adjacent bird blind along the way. The ascent continues for a short spell on the Wood Thrush Trail to the right, reaching, at 730 feet, the highest elevation in Westmoreland. The path then wends slightly to the left into a shady grove of beech trees, passes a striking ridge of granite, and encounters, as it courses downhill, a rock slide of scattered glacial boulders.

Several massive tulip poplars, their lower trunks measuring 4 feet or more in diameter, appear a few minutes later in the vicinity of a couple of foot bridges. Bechtel Lake, one of the more popular family destinations in the sanctuary, is just beyond. Poison ivy thrives in this locale, but you should also be vigilant for the turnoff to the right onto the latter segment of the Easy Loop Trail (red). This final fifth of a mile leads by a large stand of white pines (and an occasional hop horn-beam), a couple of old-fashioned outhouses, and the Neighborhood Burying Ground (its graves dating from 1824 to 1915), ultimately terminating by the nature center.

Plan to make time for a peek inside that facility. Sure, other than the bearded dragon, most exhibits are rather folksy. But look more closely at the taupe-colored, clapboard-sided building itself. This 200-year-old Colonial structure was once the Presbyterian Church in nearby Bedford Village. When the community there outgrew it, the private, not-for-profit corporation that operates Westmoreland stepped in and had it taken apart and reassembled at its current location.

## NEARBY ACTIVITIES

When we're feeling energetic, we like to combine this hike with a shorter spin through the **Arthur W. Butler Memorial Sanctuary** (Hike 3), less than half a mile away. There's also the recently created **Angle Fly Preserve**, in nearby Somers (Hike 1).

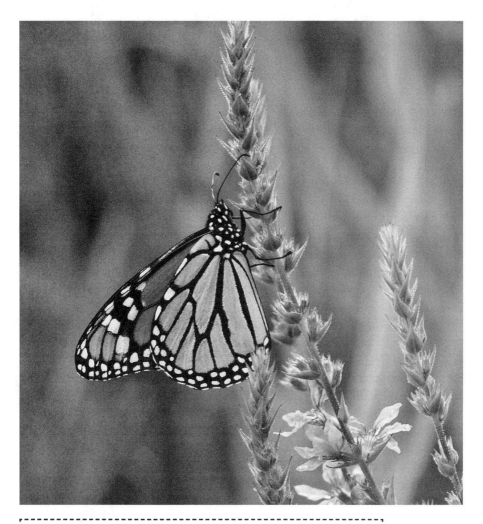

Hard to imagine that this fragile summer beauty goes snowbirding in the mountain forests of Michoacán, Mexico.

If you have a chance to freshen up after your exercise, you may want to indulge in quite a different experience: namely, a musical evening at **Caramoor** in Katonah, which is a great treat both because of its reliably splendid concerts and its gorgeous Renaissance-style setting. For programs and other details, visit **caramoor.org.**

History buffs will want to check out the **John Jay Homestead State Historic Site,** the farmhouse—maintained with period furnishings—where the first U.S. chief justice retired; it's on NY 22 in Katonah. For details, call 914-232-5651 or visit **johnjayhomestead.org.**

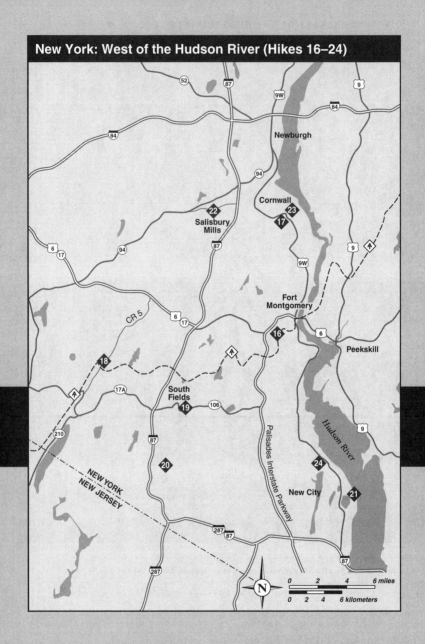

# New York: West of the Hudson River (Hikes 16–24)

Newburgh

Cornwall 23
17

Salisbury
Mills 22

Fort
Montgomery

16

Peekskill

South
Fields 19

18

New City

24

21

20

NEW YORK
NEW JERSEY

Palisades Interstate Parkway

Hudson River

| 0 | 2 | 4 | 6 miles |
| 0 | 2 | 4 | 6 kilometers |

N

# NEW YORK:
## WEST OF THE HUDSON RIVER

# 16 BEAR MOUNTAIN DOODLETOWN CIRCUIT

### KEY AT-A-GLANCE INFORMATION

**LENGTH:** 8.1 miles

**ELEVATION GAIN:** 2,346 feet

**CONFIGURATION:** Loop

**DIFFICULTY:** Strenuous

**SCENERY:** Mixed forest on steep slopes, views from the Appalachian Trail, ruins of an old mining town, and secluded cemeteries

**EXPOSURE:** Shady on slopes and in valleys, very open on ridges

**TRAFFIC:** Heavy on weekends, especially in spring and autumn

**TRAIL SURFACE:** Mostly packed dirt with some very rocky stretches, rooty in places

**HIKING TIME:** 4.5 hours

**DRIVING DISTANCE:** 37 miles

**SEASON:** Year-round, sunrise–sunset, weather permitting; possible summer closures due to fire danger

**ACCESS:** Free; dogs on leash, bicycling on paved roads, no mountain bikes

**MAPS:** At one of the visitor centers along the Seven Lakes Drive; download from tinyurl.com/bearmtnmap

**FACILITIES:** Restrooms at visitor center near Exit 17 on Palisades Interstate Parkway, along with public phone, bookshop, and more

**COMMENTS:** Bring a trail map to reduce the likelihood of getting lost on the complex network of trails. Call 845-786-2701 or visit nysparks .com/parks/13/details.aspx.

## GPS COORDINATES

N41° 18.245'  W74° 0.957'

## IN BRIEF

High country meadows, distant vistas, rugged mountain climbs, and the overgrown ruins of an old village are among the many highlights of this tiring yet delightful calorie-burner of a hike, which also features possible sightings of turkey vultures, hawks, goldfinches, red foxes, white-tailed deer—even black bears and rattle-snakes. No question: this is one of the more exciting moderate-length treks in the New York area, but a couple of challenging stretches are not for those of tender feet.

## DESCRIPTION

Bear Mountain State Park is, along with its contiguous neighbor to the west, Harriman State Park, one of the most popular nature pre-serves in the Northeast, reportedly drawing more annual visitors than Yellowstone National Park. If not for the efforts of conservationists and wealthy area landowners, though, it might not have come into existence at all. Early in the 20th century, New York state authorities floated the idea of relocating Sing Sing Prison here. That was enough to galvanize E. W. Harriman, president of the Union Pacific Railroad, and others to donate money and land toward the creation of Bear Mountain–Harriman State Parks, which were jointly established in 1914 and today total more than 52,000 acres.

- - - - - - - - - - - - - - - - - - - - - - - - - - - - - - - - - -

*Directions* ⟶

Follow I-95 across the George Washington Bridge and take Exit 74 onto the Palisades Interstate Parkway North. Leave the parkway at Exit 19 toward Perkins Memorial Drive. Go right on Seven Lakes Drive and proceed for 0.5 mile to the trailhead parking on the right.

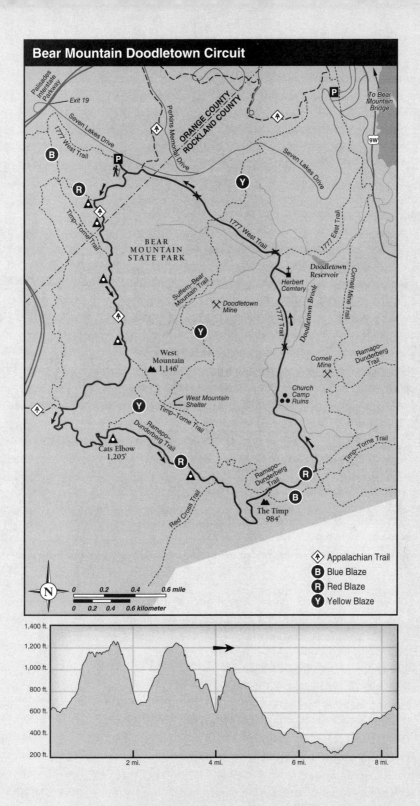

# Bear Mountain Doodletown Circuit

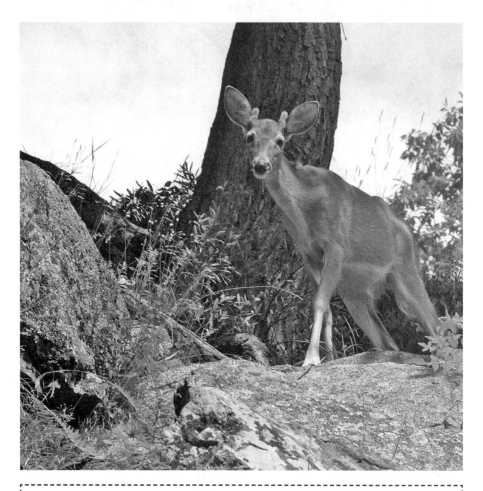

This unabashed white-tailed yearling appears very interested in our camera . . . or is it after our lunch?

Nine years after the parks' inception, the first section of the Appalachian Trail was laid down in Bear Mountain, serving as a template for later additions to this historic long trail. During the 1930s, the Civilian Conservation Corps was active in the park, constructing shelters, restrooms, vacation cabins, and roads, many of which remain intact today. It's not the period architecture, however, that draws people to the two parks like kids to ice cream. Fishing, boating, swimming, camping, picnicking, and horseback riding are just a few of the activities that make this a "something for everyone" sort of place.

Then there is hiking, and in Bear Mountain–Harriman you've got miles and miles of some of the best trekking terrain in the entire New York metropolitan region. Granite domes, rocky ravines, inspiring vistas, mellow meanderings through grassy forests, butt-busting climbs over mountaintops—whatever kind of hike you want is available here. The Doodletown Circuit, a strenuous loop of just over 8 miles, is a fine introduction to Bear Mountain's natural beauty and historic past. Begin the hike on the 1777 West Trail, by the east side of the parking lot. Follow the white-disc blazes as the path climbs over rocky, fern-speckled ground through laurels, maples, and blueberry bushes before leveling off. At that point, just a few dozen yards from the trailhead, the elongated white blazes of the Appalachian Trail (AT) appear. Jog right, off the 1777 West, now following a fairly fresh layout of the AT.

This relatively new stretch of the historic "long path" initially passes over undulating, stone-studded terrain, shaded largely by beeches, maples, and various oaks. Ignore the Fawn Trail, to the right, sticking instead with the AT as it bends left and begins snaking uphill. During its climb, the trail showcases some dramatic granite uplift, craggy outcroppings that serve as a teaser for some of this hike's many geological highlights.

You'll want to catch your breath at the first false summit, a grassy plateau more than 300 feet above the trailhead that offers a clear vista of Bear Mountain Peak and the Hudson River. The views of both are even more commanding farther south along this rising dome of granite, as the well-beaten track tacks between scrub oaks and black birch saplings, climbing still higher up a talus slope. There is little in the way of real shade during this stage of the trek, with the exposure growing as you hang a left at the junction with the Timp–Torne Trail (TT, blue blazes) and ascend a rocky knob that is more than 600 feet above the parking area.

Keep to the right of the oak growing off the knob and maneuver by a thicket of young birches on your way to still another granite shelf, this one overlooking the Palisades Parkway, a couple of colossal car lots, and the expansive hills of Harriman to the west. Continuing along the rocky ridge, which rises and falls and gives way momentarily to a lush, green saddle, you will enjoy an extension of those westward views. The trail eventually leads to West Mountain Peak at 1,146 feet of elevation. We once encountered a pretty hefty rattlesnake here, dozing by a rotted tree stump, so be careful where you step, just in case it or its offspring are still in the area.

The TT diverges from the AT a short distance from there. The first time we wrote up this hike, we recommended the left fork, which passes over a very appealing mountain meadow of scrub oaks and calf-high grass on the way to the West Mountain shelter. If you choose to go that direction, stick with the blue markings all the way to the crossing with the Ramapo–Dunderberg Trail (RD, red dot on white blazes), just beyond the crest of the Timp, where you can jog left and proceed on into Doodletown. Otherwise, for a superb workout through one of the park's more colorful areas, bear right, remaining with the AT. From initially hugging the edge of the crest, the trace drops precipitously lower, losing 550 feet in altitude before reaching a wide, level bicycle path. The AT continues downhill, but you should scoot left here, remaining on the bike path for a couple of minutes, until you hit the junction with the RD (GPS: N41° 16.891' W74° 1.306'), where you again spurt to the left.

The RD first climbs through a cluster of mountain laurel before briefly merging with the Suffern–Bear Mountain Trail (SBM, yellow blazes), near the top, only to break away to the right moments later. The singular beauty of this windswept plateau, colored by scrub oaks, chestnut snags, and long, wavy grass, might inspire you to wander off the trail and rest a bit by one of a number of large, oblong erratics. By all means, go ahead. Be sure to save time, though, for the subsequent series of viewpoints, including some that offer far-reaching vistas of the Hudson River and even Manhattan to the south. That rough-looking, wrinkly peak, by the way, visible straight ahead, due east as the track gradually drops off West Mountain, is the Timp, your next destination. Don't worry about its impregnable appearance: the route circles around to the south and scratches up the bluff over easier ground. Ignore the side trails you encounter along the way, including the Red Cross on the right, and the Blue Cross seconds afterward, sticking with the RD all the way up, and then down, the Timp. You'll switch to the TT, merging from the left, on the east side of the Timp, just as you begin to lose elevation. Swing right on it, now following the blue blazes, as the RD forges straight ahead.

After slithering through a colorful stretch of boulders and glacial debris (in about a quarter-hour of measured walking), the TT crosses a grassy forest road. Leap left there, now with the white blazes of the well-trammeled 1777. This easy, pebbly carriage lane, which passes the RD in another minute, will guide you all the way into Doodletown. The first remnant you may notice of that old community will likely be a poplar-shaded stone foundation, to the right of a confluence of streambeds. These are the remains of a dam and pool constructed by a church camp many decades ago.

Farther on is a series of old-growth maples—some with trunks measuring 4 feet across—where, not so coincidentally, a patch of pavement appears, as well as an old stone wall by the roadside. The surest indication that you are now in the heart of Doodletown is the appearance of interpretive signs marking where many houses once stood. Some residents held on until as recently as the 1960s; perhaps they were the ones who planted the irises that grow here, as well as the handful of spruce trees—conifers that are not native to Bear Mountain. The mounds and depressions on either side of the lane seem pregnant with ruins now concealed by vines and other vegetation. A driveway to the right leads to an open foundation, with several young maples rising from its core and old cooking pots littering the ground nearby. You might easily spend a couple of hours exploring the network of lanes that cut through these woods. Save time, though, for a brief side trip to the Herbert Cemetery, on a narrow lane to the right (GPS: N41° 17.702' W73° 59.867'), just after you pass two prominent pillars left of the trail. Many of the graves date to the early 1800s, their headstones standing at odd angles like teeth badly in need of an orthodontist.

Returning to the 1777, proceed for another 100 yards, brushing by a bush of pink-flowering rose of Sharon, to the trail's departure from the carriage road—a left into an overgrown thicket. This is the start of 1777 West and the route back to your car. If you would like to see the Doodletown Reservoir first, however, continue along the wide track to the T, turn right, and hang another right at the

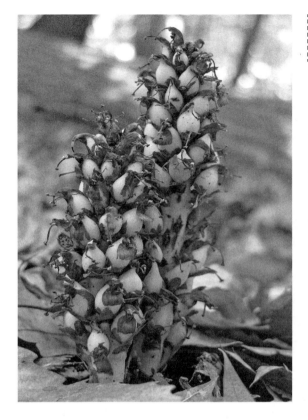

A pinecone or a corncob? No, this is squawroot, a parasite that lives off the roots of oaks and beeches.

ensuing fork, which leads in a few additional steps to the Second June Cemetery and a modest overlook of the water. Retrace your steps from there to the point where the '77 West begins and stay with that as it climbs, skips over a stream and by a ravine, and then meets the SBM at yet another T. Keep to the left, now following the white discs of 1777 on the old Doodletown Road, an unpaved avenue lined with oaks. This stretch is an active birding area, where we have seen at various times goldfinches, robins, and a red-tailed hawk. The parking area lies about 15 minutes down the trail.

## NEARBY ACTIVITIES

This all-in-one park features several lakes where boating, fishing, and swimming are popular pastimes. Family picnics and barbecues go on all summer. In winter, skiing, sledding, snowmobiling, ice-skating, and ice fishing are permitted.

Hungry hikers can soothe their appetites in the snack bar or restaurant of the historic **Bear Mountain Inn,** a rustic lodge along US 9W, where a trailside museum and zoo are also located. For details, call 845-786-2731 or visit **visitbearmountain.com.**

# 17 BLACK ROCK FOREST PEAKS TO PONDS TRAIL

## KEY AT-A-GLANCE INFORMATION

**LENGTH: 13.5 miles**

**ELEVATION GAIN: 3,115 feet**

**CONFIGURATION: Loop**

**DIFFICULTY: Very strenuous**

**SCENERY: Half a dozen summits and lakes, with lots of rock-scrambling between gorgeous vistas and dizzying depths**

**EXPOSURE: No canopy on the barren summits, but shady elsewhere**

**TRAFFIC: Often light, but summer weekends may draw the brave.**

**TRAIL SURFACE: Mix of dirt and rocks; some grassy stretches**

**HIKING TIME: 7–8 hours**

**DRIVING DISTANCE: 49 miles**

**SEASON: Year-round, sunrise–sunset**

**ACCESS: Donation suggested; pets on leash, no mountain biking or horse riding on trails**

**MAPS: Posted and available at trailhead kiosk; USGS *Cornwall*; blackrockforest.org/html-files /imagemap.html**

**FACILITIES: None**

**COMMENTS: The woodland roads provide good cross-country skiing trails in winter. The forest may sometimes be closed due to fire hazard or deer hunting (typically mid-November–early December). Call 845-534-4517 or visit blackrock forest.org for more information.**

## GPS COORDINATES

N41° 25.118'  W74° 0.639'

## IN BRIEF

Historians report that Rome was built on seven hills. That's one more than Black Rock Forest can boast of, but then Black Rock also has half a dozen bodies of water, and because it sees relatively few visitors, you are apt to have many of those features exclusively to yourself. Between the rock-scrambling to vistas and stream-hopping through swamps, you'll enjoy a great workout in a diversity of habitats that virtually guarantees wildlife sightings.

## DESCRIPTION

"Great crystals on the surface of the earth, Lakes of Light. If they were permanently congealed, and small enough to be clutched, they would, perchance, be carried off by slaves, like precious stones, to adorn the heads of emperors. . . ." It was Walden and White Ponds to which Henry David Thoreau referred, but his words seem just as applicable to the many radiant bodies of water within the Black Rock Forest Preserve. In fact, this park is so enchanting that after a few hours of tramping its high points and hidden dells, you may find yourself contemplating where to erect a cabin. Part of the reason this sanctuary is so captivatingly

------------------------------------------------

## *Directions* ———————————➤

**Follow I-95 across the George Washington Bridge and take Exit 74 onto the Palisades Interstate Parkway North. Drive 37 miles to the traffic circle and take the third exit onto scenic route US 9W North for 9.1 miles to Mountain Road. Make a right on it, and an immediate sharp right again, into a narrow tunnel leading to Reservoir Road. Continue straight for 0.1 mile to the parking area on the right.**

# Black Rock Forest Peaks to Ponds Trail

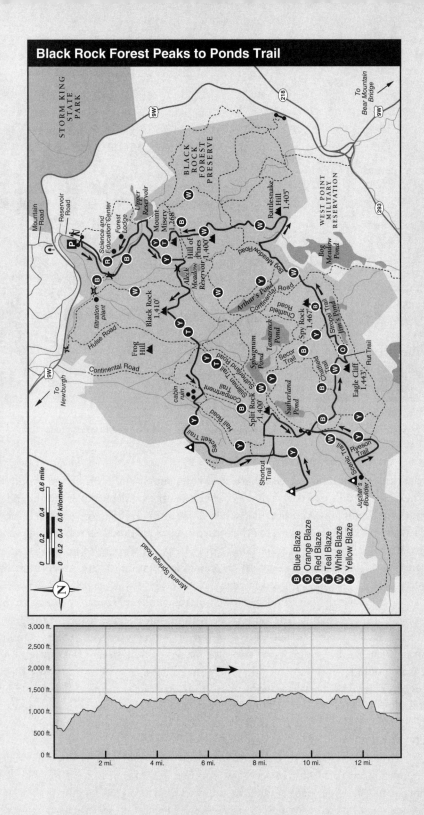

STORM KING STATE PARK

BLACK ROCK FOREST PRESERVE

WEST POINT MILITARY RESERVATION

To Bear Mountain Bridge

9W

218

293

Mountain Road

Reservoir Road

Upper Reservoir

Science and Education Center

Forest Lodge

Mount Misery 1,268'

Rattlesnake Hill 1,405'

filtration plant

Black Rock 1,410'

Hulse Road

Frog Hill

Continental Road

Aleck Meadow Reservoir

Hill of Pines 1,400'

Bog Meadow Road

Bog Meadow Pond

Arthur's Pond

Continental Road

Chatfield Road

Spy Rock 1,467'

Jim's Pond

Stropel Trail

Rut Trail

9W

To Newburgh

cabin ruin

Compartment Trail

Sutherland Road

Sphagnum Pond

Tamarack Pond

Second Trail

Chatfield Trail

Eagle Cliff 1,443'

Split Rock 1,400'

Sutherland Pond

Hall Road

Seckett Trail

Shortcut Trail

Ryeson Trail

Jupiter's Scenic Trail

Jupiter's Boulder

P N

Mineral Springs Road

0     0.2     0.4     0.6 mile

0     0.2     0.4     0.6 kilometer

N

**B** Blue Blaze
**O** Orange Blaze
**R** Red Blaze
**T** Teal Blaze
**W** White Blaze
**Y** Yellow Blaze

3,000 ft.
2,500 ft.
2,000 ft.
1,500 ft.
1,000 ft.
500 ft.
0 ft.

2 mi.     4 mi.     6 mi.     8 mi.     10 mi.     12 mi.

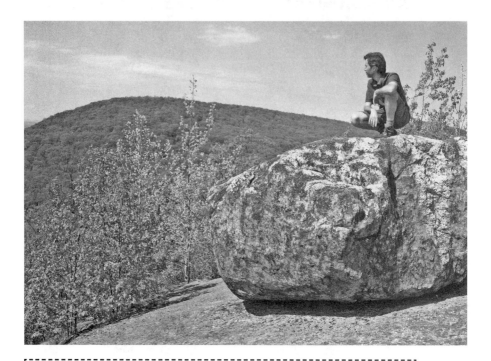

Beyond admiring the ridge views and the impressive Jupiter's Boulder, you might also spook a ledge-lurking vulture.

beautiful is its unique location between Schunemunk and Storm King Mountains, where it straddles two thriving ecosystems—the Hudson River basin and the Hudson Highlands. Additionally, while most of its 3,785 acres were set aside as early as 1928, the preserve's relative obscurity has resulted in a refreshingly unsullied domain. The miles of trails here, from broad forest roads to narrow woodland rambles, crisscross half a dozen peaks and a like number of lakes, with foot traffic surprisingly light throughout the year.

On leaving the parking lot, the red-blazed trail sinks down into a dark forest of hemlock, oak, maple, and tulip trees, with luminous ferns rising off the ground. Within half a mile the path hits bottom at a four-way intersection; continue straight across the bridge, now with blue markings. The stream to your left on the ensuing uphill grind is an auditory and visual delight that cascades noisily through several rocky constrictions. Ignore the sundry spurs as you plod along, and in 10 minutes hop straight over the little arroyo and switch to the yellow-blazed track (the blue markings cross the wider stream on your left, a spot teeming with trout lily in spring), still moving up the slope.

In another 5 minutes the yellow trail crests at a forest road. It proceeds straight on up to Mount Misery, but you turn right, saving the Misery for later. Stay with this wide, pebbly lane for the next quarter-mile, hanging a right at the wooden gate, which provides access to Aleck Meadow Reservoir. (A small swamp stream oozes under the forest road just prior to that turnoff, where purple violets and marsh marigolds bloom in May.) From this beautiful body of water, follow the path counterclockwise below the earthen embankment of the lake, gaining meanwhile a good view from the concrete bridge of the water sluicing downhill over a rocky streambed. Just as you regain a level with the reservoir (look for purple irises in late spring), the path veers right, heading upward among hemlocks, beeches, black birches, black gum trees, and innumerable boulders. This route, marked with a yellow rectangle (and the teal diamonds of the Highlands Trail), meets a T in 3 or 4 minutes and continues to the left. Then, in 60-plus seconds, it swerves to the right, trending steadily higher.

In less than a quarter-mile, the surroundings evolve from hardwoods and mountain laurel, where wild turkeys are frequently observed, to a more spartan, boulder-strapped environment. The final scramble up a steep rock face brings you to a sunny ledge, with views through spicebush to the south and of the Schunemunk range to the west. That's just an appetizer for Black Rock summit, 70 feet farther up the path, with its breathtaking panorama highlighted by the expansive Hudson as it flows under the Newburgh Bridge to Storm King Mountain, and Breakneck Ridge beyond the river. At 1,402 feet of elevation, Black Rock is not the highest peak you'll climb today, but it may well deliver the most exciting vistas.

When you have had enough of this celestial setting, chase after the rectangular yellow blazes as the Stillman Trail (ST) departs the dome, down a series of natural steps, and swings left into the mountain laurels. In 8 minutes, the ST launches left on the unpaved Hulse Road, only to jump right at a pipe gate by a four-way intersection of forest lanes. Leave the ST as it veers left immediately, remaining instead with Continental Road for 65 to 70 paces and then shift left on the Sackett Trail (SAC, yellow circles). This single-file track edges lower into a boggy, boulder-filled environment before meeting the grass-surfaced Hall Road. Steer left there and continue on Hall Road to the succeeding four-way intersection (GPS: **N41° 24.223' W74° 2.067'**), where you shift right, still on the SAC. This meandering stretch of trail passes by an old cabin ruin (not much left beyond its chimney) and hops across a shallow stream (decorated with the virginal white blossoms of meadow anemones from late April through mid-May), before arriving at an appealing ridge (prime wild-turkey habitat) with pretty fair views to the west. It ends at a crossing with the ST, where you bear right, now moving due south. In 5 or 6 minutes of negligible elevation gain, the Stillman meets a junction with the Shortcut Trail (SC, yellow triangles). Remain with the ST for now, but make a note of this crossing; you'll return to the SC later on. In another handful of minutes padding along the ridge, the ST ends at a picturesque overlook, showcasing Schunemunk Mountain to the west and the Shawangunks and Catskills far off to the right of that. With dwarf oaks providing shade, there's a subliminal beauty to this rocky perch, a beauty that is enhanced by its isolation from the more heavily trafficked parts of the preserve. Back at the Shortcut turnoff, head right and follow the yellow triangles as they lead you over the ridgeline and back to Hall Road. Spin left there, still with the triangular blazes, and when the SC ends, in roughly 4 minutes, vault right, once more on the Stillman Trail, and proceed up the slope, away from the forest lane.

On reaching the top of the hill, the ST swings left, but you should persist directly ahead on the trace, past the vernal pool to the right that turns black with wriggling tadpoles in springtime, all the way to the rock ledge vista point. This is the aptly named Split Rock, elevation 1,400 feet, a fine vantage point from which to survey Sutherland Pond, directly below, as well as the New York City skyline—if it's a clear day—while noshing on an energy-restoring sandwich. Incidentally, among the skunk cabbage of the marsh just south of the pond are sundews—rare, insect-eating plants.

Having polished off your Dagwood, hang a right on the Split Rock Trail (white blazes), and when it ends, in a minute or two, turn left onto the continuation of the Compartment Trail (CT, blue blazes), which overlaps the Highlands Trail. Stick with the CT all the way to the bottom of the slope, drifting right at the cable gate, carrying onward along the unpaved Sutherland Road. Compartment terminates at an intersection with the Arthur Trail (AT, yellow markings), to the left, but delay that turn for yet another scenic detour, persisting instead along Sutherland Road for a further 2 minutes, jumping off it to the right when the teal-indicated Highlands Trail breaks that way, uniting with the Scenic Trail (SNC, white tags) (GPS: **N41° 23.400' W74° 2.441'**). In something like 7 minutes the narrow path crosses a wide, grassy lane, long ago abandoned, and in a similar amount of time it brings you to a lichen-embedded granite shelf, well encircled by white birch saplings. From this vantage point, you have a fine vista to the west of the ridge you were treading along an hour earlier, as well as the mountains to the northwest. A neighboring shelf, just up the trail, offers a nearly identical vista. And perhaps 30 steps beyond that is Jupiter's Boulder, your final stop in this area of the preserve. The views here are much the same as those you've just experienced, with slender black birches supplanting their paler cousins, but the presence of the giant erratic, Jupiter's Boulder, right in the center of this outpost, lends the scene an air of high drama the two previous spots lack.

On completing your orbits around Jupiter, fly back to the junction with the grassy forest lane and launch yourself to the right, onto the little-used Ryerson Trail (yellow rectangles). Tempting as it may be to keep ambling along this gardenlike path, Ryerson tacks to the left in less than a minute—and you should follow it. A rapid descent ensues through a mature, rock-studded forest, where the canopy is so dense that very little grows on its floor (although we once encountered a racer snake here, which vibrated its tail among the dry leaves, creating a menacing, misleading rattling sound, before zipping away under some brush), culminating in a left turn onto another seldom-traveled forest road. This wide route, which is surprisingly open to the sun, smacks into the gravel-surfaced Jim's Pond Road in about 200 yards, at which point you heave to the left. The turnoff you previously took onto the SNC, now on your left, arises quite quickly, and 150 yards beyond that is the junction with the AT. Jag right there, now following yellow blazes. Large rocks,

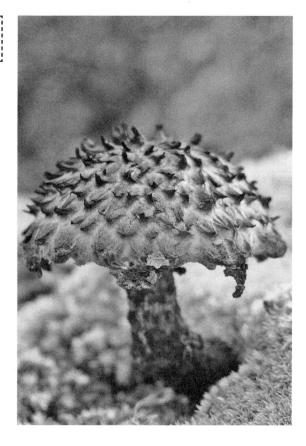

wooden planks, and a stretch of boardwalk help ease your way through this splendid swampland, which is succeeded by a break to the left, once again onto the SNC (white blazes). Persevere on this meandering route for about a half-mile, bolting right at the emergence of the Chatfield Trail (blue swatches), only to launch off of that when you meet a blue-blazed spur on the right. This detour forges into a jumble of rocks, at which point you should scale the large, rounded Sisyphean boulder, the highlight of Eagle Cliff, at an altitude of 1,443 feet.

This vertigo-inducing aerie projects precariously from the ridge and is so isolated you might actually see an eagle or (more likely) vulture roosting on it. The fabulous views swoop from the north to east to south, with Jim's and Wilkins Ponds serving as focal points below, while the denuded hill to the southeast, pocked with rusting military vehicles, is part of a United States Military Academy training area. Wander down the orange-blazed spur to the east, along the length of this sensational ledge, and slip off the rocks in 300 yards. Trot left when the spur merges with a yellow-marked route, and pivot to the right as those yellow indications collide again with the Scenic Trail. In 8 minutes, a blue-blazed trace on the left, indicated by a cairn of stones, rapidly hits Spy Rock, a romantic nook shaded by a lone pitch pine. This is the highest point in the park, at 1,467 feet, but the views are limited. Moseying onward, the SNC soon arrives at a staggered four-way intersection, requiring a dogleg first to the right and then to the left to carry you straight on. About 4 minutes beyond a yellow-blazed trace to the left (which leads over the rocky ridge to Arthur's Pond), the SNC staggers right, off the forest road.

From initially losing elevation, the trail soon starts to churn upward, sputtering to the pinnacle of Rattlesnake Hill (1,405 feet) in about 15 minutes. This granite shelf is coated with pale-green lichen, like barnacles clinging to the hull of a ship, and fringed with pitch pines. Visible through the latter is Bog Meadow Pond, where you may see people boating. Don't fret too much, though, about encountering Rattlesnake Hill's namesake reptile: the most exciting animal we've encountered here is a scarlet tanager chirping musically at the setting sun. Walk directly across the dome and pass into the tangle of mountain laurel, with a couple of similar knobs succeeding this first one as the path keeps to the west side of the ridge. From there, a 2-minute descent brings you to an intersection with a forest road, which the White Trail crosses diagonally. Then it's back to higher ground, meandering through an impressive spar of stony uplift. In little more than a minute, you near the top of the rise, with the boulders giving way to a grassy sward.

As with the previous peak, you may wonder about the name of this sun-exposed crest, Hill of Pines (1,400 feet), on observing that the two or three pitch pines growing here are greatly outnumbered by oak and spicebush. Justification for that moniker grows as the SNC descends through an increasing number of hemlocks. The rocky trail, which doubles as a streambed in wet weather, swerves toward the northwest as it nears the bottom of the gulch, crossing a blue-blazed path when it reaches a natural rock garden, with a superabundance of boulders and stones littering the terrain. When the SNC ends by the base of the next ridge, switch to a yellow-and-teal-blazed track and bear to the right, instead of legging it straight up the lower part of the hill.

Pick your way carefully through this boulder field and gradually climb the steep heap of rocks known as Mount Misery. (In this case at least, there is no mystery surrounding the name.) You may have been higher today, but this ascent is probably the most arduous. Soon enough, though, the hard, eluvial turf changes to grass and a more gentle approach, delivering you at last to a very pretty knoll. There are great views to the west, including of Aleck Meadow Reservoir and Black Rock Summit, where you were hours ago, as the trail lunges to the far edge of the peak and sticks with the ridge for several minutes. And then it's sharply downward, and in 5 minutes you arrive at the same crossing with the forest road you were at near the start of the hike. Although you can continue straight with the yellow blazes and retrace your earlier steps back to the parking area, we prefer the easier return via the dirt road, to the right, passing Upper Reservoir along the way.

## NEARBY ACTIVITIES

You may have caught a glimpse—or an earful—of some military activity from one of the southern ledges at Black Rock Forest. Indeed, the **United States Military Academy** at West Point is just a few miles south of this preserve. For details on the academy's museum, events, or parade schedules, call the visitor center at 845-938-2638 or visit **usma.edu**.

# FITZGERALD FALLS TO LITTLE DAM LAKE (APPALACHIAN TRAIL)  18

## IN BRIEF

Near the start of this exciting trek lies Fitzgerald Falls, a waterfall so dynamic that you may wonder what could possibly follow as an encore. Don't worry: high drama is the norm for a wild stretch of trail that is generously peppered with rocky vistas and rugged gorges, in addition to a bayou boardwalk and romantic lake. Just remember to slip an extra apple into your day pack, because this hike requires plenty of stamina.

## DESCRIPTION

By most standards, an elevation gain of 450 feet hardly puts one at risk of a nosebleed. But when that feat is accomplished six times in a single outing—accompanied by corresponding losses in altitude—you may begin to wish that Tenzing Norgay had come along to carry your box of Kleenex. This out-and-back trek from Fitzgerald Falls to Little Dam Lake involves a

---

## Directions →

Follow I-95 across the George Washington Bridge to NJ 4 West onto NJ 17 North. Continue 15 miles, then merge onto I-287 North. After 0.5 mile switch to I-87 North for 1.4 miles to Exit 15A (Sloatsburg), and head north on NY 17. Proceed for 7.3 miles, then go left onto NY 17A West. For the shuttle option, drive one car 3.1 miles, then turn left on Benjamin Meadow Road, followed by a right on Bramertown Road. After 0.9 mile, make a left on East Mombasha Road. Continue for a half-mile to a small parking space on the right, where the white AT blaze is visible on both sides of the road. For trailhead parking, drive the second car back to NY 17A, go right on it for 4.3 miles, and make a right onto Mountain Lakes Road/CR 5. Follow it for 3.7 miles to a small parking lot on the right.

## KEY AT-A-GLANCE INFORMATION

**LENGTH: 11.2 miles (6.2 miles with shuttle-car option)**

**ELEVATION GAIN: 2,618 feet (out-and-back)**

**CONFIGURATION: Out-and-back**

**DIFFICULTY: Strenuous**

**SCENERY: Vertically zigzagging path takes in cooling falls, hemlock forests, challenging rock scrambles, peaceful lakes, and awesome vistas.**

**EXPOSURE: Plenty of shade, except for grassy sanctuary and several bald summits**

**TRAFFIC: Often light, but the AT has many faithful fans and thru-hikers.**

**TRAIL SURFACE: A hearty cocktail of rocks, dirt, grass, and granite ledges**

**HIKING TIME: 6.5 hours**

**DRIVING DISTANCE: 45 miles**

**SEASON: Year-round**

**ACCESS: Free; no bicycles, no horses, no motorized vehicles**

**MAPS: USGS *Schunemunk***

**FACILITIES: None**

**COMMENTS: You and your hiking boots had better be in good shape to accomplish three major ascents and descents in each direction.**

## GPS COORDINATES

N41° 16.416' W74° 15.259'

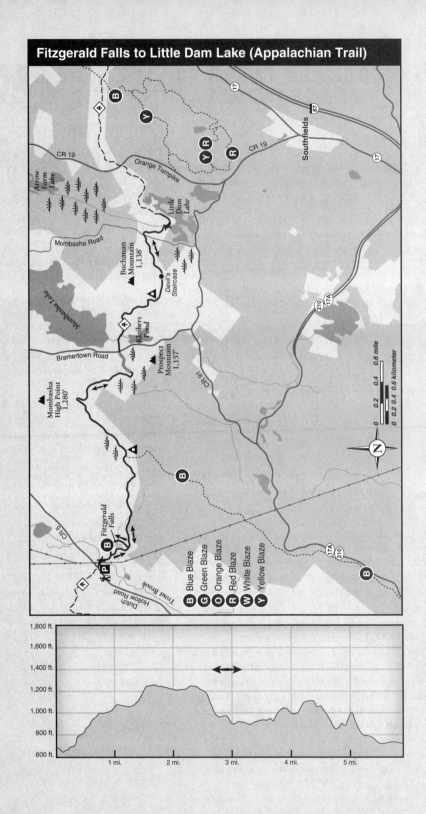

# Fitzgerald Falls to Little Dam Lake (Appalachian Trail)

heart-pounding effort in climbing three significant peaks. And while the vistas from a couple of those birds' nests are the stuff that dream hikes are made of, some of the more terrestrial sights along the way have an even splashier impact.

The most obvious of those is Fitzgerald Falls, near the start of the jaunt. This sensational waterfall sets the tone for a highly scenic stretch of the Appalachian Trail (AT, white blazes), one so visually exciting and physically challenging that there is hardly ever a dull moment. The path initially descends off the east side of the road into a power-line break. On crossing that, it skips over a bridge and enters a cool, dark hardwood and hemlock forest. The AT slowly meanders uphill away from the stream, Trout Brook, skipping by, as it does so, the end of the Blue Falls Bypass Trail (blue blazes, to the left). Do the easy hopscotch across the seasonal flow, bearing straight ahead, past a fine display of craggy traprock talus to the left, before arriving at the foot of Fitzgerald Falls.

You may wonder on gazing up at this tremendous cascade—with its dramatically high pour-off producing a deafening roar and wafting clouds of mist—where the hike can possibly go from here. The answer, in a word, is *up*. The trail scales a series of well-crafted steps fashioned into the rocky bluff, just to the right of the crashing waterfall. This setting is nearly as thrilling seen from above, where the stream froths with whitewater as it approaches the edge. The AT grows steeper as it launches into the heart of the hemlock forest, its floor scored by lichen-and-moss-coated rocks. Breaking up the climb are three fun stream fordings sandwiched around a crossing with a forest road, after which the path hits a false summit by a tumbledown wall. Just after that first stream, by the way, you'll find the other end of the Blue Falls Bypass Trail, which you may want to take on your return.

Gradually, the AT drifts out of the hemlock hamlet into a concentration of maples, with a nucleus of old walls running nearby. It may be a bit rocky underfoot, but the hiking is easier for the time being as the ground alternates between a gentle rise and a steady descent. About 10 minutes into the latter, you bottom out and start gaining elevation again, with some seasonal arroyos percolating alongside the path. Indeed, the trail itself has come to resemble an ancient streambed—or a massive moraine field. The appearance of mountain laurel signals the advent of another steep climb, this time through a beautiful boulder-filled gorge. The culmination of that effort is a rocky knob, well shrouded in scrub oaks and blueberry bushes, with an AT register attached to a tree. On signing in once, we read that a previous hiker had seen a black bear on the blue-blazed track to the right—a side trip down that yields, in 150 feet, a great view to the west and south from a granite ledge.

If it is warm weather, you may hear what sounds like the chirruping of yellow-shafted flickers as you continue on the AT. That tuneless melody is actually the mating call of frogs in the vernal pond through the spicebush to the left. For the next few minutes, the path overlaps the rocky plateau, a composition of pudding-stone and other conglomerates, as it climbs ever so slightly to the second knob. This rocky dome is Mombasha High Point, which sits at an elevation of 1,280

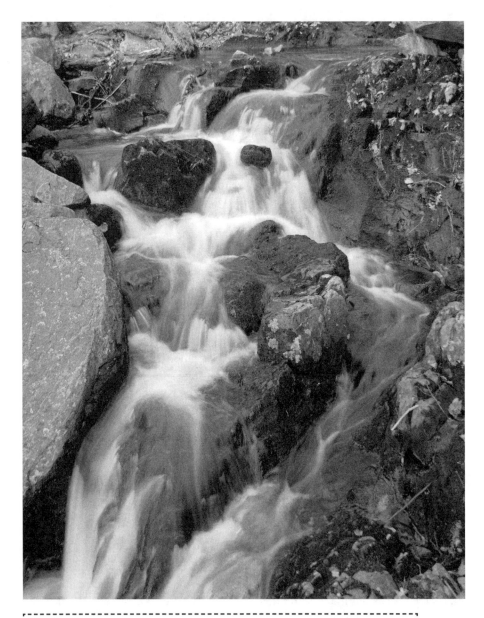

You'll have to follow the trail above Fitzgerald Falls to reach this cascade, where the stream begins its pour-off.

feet—more than half of those being above the trailhead. Take a breather and enjoy the 360-degree panorama, with Mombasha Lake glimmering below to the east.

The descent that ensues (there's *always* a descent after such a viewpoint, isn't there?) begins rather tentatively, with a scramble over rocks by the edge of the ridge, but you gain momentum on exiting the boulder field and grove of pitch pines. In a dozen minutes, the path flattens out at the level of the lake and cruises straight through a four-way intersection. Ignore the unblazed trace to the left after the crossing, staying with the well-marked AT as it slides off a stone shelf and continues to lose elevation, passing meanwhile through a second four-way junction. You are now approaching an attractive swamp, with hefty boulders and thick clusters of laurel all around. A fun succession of wooden planks serves as an introduction to a lily pond. On departing this area of white birch, beech, maple, oak, and sheep laurel, a second, longer set of duckboards carries you to an open field of low-lying scrub. Described by some as a butterfly preserve, this sun-exposed expanse is no less attractive to a rich array of birds (come to think of it, birds do eat butterflies, don't they?), so you may want to keep your field specs handy.

The AT crosses Bramertown Road here, hopping over a short bridge and reentering the forest. After fording a seasonal stream via a handful of stepping-stones, it is back into a climbing mode, this time steeply up the rocky, fern-flavored hill. In 3 minutes of chest-thumping effort, the slant grows less severe, until the fickle path starts to lose altitude, spinning into a laurel and hemlock hollow clenched within the jagged teeth of a watery ravine. To describe this primeval landscape of fractured and fissured granite as "dramatic" or "impressive" would be to damn it with faint praise. There will be plenty of time to think of your own superlatives as you pick your way, rock by rock, to the top of the bluff. Once that fun scramble is over, the ground levels off as the AT hugs the edge of the ravine and overlooks the abyss. This idyllic setting, part of Buchanan Mountain, persists for several hundred yards, ultimately reaching a shelf at the south end of the peak with vistas extending far to the south and east. As beautiful as this spot is, the knoll off the path behind you is no less enchanting and provides the possibility of a private place in which to read, sketch, or woo your sweetheart, out of sight of other hikers.

Directly after that, another descent commences, steadily accelerating until you bottom out by a couple of seasonal streams. Look for jack-in-the-pulpits as you jump over those, and the two arroyos that follow during the next rocky ascent. If you took pleasure in the previous ravine romp, you'll love this one—it packs an exhilarating, ankle-challenging scramble up the Devil's Staircase, a rugged slope of rubble. This is a different chunk of the same Buchanan Mountain you were on a short time earlier, with a splendid view of Little Dam Lake from the crest. When you've regained your stamina and wearied of this wonderful locale, resume walking to the east, staying with the path on its downward trajectory. In 7 minutes and after a loss of 300 feet, the AT meets a road, slips over the blacktop, and proceeds into the woods.

The moss-sided track meanders from east to southeast, mildly descending, in 5 minutes, to a narrow footbridge. The swamp to the left is a haven for waterfowl, while Little Dam Lake to your right is favored by shutterbugs. No wonder, given the appealing look of the rock-lined lakeshore, attractively fringed with mountain laurel, hemlock, and scrub oak. The AT hooks to the left, through a clutch of laurel. For a moment the water is hidden, until the vegetation parts and you gain a view across the lake of a prominent rock face jutting out from the opposite shore. This is

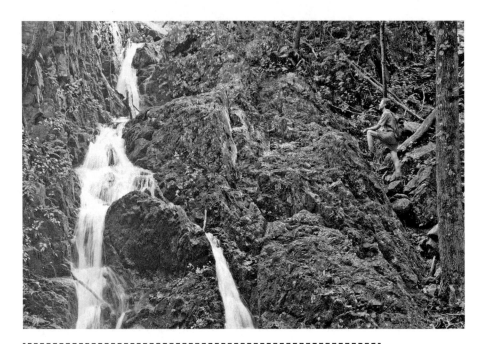

You're not in the Amazonian rainforest, but the misty spray of Fitzgerald Falls feeds a lush environment.

the turnaround point of the trek (GPS: **N41° 15.858' W74° 11.391'**), although obviously you should feel free to explore the vicinity before doing so.

It will likely require 10 to 15 minutes of stiff climbing from the road to reach Buchanan's second crest, and an additional 15 minutes to hit its first peak. Remember as you scramble down their far sides, where the afternoon sun warms the rocks, to inspect the hidden nooks for rattlesnakes prior to planting your feet or hands. Some out-and-back linear hikes can seem tedious on the back half as you pass through familiar terrain. Not here, not with so stark a reversal of ascents and descents, and the effort required to handle them. Even the sloping hemlock forest that you ambled through on your approach to the top of Fitzgerald Falls assumes a special, almost mystical aura when seen in the waning light of day.

## NEARBY ACTIVITIES

At the **Museum Village of Old Smith's Clove,** in Monroe, visitors are taken back to the 19th century. Costumed interpreters demonstrate crafts, and exhibits include a natural-history museum, a schoolhouse, a drugstore, and lots of Americana. Call 845-782-8247/8248 or visit **museumvillage.org** for details.

# HARRIMAN HIGHLANDS TRAIL  19

## IN BRIEF

How hardy are you? The answer to that question will determine how far you penetrate into this fabulous wilderness wonderland of rocks, meadows, and far-reaching vistas. Granite domes exuding a flavor of the far west are just one highlight. Others involve glacial gorges, mining ruins, a couple of laurel-fringed ponds, and beauty that never stops.

## DESCRIPTION

You don't have to be an über-hiker to enjoy hoofing it around the woods of Bear Mountain and Harriman State Parks. Of the miles of trails that run seamlessly through their backcountry, there are a handful that are flat and relatively easy. We're not going to talk about those, though, because, frankly, that's not why we go there. These are parks where serious hikers and outdoors enthusiasts can take blister-busting treks to granite aeries, tromp from one end of a forest to another without meeting many other souls, and thread through serrated gorges that both humble and inspire at the same time.

The Harriman half of this dynamic duo of parks owes its name—and its existence—to

---

### Directions

Follow I-95 across the George Washington Bridge to NJ 4 West onto NJ 17 North. Continue 15 miles, then merge onto I-287 North. After 0.5 mile switch to I-87 North for 1.4 miles to Exit 15A (Sloatsburg), then head north on NY 17. Drive about 7.3 miles and ascend onto the entrance ramp for NY 17A, on the left. Turn right at the stop sign in 0.1 mile, then right again onto CR 106. Follow it eastward for about 3.4 miles. A few parking spots are available on the left side of the road.

---

### KEY AT-A-GLANCE INFORMATION

**LENGTH:** 11.3 miles

**ELEVATION GAIN:** 2,514 feet

**CONFIGURATION:** Balloon

**DIFFICULTY:** Strenuous

**SCENERY:** Fascinating mix of polished rock tables, blueberry and laurel patches, mysterious mines, marshlands, bald glacial ridges offering panoramic views, dense lowland forests, and sparse mountain vegetation

**EXPOSURE:** Shady in the valleys, open on ridges and grasslands

**TRAFFIC:** The higher you climb, the lonelier it gets.

**TRAIL SURFACE:** Very rocky

**HIKING TIME:** 6.5 hours

**DRIVING DISTANCE:** 37 miles

**SEASON:** Year-round, sunrise–sunset

**ACCESS:** Free, except for parking in major-use areas; pets on leash not exceeding 6 feet, no mountain bikes

**MAPS:** At Reeves Meadow visitor center, on southern end of Seven Lakes Drive; USGS *Popolopen Lake*

**FACILITIES:** No water or restrooms on trail

**COMMENTS:** Like adjacent Bear Mountain State Park, Harriman is best explored with a detailed map to reduce the likelihood of getting lost. For further information, call 845-786-2701 or visit nysparks.com /parks/145/details.aspx.

## GPS COORDINATES

N41° 13.819'  W74° 8.394'

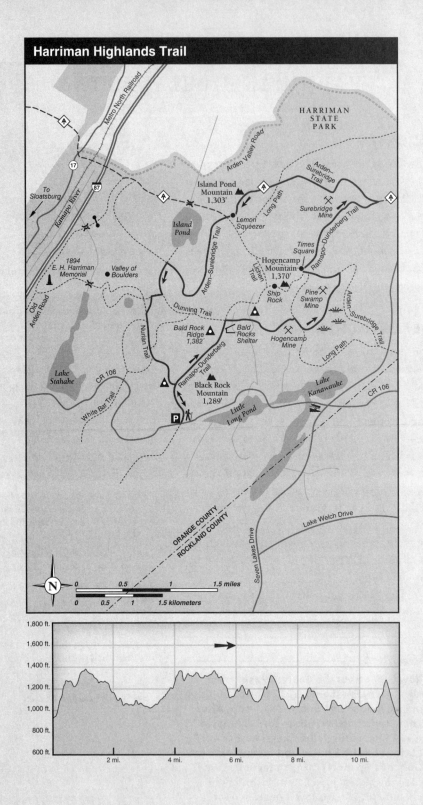

# Harriman Highlands Trail

E. W. Harriman, erstwhile president of the Union Pacific Railroad. He spearheaded the effort to preserve this area of the Empire State from developers who, among their other planned "improvements," wanted to relocate Sing Sing Prison to neighboring Bear Mountain. E. W. donated both money and land toward the creation of Bear Mountain and Harriman, which were jointly established in 1914 and today total more than 52,000 acres.

Look for the red-dot-on-white-blazes of the Ramapo–Dunderberg Trail (RD) by the lower of the two small parking slots, and plan to stick with this for the first mile of the 11.3-mile jaunt. For 50 yards, the RD tapers downhill near the road before swerving up, up, and away to the left along a well-worn, rocky trace. In 5 minutes you'll be among boulders and laurels, but even then the climb is just beginning. Ten more minutes of hearty exertion sends you through blueberry bushes, beech trees, maples, oaks, and many, many lichen-stained rocks, right to the top of the craggy ridge.

Well, almost. The final assault to the crest requires a bit of hand-over-foot clambering to surmount a few good-size slabs of stone. That bit of fun concluded, you'll be rewarded with spectacular views from an unspoiled, grass-plumed plateau. Rest a moment in this rarefied atmosphere, as you've just notched the most sustained climb of the hike. Keep in mind, though, that there's plenty more to come, with your cumulative elevation total topping out at an energy-sapping 2,500 feet. For several hundred yards, as you proceed due north along the RD among the birch saplings and oaks, the path hops from one polished crest to the next, shifting first northwest, then northeast, succeeded by a hard move to the east. If there were snowcapped mountains beyond these rugged domes, one might mistake this perch for a granite throne high in the Sierra Nevada. Unlike at the latter, though, bears breaking into cars is as yet unheard of in this park.

A half-hour of steady walking delivers you to Bald Rock Ridge, the highest point in Harriman at an elevation of 1,382 feet, with a fine vista to the northeast of Black Rock Mountain. Persevere along the RD as it snakes to the left of a backpacker shelter built in 1933, enduring evidence of the Civilian Conservation Corps's masonry skills. Also enduring are the scars of a wildfire, with numerous snags dotting the immediate surroundings. In a few minutes, you'll meet the Dunning Trail (DT, yellow blazes), where you should veer right. The ensuing descent, initially through waist-high scrub, is quite gradual, showcasing in the process the broad extent of the rocky plateau. After merging with an old forest road, remain with the DT as it trends toward the northeast, passing an unblazed path on the right. Another 5 minutes brings you to a reed-filled marsh, where such birds as yellow-shafted flickers, slate-colored juncos, and Eastern bluebirds occasionally cavort by the water. This pretty, pastoral area has recovered well from its time as a beehive of iron mining during the mid-to-late 1800s. Relics of that era linger on in the vicinity, though, in the slag heaps you see, and a series of old pits to the left of the trail. Stick with the yellow markings as the Long Path (LP, aqua blazes) joins the track from the left, then splits right in a few steps. The

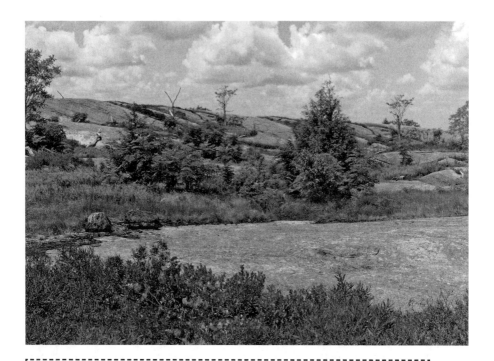

The domelands of Yosemite National Park have nothing on the granite highlands of Harriman.

succeeding body of water, opposite yet another mine, is well flanked by hemlocks and serves as home to a couple of beaver lodges. The DT ends just beyond that, once you've passed the pond. Your route, the Arden–Surebridge Trail (ASB, red triangle on white marking), lies to the left, on the near side of the stream, though a short hop across that flow brings you to still one more mine (GPS: N41° 15.047' W74° 6.728'), the most sizable along this stretch.

Now heading uphill on the ASB, the LP reemerges from the left just as you hit Times Square, a major intersection where you will find boulders, laurels, and hemlocks rather than neon lights and Yellow Cabs. Before switching from the ASB to RD, a hard right by the boulder, be sure to double-check your bearings; we have encountered more perplexed people at this tricky crossing than anywhere else in the park. From this point to where you connect with the Appalachian Trail (AT, long white blaze), the path zigzags from the base of one rocky knob to another, following an extension of the ridge you were treading along earlier. Be careful as you drop down off the second hill, by the way, as the steep angle of the north-facing granite can be treacherously slick in icy or wet weather.

Swing left on meeting the AT, at the midpoint of the fourth rise, and hang with that all the way through the Lemon Squeezer. En route to that jagged clenched fist of a ravine, the AT sinks into a hemlock-shaded area of yet more iron mines; be sure to steer left with the white slashes just before the stream there.

Your crossing comes in a few minutes—look for a fallen tree to use as a bridge if the water level is high—with the ensuing ascent to a beech-and-oak grove followed by—that's right—another loss of elevation. The AT then branches left, leaving this rocky pour-off of a trail, eventually running into a signed intersection with the LP. Continue straight, still with the AT, as the path soars up a grassy slope, passing, at its second apex, the foundation stones of E. W. Harriman's summer cottage (GPS: **N41° 15.710' W74° 7.834'**). Now rolling downhill, use caution as you sidle through the boulders of the Lemon Squeezer, a fun-but-hazardous bit of hand-to-hand maneuvering. Once through those fractured, fissured megaliths, hang a right, still adhering to the white bars of the AT, along with the red triangles of the ASB, which have only now reappeared.

Moments after leaving the Squeezer, just as the track levels off, dog it to the left with the ASB as it veers away from the AT. That's Island Pond, a glacial kettle hole, visible to the right as you descend in a southerly direction. Bear right on the ASB when a narrow forest road breaks left, and prepare for another lengthy climb, this one topping out at 1,200 feet by Tomahawk Rock, an oblong erratic crowned with ferns. (We spooked a herd of half a dozen deer here our last time through.) From this crest the path bends toward the west and begins an inexorable descent through mountain laurels and hemlocks, eventually reaching an unblazed forest road. Jag left on this wide route, departing from the ASB, and persist with it past the emergence of the yellow blazes of the DT, keeping to the left as the latter break right. Seconds after that, the white markings of the Nurian Trail (NT) surface from the right, joining the forest road. When they hop off it to the left a few seconds later (GPS: **N41° 14.737' W74° 8.826'**), hop with them, returning to the shade of the forest. Stay faithful to the Nurian past its overlap with the White Bar Trail, all the way back to where it meets the RD, at the peak of the first dome you conquered, 6 hours earlier. Your approach to this fork will be heralded by the NT swinging left at the base of the sizable monolith, up a few crude stone steps by a jumble of logs. This stretch calls for some dexterous scrambling before the white blazes end at a scrub oak and a junction with the RD. To return to the parking area, jog right and stick with the RD as the path begins its descent.

# NEARBY ACTIVITIES

Here's a cultural trip best done before the lengthy hike: **The Hermitage** (a National Historic Landmark), in Ho-Ho-Kus, New Jersey, originally built in the mid–18th century, was later transformed into a superb example of Gothic Revival architecture. George Washington stopped by during the Revolutionary War, and rooms are still furnished with Victorian antiques and more. For details, call 201-445-8311 or visit **thehermitage.org.**

# 20 HARRIMAN SEVEN HILLS LOOP

## KEY AT-A-GLANCE INFORMATION

**LENGTH: 9.8 miles**

**ELEVATION GAIN: 2,078 feet**

**CONFIGURATION: Loop**

**DIFFICULTY: Moderate to strenuous**

**SCENERY: Pristine hills, bald glacial ridges, great views, ruins, boulder fields, and a peaceful lake**

**EXPOSURE: Canopy cover alternates with exposure**

**TRAFFIC: Very popular area of the park: Pine Meadow Lake attracts swimmers and fishermen; the higher ledges are solitudinous.**

**TRAIL SURFACE: Rocky ledges, grassy patches, roots**

**HIKING TIME: 5.5 hours**

**DRIVING DISTANCE: 30 miles**

**SEASON: Year-round, sunrise–sunset**

**ACCESS: Free; pets on leash not exceeding 6 feet, no mountain bikes**

**MAPS: Reeves Meadow visitor center at trailhead; USGS *Ramapo***

**FACILITIES: Restrooms at trailhead**

**COMMENTS: For further information, call 845-786-2701 or visit nysparks .com/parks/145/details.aspx.**

## GPS COORDINATES

N41° 10.428' W74° 10.126'

## IN BRIEF

Don't be fooled by the "moderate to strenuous" rating of this hike—it is far easier than the cumulative elevation gain and overall length might suggest. That's not to say it will be a walk in the park. But for a relatively modest effort, you can expect miles of dome-top ridges, otherworldly vistas (including a glimpse of the Manhattan skyline), a historic ruin by a pristine lake, and hours of backcountry seclusion in which you're more likely to see deer or bears than too many other hikers.

## DESCRIPTION

Once, a long, long time ago, we delved into this section of Harriman State Park and came away distinctly underwhelmed. It wasn't simply that we found the trails too easy; there was also an absence of that sense of awe one experiences from, say, the views atop the bluffs at Claudius Smith Den, or the high drama of the clenched-fist passage through the rocky outcropping of the Lemon Squeezer. Other trails offered the promise of padding through remote woods undisturbed by our fellow hikers, of being far away from everyone else. Not so this Seven Hills area, where on most weekends scores of cars clog the parking lot at the Reeves

-------------------------------------------

### *Directions* ⟶

**Follow I-95 across the George Washington Bridge to NJ 4 West onto NJ 17 North. Continue 15 miles, then merge onto I-287 North. After 0.5 mile switch to I-87 North for 1.4 miles to Exit 15A (Sloatsburg), then head north on NY 17. Drive 2.5 miles and turn right on Seven Lakes Drive. Proceed for 1.5 miles and turn into the Reeves Visitor Center parking lot, on your right. There is overflow parking along the road.**

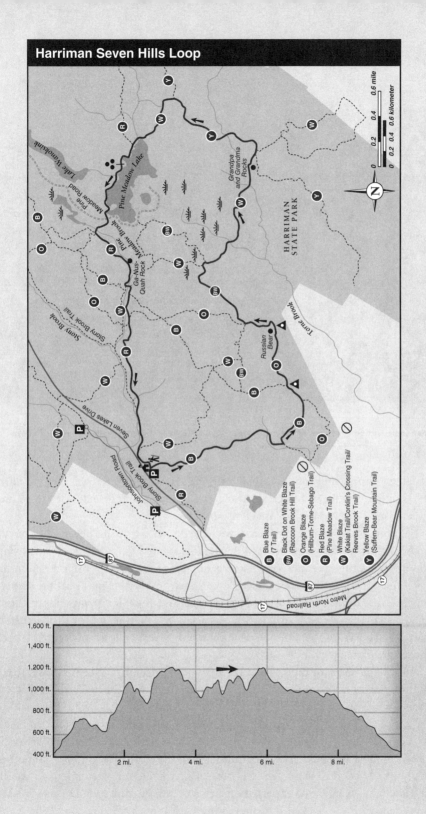

# Harriman Seven Hills Loop

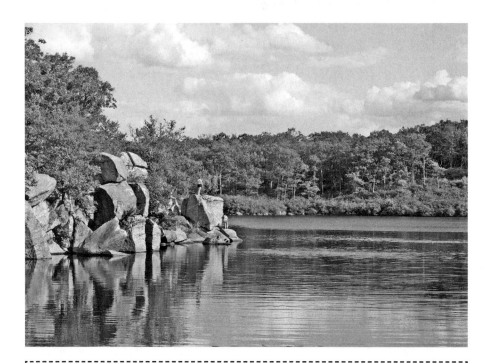

**The 5-mile round-trip to Pine Meadow Lake does not deter overheated city dwellers in need of a swim.**

Meadow visitor center, often spilling onto the shoulder of the road. There is nothing quite like hordes of hollering strangers flooding the forested aisles to shatter the illusion of getting away from civilization.

With the passing of many years, we thought we'd give this Seven Hills circuit another try. And you know what? We soon discovered that we were dead wrong. Not only does this 9.8-mile loop provide numerous chances to lose oneself in the backcountry, it also includes some of the most breathtakingly beautiful scenery you are likely to find anywhere in Harriman, and enough up-down-and-up climbing, for a cumulative gain of 2,078 feet, to satisfy a Marine Corps drill sergeant. From being a part of the park we once shunned, Seven Hills is now one of several that we gravitate to.

With your back to the kiosk at the Reeves Meadow visitor center, walk to the opposite side of the parking area and search for the path, which lies about four car spaces shy of the far end of the lot. Look for the red-square-on-white-blazes of the Pine Meadow Trail in the relatively open successional field, where a few fruit trees and a couple of cedars grow (as well as clover, cow vetch, and other wildflowers in season). Almost immediately the path leads into the cover of the forest, composed mostly of hardwoods and birch, with too many hemlocks succumbing to woolly adelgid blight. As might be expected of such a popular hiking spot, the trail is heavily eroded, with the packed dirt alternating with loose rocks and unwieldy roots. Fear not, you'll soon be putting this unpleasant stretch behind you.

Soon, as in a couple or 3 minutes. That's how long it should take to get to the T, where you turn left onto the Seven Hills Trail (SHT, blue square on white blazes), as Pine Meadow veers off to the right. Traipsing uphill among ferns and hardwoods, along with a smattering of pines, the SHT is three-person-wide for now but will gradually narrow to single-file. Plan to remain with this trail for the next 1.4 miles, as it draws you across seasonal streams and vestigial riverbeds, through the wonderful sort of glacially wracked scenery so typical of Harriman.

In about 30 minutes of circuitous hiking over pleasantly undulating terrain, the SHT arrives at a junction with an orange-blazed path. The latter begins here and heads to the right across an attractive, slightly overgrown grassy patch, but you should bear left, still on the SHT, as the track begins a steady, somewhat steep ascent over rock-pocked turf. The rubble lessens as you near the ridgetop, with the landscape evolving into a visually appealing blend of tall grass and giant erratics. At this stage, with the crest of the ridge still ahead, the Hillburn–Torne–Sebago Trail (HTS) joins the SHT from the right, the two paths overlapping as you continue straight.

In perhaps 5 minutes of rambling through a delightful, boulder-strewn area, the two trails separate, with Seven Hills breaking left, the orange-blazed HTS going right (more straight, actually). Shift to the HTS here, but before doing so be sure to head up the short trace to the right to Torne View, where the wavy plateau of bedrock, dotted with cedars and scrub oaks, is at least as impressive as the expansive vista. From this point the HTS descends a tad, then climbs back up to the fractured granite setting of the ridge, meandering for a spell among numerous eye-fetching erratics. The ensuing, more decisive descent draws you to a seasonal stream, where you may need to scour the thickly wooded surroundings to spot the continuation of the trail. Although it appears to persist northward across the stream, the HTS actually hooks to the right, passing over a rickety bridge, then doglegs back to the left, resuming its course to the north.

Having successfully leapt that hurdle, your next move is back uphill, this time in a grinding ascent up the face of the Russian Bear, a blunt, scree-covered cliff face. The reward for what is perhaps the most physically demanding stage of the hike? A superlative view—not just of the Orange & Rockland Utilities compound in the foreground, but also—if the weather is clear—the Manhattan skyline far off in the distance. On leaving that vista point, the ascent eases considerably, as the trail traipses through a highly scenic setting of grass-fringed fractured rocks, along with a fair share of blueberry bushes. Don't get too absorbed by this lovely environment, however, as the subsequent intersection, a four-way crossing with Raccoon Brook Trail (RB, black square on white blazes), is easy to miss, primarily because in this relatively treeless environment, the junction with the RB is marked by a blaze painted on a low rock.

To cut the hike short by several miles, continue straight on the orange-blazed HTS all the way to its meeting with the Pine Meadow Trail, and skip down four paragraphs to resume the narrative. Otherwise, for even more sensational scenery, turn right on the Raccoon Brook Trail. The spectral beauty of this ridgeline romp is briefly interrupted when the RB drops into and scoots across a gas-line cut. But all too soon, having risen out of that gully, the path dives sharply off the craggy ridge. After bending right at a junction with an unblazed forest road, the Raccoon zigzags first east-southeast (uphill), then east-northeast (trending downhill), passing all the while among head-high laurels and a dizzying assortment of boulders. Almost imperceptibly, the Kakiat Trail (KT, white markings) merges from the left, overlapping the RB for about 30 yards. When the RB and its black-dot blazes finally break away to the left, be sure to bear right, sticking now with the Kakiat.

The ensuing stretch of the hike is one of the more challenging, largely because of the haphazard distribution and maintenance of blazes. But while it is difficult from a route-finding perspective, it is also highly rewarding, both because of its relatively untrammeled state and for the high drama of its glacially scoured environment. On meeting a forest road (doubling as a horse trail) subsequent to a steep descent, the KT doglegs first left, then quickly right, darting back into the laurel thicket. Gradually, as the bedrock trail surface is replaced by moss, roots, and loose stones, and the oak and chestnut trees become more numerous, the KT arrives at yet another seasonal stream. You'll need the sharp eyes of a Vegas dealer to spot the white blazes here, as they hop into the shallow gully and climb out again on the stream's north side (*not* to the right along the rock fin, as appears to be suggested by the worn trace). The short uphill clamber culminates in a brief brush with the gas-line cut, which the KT skirts to the left. The highlight of this piece of trail, which has woven around its share of fractured domes, pointed rocks, and granite uplift, comes near its end (for you), at Grandpa and Grandma Rocks, a debris field of colossal erratics, with the word KAKIAT stenciled onto the side of one of the more massive specimens.

A few minutes of additional walking brings you to a short overlap with the Suffern–Bear Mountain Trail (SBM). Turn left on the SBM and follow its yellow blazes for the next half-mile, until you reach Conklin's Crossing (CC), an intersection marked by an enormous boulder. (For the sake of brevity, we will curtail further descriptions of a ground corrugated by the marvelous eye candy of craggy uplift and glacial detritus, which runs with few interruptions from much earlier in the outing, right through the SBM to well after the termination of the CC.) Turn left on the white-blazed CC, and in short order you will hit the southern foot of Pine Meadow Lake. On descending toward the water, bear right (the trace to the left peters out), making a counterclockwise circuit around the east side of the lake. Conklin's Crossing ends at a T, by a couple of rusty pipes that date to 1934, when the Civilian Conservation Corps (CCC) had a camp in the vicinity. Swing left, onto the Pine Meadow Trail (PMT, red square on white blazes), the same path on which you began your hike so many hours earlier.

From one inviting opening onto the lake to another, sandwiched around a rock-studded meadow, the PMT eventually arrives at a waterside cabin ruin, its imposing stone foundation flaring outward at its base. This, too, is a remnant of the CCC camp, not the Conklin cabin site listed on some maps. The Conklins, incidentally, made their home in this locale from 1779 until 1935, when flooding caused by the creation of Pine Meadow Lake drove them out. (The family cemetery lies in the woods to the west of the far shore.)

Plan to remain with the PMT all the way back to the trailhead. This can be somewhat tricky once it crosses the unpaved forest road on leaving the lake, due to the great number of social trails and other access routes that cut through the understory. An extra hazard involves occasional flooding of the path, typically in early spring. Well-positioned stepping-stones and a couple of strategically placed bridges will get you through the worst of that, though it's still possible you'll end up with wet feet. In fact, wet feet may be the desired outcome when you reach Ga-Nus-Quah Rock, shortly after passing a stone-buttressed foundation. To the left of the trail, Ga-Nus-Quah Rock is actually a cataclysm of rocks where the stream that's been paralleling the PMT passes through a constriction of slickrock boulders, making for a very appealing wading hole. Subsequent to that sylvan setting is a complex nucleus of trail crossings: just stick with the red-square-on-white markings and you'll be fine.

Once the PMT has devolved to the condition of an ancient riverbed, complete with a deplorable amount of loose stones underfoot, it passes some old stone steps that lead, on the left, to a tumbledown barbecue pit. Yes, another indication that the CCC was once here, too. And then, also on the left, the orange blazes of the Hillburn–Torne–Sebago Trail emerge, joining the PMT (only to forge back into the woods to the right in about 60 yards). Aside from the shifting rubble underfoot, the remainder of the hike is relatively easy, and in about 1.2 miles of fairly level walking, you'll be back at the Reeves Meadow visitor center.

## NEARBY ACTIVITIES

The opening hours of **Bellvale Farms Creamery,** in Warwick, coincide perfectly with the hiking season. Curious what Barn Boots or Calf Trax tastes like? This award-winning dairy farm makes more than 50 basic and complex ice-cream flavors that would convince even the toughest AT thru-hiker to make a detour. And while you're indulging, remember to say "hi" to the Holstein herd. Check it out at **bellvalefarms.com.**

# 21   HOOK MOUNTAIN HEIGHTS

## KEY AT-A-GLANCE INFORMATION

**LENGTH: 5.8 miles**

**ELEVATION GAIN: 1,243 feet**

**CONFIGURATION: Loop**

**DIFFICULTY: Strenuous**

**SCENERY: Dense hardwood forest, a rock-strewn ridge, and an extended stretch along the shore of the Hudson River**

**EXPOSURE: Well-shaded, except for a few open summits; morning sun along the river**

**TRAFFIC: Very light midweek but can get crowded on summer weekends**

**TRAIL SURFACE: Packed dirt, granite bedrock, crushed cinder**

**HIKING TIME: 3 hours**

**DRIVING DISTANCE: 25 miles**

**SEASON: Year-round, sunrise–sunset**

**ACCESS: $8 parking fee; pets on leash not exceeding 6 feet, no mountain bikes. Nyack Beach Sate Park has wheelchair-accessible trails.**

**MAPS: Posted for sale at park office in parking field 2; USGS *Nyack***

**FACILITIES: Restrooms at Nyack Beach State Park, 4 miles into the hike**

**COMMENTS: For further information, call 845-286-3020 or visit nysparks .com/parks/81/details.aspx.**

## GPS COORDINATES

N41° 8.634'  W73° 54.746'

## IN BRIEF

Breathtaking vistas of the Hudson River from a traprock ridge 702 feet up are just one reason to choose this excellent hike. Another is the extended promenade alongside the water on the back half of the loop. Add to that an assortment of plants that might leave a botanist slack-jawed with wonder, and we're willing to bet that after one tour of Hook Mountain, you too will be hooked.

## DESCRIPTION

Hook Mountain, situated along the Hudson River at the lower end of the Palisades, owes its name to the Dutch settlers who dubbed it Verdrietege Hoek ("Sad Corner"), because this perilous stretch of the Hudson claimed many lives. What was sad for the Dutch very nearly became sadder still for the mountain itself. That's because after its historical peak during the Revolutionary War, when the crest served as both a signaling point and a sanctuary for patriots, Hook Mountain became a focus of various development schemes. By the 1830s, for instance, nearby Rockland Lake was the site of a thriving ice industry, and the Knickerbocker Ice Company, with more than 2,000 people on its payroll, used the Hook to

------------------------------------------------

### *Directions* ⟶

**Follow I-95 across the George Washington Bridge to Exit 74, and merge onto the Palisades Interstate Parkway North. Drive to Exit 4 and merge onto US 9W North. Continue to follow it for 11.3 miles to the park entrance. Go right, then left on Rockland Lake Road. Proceed 1 mile, past the park office and parking field 2, to Landing Road. Turn left on it and park on the right side after 0.1 mile.**

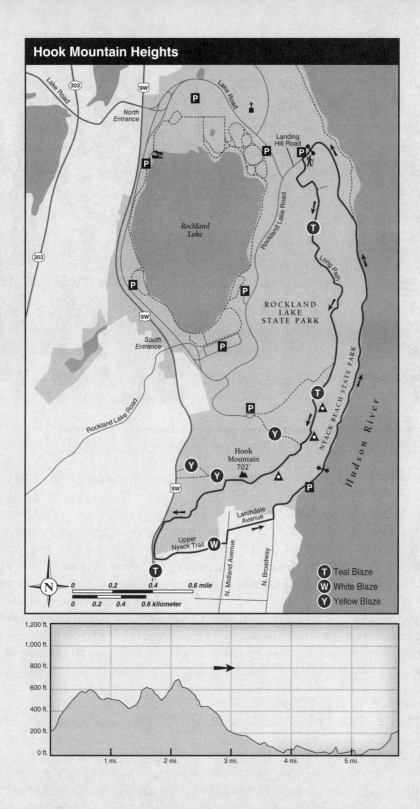

# Hook Mountain Heights

T Teal Blaze
W White Blaze
Y Yellow Blaze

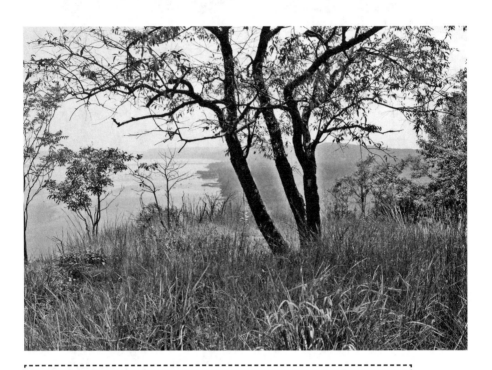

A lush picnic meadow is not exactly what you expect to find atop a volcanic ridge, and the panoramic view is worth the climb as well.

run cakes of ice down to the Hudson River to awaiting transport ships. That was just in winter. Summertime placed other pressures on the promontory: brickyards in Haverstraw plumbed the Palisades for clay, leaving behind pockmarked ground and land denuded of trees. In 1846 alone, Hook Mountain and, to the north, the Tors were stripped of 11,000 cords of wood, fuel used to power the brickyards' furnaces. An even worse threat, however, was posed by the 31 quarries operating in this area of the Hudson that used rock-crushing machinery and dynamite to reduce awe-inspiring monoliths to heaps of gravel. George Perkins, head of the Palisades Parks Commission, spearheaded a grassroots campaign to save the bluffs, convincing wealthy patrons (including the Harriman and Rockefeller families) to donate to the cause. Thanks to his efforts Hook Mountain was saved, and today, after years of augmenting the holdings, the state park totals 676 acres of mostly undeveloped woodland.

On exiting your car, walk to the kiosk on the east side of the parking area and pick up the teal blazes of the Long Path (LP). Follow them to the right, passing a series of concrete foundations as the trail heads south, and plan to remain on the LP for most of the first half of this hike. The 1,243 feet of elevation you gain on this trek (the bulk of it on the LP) begins gradually, with so gentle a slope you may feel like you're climbing a series of low steps, albeit grass-covered ones. The easy grade of this stretch owes to an overlapping of the LP with some of the old forest roads that once coursed through here.

You'll see evidence of those road constructions early on, as you amble past a series of magnificent old retaining walls, in which the remaining stonework is still so solid it could serve as a sidewalk. The tranquility and relative solitude of this setting are in striking contrast to that time, more than a century ago, when the hill was barren of trees and 3,000 men traversed the lanes, hollering greetings to each other as they hauled wood and clay or transported ice.

The views of the Hudson River are rather limited when you reach what seems to be the crest of the ridge, given that the LP lies in a grooved track, with higher ground (basaltic diabase, actually) on either side of it. Keep plugging onward, and as the forest road makes a hairpin turn to the left, stick with the teal blazes of the narrower path to its right. Within a minute of scaling this, the steepest section of the trail thus far, you will be on the true spine of the ridge. Stick with the LP as it arcs to the right, southbound, and then bear left on the spur, 10 paces ahead. This short conduit leads to a rocky shelf of an overlook, where you can enjoy your first unobstructed vista of the river.

More—and better—panoramas await farther down the LP. The ridge peaks at a fine formation of basaltic traprock, a grass-fringed, sun-exposed spot that towers 702 feet above the Hudson. The next viewpoint, while lower, is even more stunning and offers glimpses, from its basaltic terrace, of both the river and an extended patch of shore-side real estate, including much of Upper Nyack to the south. Because of the sheer drop of several hundred feet, by the way, you'll want to keep a keen eye on any little ones who may have accompanied you to this point. The same holds true of the ensuing stretch as it drops down over a ragged, rock-filled bit of trail. Once by the worst of that debris, the path forks, with a yellow-blazed route edging to the right. Unless you'd like to bail out back to Rockland State Park, bear left, sticking with the teal tags.

From this dip, the LP resumes its uphill surge, continuing to adhere to the Palisades' ridgeline. Though the trail is much overgrown here in summer by vines and various weeds, you may spy such plants as asters, yarrow, butter-and-eggs— even yucca. Prickly pear cacti grace the next peak, a visual reinforcement of how hot this sun-struck spot can get in the warmer months. Another fork lies just below this crest, once you're past a scree-filled patch. Keep left, on the LP, and in a few minutes the trail levels off and merges with another forest road.

Look for the three white blazes of the Upper Nyack Trail on a tree to the left, just as the path narrows to single-file. Turn there, finally departing the LP. After snaking downhill among black birches, the Upper Nyack Trail enters an undeveloped berm of trees, a linear swamp hemmed in by a residential neighborhood on one side, a paved road on the other. (Look for the blue-violet flowers of lobelia in summer.) Once across a couple of duckboards, the trail spits you out on North Midland Avenue. Look to the left for a white blaze painted on the back of a street sign and head that way.

Continue straight on this paved road, bypassing the first left (which leads to a housing development), till you reach the stop sign by a dark-brown log cabin, one of several buildings within the domain of Marydell Faith and Life Center, a Christian retreat and conference facility. Swing right here, on Larchdale Road, and stick with it all the way to the next stop sign, where the white blazes (painted on telephone poles) direct you to the left. The Hudson River should now be on your right, while the Palisades tower impressively, imposingly, directly ahead and above.

The white blazes end in about 250 feet, at the entrance to Nyack Beach State Park. Veer sharply right at the gatehouse, heading toward the beach. You'll encounter some picnic tables as you draw closer to the water, and a stairway leading to the shore across from the stone office building. The park road ends by an enormous structure (last chance to use the restrooms!), even as the pavement continues to flank the Hudson's western shore. Mosey ahead on what is now a multiuse walkway, the asphalt eventually devolving to cinder in much the way that the sycamores lining the promenade yield to sumac and other scrub. Note the massive boulders and heaps of talus to your left: some of this debris has fallen from the towering bluff, and much was left behind when the quarries closed.

Eventually, after about 1.25 miles of riverfront rambling, patches of pavement resurface, just as the path begins a gradual ascent. Ignore the two successive spurs to the left when the path levels off, then go left at the third junction (about 35 paces from the second spur), remaining with the main track. (The right option at this wishbone fork descends toward the Hudson and leads to the Haverstraw Trail in 3.5 miles.)

Stick with the road as it doglegs around a brownstone building, disregarding the unpaved track on the left, and meander with it, eventually gaining modest elevation. Four minutes after putting the brownstone residence behind you, the parking area should come into view.

## NEARBY ACTIVITIES

**Rockland Lake State Park,** just west of Hook Mountain, is no longer a center of ice production, as it was for much of the 19th century. Rather, it's the nucleus of a great range of recreational activities, and an ideal destination in its own right. In addition to a pair of Olympic-size pools and a handful of tennis courts, the park features picnic grounds, a paved fitness path, and fishing in its namesake lake. Winter activities include cross-country skiing and both sledding and tobogganing. For more information, call 845-268-3020 or visit **nysparks.com/parks/81/details.aspx.**

# SCHUNEMUNK MOUNTAIN RIDGE LOOP 22

## IN BRIEF

Some hikes balance a number of attributes, providing a razzle-dazzle of experiences. Then there's Schunemunk Mountain. After a grueling gain of nearly 1,000 feet right at the outset, you'll enjoy several miles atop a double ridge, with nothing but views to distract you. Views north to the Catskills, west to Kittatinny Ridge, east to the Hudson, and to the south— well, you get the idea: for views better than this, you'd have to sprout wings. The autumn leaf-peeping is heaven-sent, and for sensational highland scrambling from one puddingstone knob to another, this one is hard to top.

## DESCRIPTION

Remember the fable about the grasshopper and the ant? Good, because the tiring, knee-buckling haul up the slope of Schunemunk Mountain is best approached with the steady pluck of a pismire rather than the short-lived, "be happy" attention span of a leaf-eating locust. The 1,000-foot vertical gain at the outset of this hike is indeed draining, but once that is out of the way, you'll have several miles of ridgetops to ramble along, with views that never stop and only a modest amount of additional exertion required.

- - - - - - - - - - - - - - - - - - - - - - - - - - - - - - - - - - -

## *Directions* ———————————→

**Follow I-95 across the George Washington Bridge to NJ 4 West onto NJ 17 North. Continue 15 miles, then merge onto I-287 North. Drive to Exit 16 and merge onto NY 17 West. After 4.5 miles take NY 208 North via Exit 130. Continue 3.2 miles and veer right on Clove Road. Proceed 4.4 miles and go right onto Otterkill Road. The parking lot is 0.8 mile farther, on the left side.**

### KEY AT-A-GLANCE INFORMATION

**LENGTH: 9.2 miles**

**ELEVATION GAIN: 2,223 feet**

**CONFIGURATION: Balloon**

**DIFFICULTY: Strenuous**

**SCENERY: Steep ascent leads to double ridge, separated by a brook and a swamp, yielding several 360-degree vistas on top of conglomerate bedrock, surrounded by dwarf growth of pitch pine and oak.**

**EXPOSURE: Shaded ascent, exposed ridge loop**

**TRAFFIC: Popular venue in spring and fall**

**TRAIL SURFACE: Rock-studded dirt, some grassy patches, and bedrock**

**HIKING TIME: 6 hours**

**DRIVING DISTANCE: 53 miles**

**SEASON: Year-round, sunrise–sunset**

**ACCESS: Free; no pets, no bicycles, no motorized vehicles**

**MAPS: USGS *Cornwall-on-Hudson***

**FACILITIES: None**

**COMMENTS: Wear good hiking shoes with decent traction. Binoculars will help with identifying distant landmarks and soaring birds. In winter, blazes and cairns may be snow-covered. For more information, call 518-690-7850 or visit tinyurl.com /schunemunkpreserve.**

## GPS COORDINATES

N41° 25.543' W74° 6.096'

# Schunemunk Mountain Ridge Loop

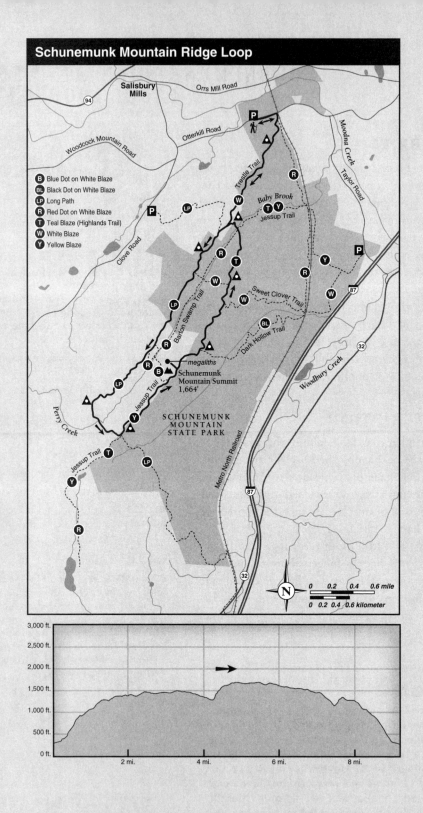

**Legend:**
- **B** Blue Dot on White Blaze
- **BL** Black Dot on White Blaze
- **LP** Long Path
- **R** Red Dot on White Blaze
- **T** Teal Blaze (Highlands Trail)
- **W** White Blaze
- **Y** Yellow Blaze

Salisbury Mills

94

Orrs Mill Road

Woodcock Mountain Road

Otterkill Road

Moodna Creek

Taylor Road

Trestle Trail

Baby Brook

Jessup Trail

Clove Road

87

Sweet Clover Trail

Barton Swamp Trail

Dark Hollow Trail

Woodbury Creek

32

megaliths

Schunemunk Mountain Summit 1,664'

SCHUNEMUNK MOUNTAIN STATE PARK

Jessup Trail

Perry Creek

Metro North Railroad

87

32

N

0    0.2    0.4    0.6 mile
0  0.2  0.4  0.6 kilometer

3,000 ft.
2,500 ft.
2,000 ft.
1,500 ft.
1,000 ft.
500 ft.
0 ft.

2 mi.    4 mi.    6 mi.    8 mi.

Geologists enthuse about how the rocky substrate of Schunemunk is far younger than the underlying base of the Hudson Highlands, and that its uplifted fins of rock are compressions of shale and sandstone dating to the Ordovician and Silurian Eras. The brittle layer of conglomerate that crowns this formation is more eye-catching still, being stained reddish-mauve in places—most notably along Schunemunk's summit ledge—by an iron-based hematite and larded with eggs of quartzite, compressed and fossilized sand from the beaches of an ancient sea. That this puddingstone is an extension of the Devonian strata is probably of interest only to specialists. What you *should* keep in mind, though, is that during an outing on May 22, 2002, one hiker was killed and two others injured when a rockslide occurred on the hill they were bushwhacking up. We suggest, therefore, that you stick to the blazed trails and think twice about bringing bantamweight walkers on this challenging trek. Timber rattlers, hidden within the folds and crannies of the rocks, are another hazard you may encounter in the 2,400-acre preserve, which became a state park in 2001.

This sensational jaunt begins 0.1 mile east of the parking lot, as you near the railroad trestle. Cross the road, head into the forest on the worn trace, marked discreetly with white blazes, and march uphill under the cover of maple, oak, black birch, box elder, and hemlock. Stay with this moss-sided Trestle Trail (TT) as it breaks to the right in a minute and soars on up the slope. Shortly after passing a red-blazed path to the left (which leads to the top of the trestle), the TT levels briefly in a thinly treed, appealingly grassy area. All too soon the sharp ascent resumes, although the worst of the climb should be behind you within a half-hour or so. Some traces along the way deliver glimpses of the valley below, with a few of the better ones offering up a fair piece of the Hudson River, the Hudson Highlands, Storm King Mountain, and even the sculpture garden of its namesake art center.

Moving along, the slope, which is crowded by blueberry bushes, continues to rise for 3 more minutes until the TT ends at a junction with the Barton Swamp Trail (BST, red dot on white blazes). Turn right and climb up the face of the slanted rock, clinging to the blazes as they flow over the north end of this conglomerate platform, arriving soon at a three-way intersection. Proceed straight onward, now on the Long Path (LP, aqua markings), hugging the rocky western ridge of the twin-crested Schunemunk Mountain, which is creased down the middle, like the crown of a homburg, by the cool, shady Barton Swamp. *Schunemunk,* incidentally, is a Lenape Indian word that denotes either "ancestral fireplace" or "excellent fireplace," depending on the translator; if you tackle this sparsely treed hilltop in summer, the meaning takes on a cruel irony.

Traipsing along Schunemunk's western rim, which is a couple hundred feet lower than the eastern ridge to the south, you are at eye level with vultures and hawks. You're also enjoying no end of spectacular vistas as the trail zigzags around stunted pitch pines—some more than a century old—and mountain laurel, with innumerable blueberry shrubs (rich with berries mid-to-late July) covering the

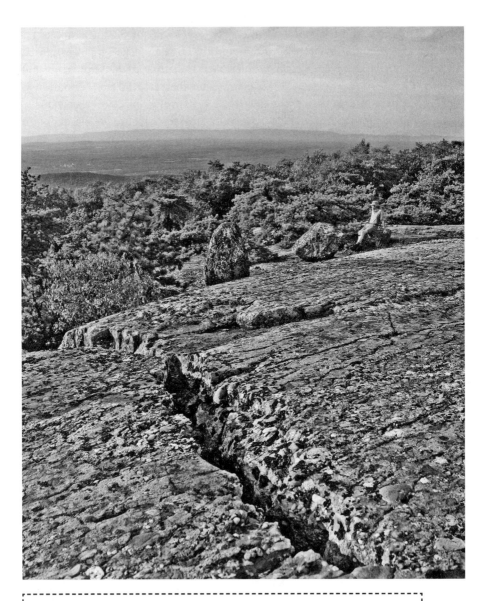

Once you reach the double-ridged summit of Schunemunk Mountain, a few spots offer stellar 360-degree vistas.

ground. Keep going straight at the junction with the Sweet Clover Trail (SCT, white blazes) on the left and at the subsequent crossing with a forest road, adhering to the rises and dips of the puddingstone plateau. Its general trend is toward the southwest, but occasionally the LP pulls a surprise by darting to the right, to the edge of the ridge. An additional surprise, which we have been fortunate enough to discover only once along this stretch, is the presence of round-headed cordyceps, an exceedingly rare form of mushroom.

Steer right (still on the Long Path) on meeting the turnoff to the left for the Western Ridge Trail (WRT, blue dot on white blazes)—unless you'd like to cut a mile or two off the hike. In another 90 seconds, just as the BST reappears, you will have to dogleg left, then pivot quickly to the right, to keep to the LP. We had the spit scared out of us here years ago by the sudden slithering of an Eastern fox snake, which we briefly mistook for a venomous rattler. A few cairns mark the route over the broad bedrock.

Gradually, the LP arcs to the southwest, dipping down into Barton Swamp, a shady notch of hardwood trees and vernal streams. Lope left on reaching the forest road, then left again in about 30 seconds at the next crossing. Hang a right in 25 strides, now leaving the wide lane, and proceed through the swamp, hopping over the moss-sided Baby Brook and another forest road, to the base of the talus slope. The first time we did this, we looked hopefully to the left and right before realizing that the trail does not indulge in any sidewinding switchbacks. That's right: the LP surges straight up, over the steepest part of this sandstone-and-shale debris. Happily, a false summit surfaces as a rest stop about 6 minutes up the rock heap, and in another minute, you should reach the shoulder of the bluff, with a 5-foot-high step to the next level. The edge of the east ridge is just a short scramble from there.

Follow the cairns over the slanting slab of conglomerate to the junction with the Jessup Trail (JT, yellow markings), turning left on the latter as it flies higher up the rock. The views are superb when you reach the top, spanning every direction but northeast. Save your film, though: the best is yet to come. The JT, which is overlapped here by the Highlands Trail (HT, teal diamonds), continues to gain ground as it scales another cataclysm of boulders, with the fractured rocks giving way to a bald knob. A stunning, prolonged platform of conglomerate succeeds that, and then the clearly marked blazes drift higher, meandering from one side of this extended shelf to the other, always sticking—like stink on a skunk—to the highest part of the ridge.

A couple of minutes after passing the other end of the WRT (with its blue-dot blazes), the JT comes to the modest peak of Schunemunk, identified by a marking on the rock that notes where a fire tower once stood. From this attractively barren spot, a hair less than 400 feet above the base of the talus slope you maneuvered through half an hour earlier, you can see the Catskill Mountains to the north, and even the needlelike monument at High Point State Park, far away in northwestern New Jersey. A second painted inscription, a minute's walk from the first (GPS: N41° 23.556' W74° 6.964'), indicates the way to the Megaliths, north over the bedrock. In less time than it takes to boil a quail egg, square white blazes draw you to this fascinating, spectacular formation, where colossal slabs of conglomerate have fractured and dropped off the main plateau, resembling a major section of an interstate highway after an earthquake.

Back on the JT, the yellow blazes are somewhat faded from this stage onward (with the teal ones of the HT even more spotty). Heave to the left in about

The round-headed cordyceps has been credited for the outstanding performance of some Chinese runners, but its effect on hikers remains unknown.

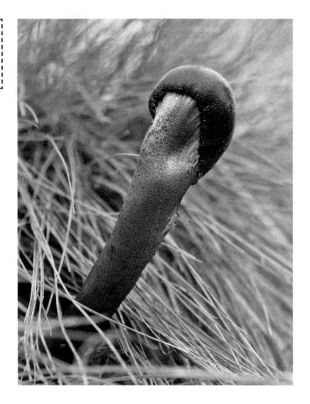

5 minutes as the path bends that way on meeting the Dark Hollow Trail (black dot on white square). About 15 minutes later, the SCT merges from the right as the main trail drops into a small gully. Are you tired of vistas yet? Atop the succeeding ridge node is yet another Hudson River backdrop, one that is certainly a bell-ringer. But if you are here in early to mid-June, try scanning the pitch pine and laurel–shaded ground, too, for pink lady's slipper orchids.

Having descended a slanted rock, the SCT breaks to the left, leaving the main track. Bear right, eastbound on the JT, still accompanied by an occasional teal blaze of the HT. Very soon the JT finally leaves the ridge, departing this wonderland of puddingstone. When it veers right at the buggy Baby Brook, you should proceed straight with the red dots of the BST (the BST also goes left here). This culminates in the last climb of the day, a rugged assault on the splintered side of the west ridge, atop which you jog right, again on the white-blazed Trestle Trail. Stroll quietly during the leisurely descent back to the road, and you just might spy a wild turkey or white-tailed deer, both of which roam these woods.

## NEARBY ACTIVITIES

For a closer look at the colorful shapes you admired from atop Schunemunk Ridge, plan to explore **Storm King Art Center,** in Mountainville. Modern sculptures by internationally renowned artists are exhibited in a splendidly landscaped outdoor environment. Visit **stormking.org** for detailed information, or call 845-534-3115.

# STORM KING SUMMIT TRAIL  **23**

## IN BRIEF

Few hikes manage to blend a rocky, mountainous setting with dynamite views while still being easily accessible from a major highway. Storm King is one of those, delivering a quick payoff in panoramas nonpareil of the majestic Hudson River and surrounding hills from a series of rough, romantic granite domes. Its handy proximity to US 9W makes this short circuit immensely popular, but there is enough viewing space atop the many domes for everyone to have a blast.

## DESCRIPTION

Raise the topic of Storm King with your culture-minded friends, and they're likely to respond with enthusiasm, going on at great length about the beautifully landscaped art center in Mountainville, where modern sculptures by internationally renowned artists are displayed in a splendidly manicured outdoor environment. Those of your cronies who are more comfortable clad in hiking boots than tasseled loafers will probably be no less enthusiastic, though their raves will touch on the outdoor sculptures wrought by Mother Nature from the glacial rocks that compose the eponymously named peak. Storm King Mountain, which hovers over the Hudson River like a

---

## Directions ⟶

**Follow I-95 across the George Washington Bridge to Exit 74 and merge onto the Palisades Interstate Parkway North. Drive 37 miles, enter the traffic circle, and take the third exit onto scenic US 9W. Proceed for 8.6 miles to a large, open parking lot on the right, on a hilltop in a bend of the road. If you come to Mountain Road, you've gone too far.**

---

**ⓘ KEY AT-A-GLANCE INFORMATION**

**LENGTH:** 3.8 miles

**ELEVATION GAIN:** 1,678 feet

**CONFIGURATION:** Figure-eight loop

**DIFFICULTY:** Moderate to strenuous

**SCENERY:** A quick, steep climb is rewarded with a rapid succession of open vistas overlooking the Highlands and the expansive Hudson River.

**EXPOSURE:** Partially exposed in the first half, more canopy in the second part

**TRAFFIC:** So popular a destination, you may have trouble finding a seat on the rock viewpoints, especially on weekends.

**TRAIL SURFACE:** Rocky scrambles alternating with dirt and grass

**HIKING TIME:** 2.5 hours

**DRIVING DISTANCE:** 54 miles

**SEASON:** Year-round, sunrise–sunset

**ACCESS:** Free; pets on leash, no motorized vehicles

**MAPS:** USGS *West Point*

**FACILITIES:** None

**COMMENTS:** The north-facing Stillman Trail can be dangerously slick with ice in winter and is best avoided when hiking in snowy conditions. Be aware that deer hunting is allowed. Call 845-786-2701 or visit nysparks .com/parks/152/details.aspx.

**GPS COORDINATES**

N41° 25.388'  W74° 0.067'

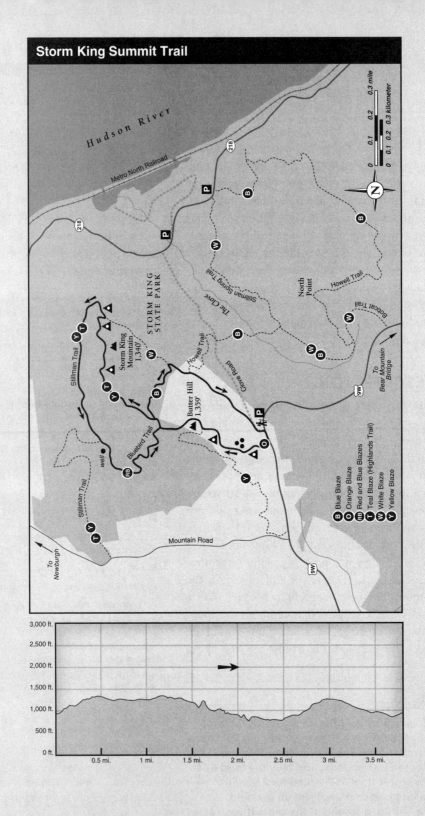

# Storm King Summit Trail

Hudson River

Metro North Railroad

218

218

P

P

P

W

Stillman Spring Trail

The Clove

STORM KING STATE PARK

Storm King Mountain 1,340'

Stillman Trail

Y

T

T

Y

W

B

well

Bluebird Trail

RB

Stillman Trail

T

Y

To Newburgh

Mountain Road

North Point

Howell Trail

Bobcat Trail

W

To Bear Mountain Bridge

9W

B

W

B

B

Howell Trail

Clove Road

Butter Hill 1,359'

P

Y

North

B Blue Blaze
O Orange Blaze
RB Red and Blue Blazes
T Teal Blaze (Highlands Trail)
W White Blaze
Y Yellow Blaze

9W

0 0.1 0.2 0.3 mile
0 0.1 0.2 0.3 kilometer

3,000 ft.
2,500 ft.
2,000 ft.
1,500 ft.
1,000 ft.
500 ft.
0 ft.

0.5 mi.  1 mi.  1.5 mi.  2 mi.  2.5 mi.  3 mi.  3.5 mi.

celestial helicopter, is indeed a spectacular hike, one that combines breathtaking vistas of the Hudson with trail-side scenery that is appealingly rocky and rough-hewn, all within a very short distance. The one catch: this double loop involves a cumulative elevation gain of 1,700 feet in less than 4 miles, with most of it coming in short, spirited bursts. Yet with so many viewpoints along the way, you may not even notice the effort.

Meanwhile, reports of live munitions impregnating the ground—dangerous detritus dating back to World War I, when the neighboring United States Military Academy used the area for artillery practice—appear to be old news. The state closed the park for three years a while back to allow the Army Corps of Engineers to clear the ordnance, and for some time now Storm King's 1,900 acres have been open for recreation. That said, bushwhackers and rock climbers should be especially cautious when venturing more than 25 feet from the trail.

Walk to the far left (or north end) of the parking lot and look for orange blazes as you near the highway. Enter the woods there and scramble up the slanted bedrock, under a mantle of maple, oak, and sheep laurel. This jaunt gets going with a jolt, like a morning gargle of Turkish coffee, zigzagging up a steep slab of granite. In 5 heart-pounding minutes, as you near the crest of the first hill, the ruins of an old cabin appear, with three stone pillars aligned in front of the foundation. This is all that's left of Spy Rock House, the summer home of Edward Lasell Partridge, a Big Apple physician who was a member of the Palisades Interstate Park Commission during the first half of the last century. In that position, Partridge helped lead the drive that preserved much of the Hudson Highlands.

The trail shifts to the left of the ruin and circles behind it toward the east, losing a touch of elevation before darting into a jumble of rocks. In a few seconds the upward trend resumes, scaling the ridge through the cleft between two boulder-wracked peaks, passing among mountain laurel, black and white birch, scrub oak, and pitch pine in the process. Catch your breath at the first knob of this bald dome (a.k.a. Butter Hill), 358 feet above the trailhead, while absorbing the great view of the western hills, as well as the neighboring Black Rock Forest and US 9W to the south. Next up is Butter Hill's crest, 3 minutes farther to the east and 50 feet higher. On the way to that spicebush-bordered summit, the orange blazes expire, replaced by yellow-and-teal ones emerging from the left (be sure to keep to the right). The small amount of scrub fringing the dome is not enough to interfere with the stellar 360-degree panorama, highlighted by the Hudson River flowing like a small sea from beneath the Newburgh Bridge to the north, growing larger and wider as it approaches Storm King.

On leaving this sun-exposed crow's nest, the narrow path glides north along the rocky ridge, arriving at a fork in a couple of minutes. Bear right, still with the yellow-and-teal blazes, ignoring the Bluebird Trail (BT, red-and-blue vertically divided markings), and in a moment you will pass the Howell Trail (HT, blue blazes) on the right. The track treads through fairly level terrain for several minutes, with Storm King peak dead ahead and the attractive granite-and-scrub-oak setting

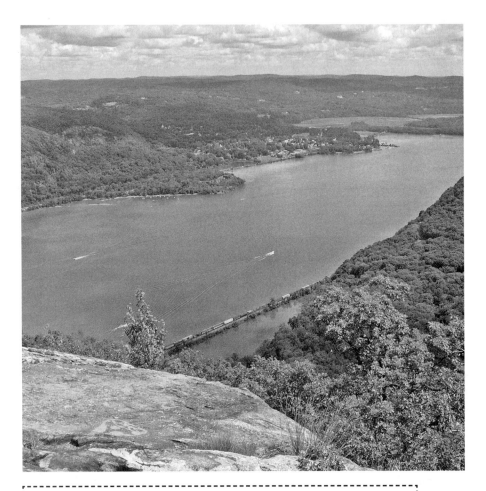

Storm King Mountain offers splendid Hudson River scenery, with Metro North trains a part of the entertainment.

common to the Hudson Highlands all around. After jogging slightly right—then left—by a stand of hemlocks, the path starts to gain ground, grinding upward over bedrock. The following plateau is more tree-covered, most notably by chestnut oaks and pitch pines, but the view north of the Newburgh Bridge is no slouch.

Continuing east toward the Hudson River, you drop into a saddle between the last rise and Storm King peak. That lull is finished in about a minute, when you come to—and must scale—a large, slanted rock face. The vista spot above that opens up in a few paces to a magnificent image of the Hudson flowing directly toward you, with an extension of the Highlands hulking dominantly across the river. Look closely and you may see boats, like little specks of foam, puttering around on the water far below. You should also be able to spot Pollepel Island, about a thousand feet off the far shore. During the Revolutionary War, colonists anchored 12 wooden bulwarks in the rocks beneath the rapidly flowing water between Pollepel and Plum Point, on the left bank of the river. These emplacements were connected by an enormous wooden chain and topped with steel spears, a *cheval-de-frise* intended to puncture the hulls of British ships sailing up the Hudson. The gambit failed, as the British used flat-bottom barges to maneuver upriver, where they burned the town of Kingston to the ground in 1777.

If you brought field specs along, take a closer look at Pollepel Island. Rising high out of the scrub growth is the grandiose ruin of Bannerman Castle, dating from 1901 to 1918. Designed by Francis Bannerman, an arms dealer, partly as a summer home and in part to house the munitions he purchased as military surplus from the federal government, the five-story baronial estate promptly fell to pieces after being acquired by the Taconic Parks Commission and New York State in 1967. Attempts are now being made by the Bannerman Castle Trust to stabilize the edifice and restore some of its paths, with boat trips there from Newburgh offered on weekends during the summer.

The environment becomes more corrugated as you shuffle along on Storm King Mountain, with additional viewpoints enticingly accessible through the laurel and beech saplings along the way. The most dramatic vista, moments away, is actually a bit lower than several of the earlier ones. No matter—from this jutting spar of a rocky perch, you have a dizzying glimpse of the choppy Hudson River as it eddies and swirls beneath you. When Persian poet Omar Khayyam penned the words "a jug of wine, a loaf of bread—and thou, beside me singing in the wilderness," it is hard to believe he didn't have this locale in mind, even though the new world of North America was still five centuries away from being "discovered." When you've had your fill of seraphic visions, as well as the wine and bread, carry your song and sweetheart onward, down to yet another rocky vantage point as the track loops southward.

In a few minutes, the descent accelerates and the path meets a junction, with the yellow-and-teal markings shifting left on the Stillman Trail (ST, which connects with the BT in a bit), while white blazes branch to the right. The circuit continues to the left, though if you are tired of breathtaking vistas or would like to quit early, you may head right and return directly to the car lot. For the first several steps the ST hugs the contours of a rocky lower ridge, showcasing the Hudson all the while. Gradually, though, it begins to descend along the north side of Storm King through an environment shrouded in hemlocks and mountain laurels, where the rocks and logs are covered in moss. After the second set of switchbacks, about 15 minutes into the descent, the ST encounters the Stillman Bridge, a log-and-plank construction that had grown rotten and precarious over the years and will probably have been replaced by the time you undertake this hike.

About a minute down from the bridge, the path passes under some old-growth hemlocks and slips easily through an impressive boulder field, at which point the ST breaks right, with the BT—your route—spurting in the opposite direction (GPS: **N41° 25.979' W74° 0.167'**). That rounded, oversize hydrantlike construction of fieldstones and concrete just a few yards downhill of the intersection, by the way, is the site of an old well, with a sizable cabin ruin cloaked among the trees just beyond. Stick with the red-and-blue blazes as they draw you steeply uphill, through hemlocks and mountain laurels, slithering toward the southeast, then the southwest, before abruptly hitting a T. Jag left on the wide, grass-surfaced forest lane, still with the red-and-blue tags. Moments after skirting a massive moraine field, the trail soars uphill, payment now coming due for all of that easy touring down the Stillman, and in 10 or so minutes of having your lungs Hoovered by the effort, the BT crests at a notch between the spires of Butter Hill and Storm King. Zig left, chasing the same yellow-and-teal tags of earlier, and in less time than it takes to read this, you will zag right, onto the HT (blue blazes). This stretch brings you over the wrinkled crown of Storm King's cranium, delivering further sensational vistas in the process, before corkscrewing downhill to its junction with the aforementioned white-tagged trail.

The white blazes bound left, back to the intersection with the ST, but you should hang a right here, stumbling along with the HT's blue markings. In another 5 minutes, those blue blotches break left, indicting the spur to the Crow's Nest. Ignore that turn, remaining straight on the (now) unblazed track. This path overlaps an old forest road, with a retaining wall supporting its left side. As it begins to rise, the boulder field peppering the slope above draws closer, until the moraine and jumbo rocks are all around—a colorful clutch of chaos, frozen in place. That is succeeded momentarily by a rusting refrigerator and a couple of tires to the left of the trail, which unofficially mark the imminent end of the hike. Storm up the steep hill ahead, then hang a left at the crest by the low, long erratic. Out in the open of a grassy berm, the parking lot is a few paces to your right. If, on unlocking your vehicle, you find that you still have energy to spare, well, why not drive over to Mountainville and that other Storm King, just to see how man's sculpturing efforts compare with Mother Nature's?

## NEARBY ACTIVITIES

You may have caught an earful of some military activity in the area. Indeed, the **United States Military Academy** at West Point is just a few miles south of this park. For details on the academy's museum, events, or parade schedules, call the visitor center at 845-938-2638 or visit **usma.edu.**

Did the glimpse of the castle on Pollepel Island pique your interest in this state-owned land? Kayak and boat tours there run on weekends from mid-June through October. For details, call the Bannerman Castle Trust, 845-831-6346 or visit **bannermancastle.org.**

# TORS' THUNDER TOUR 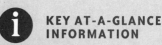 24

## IN BRIEF

While the struggle years ago to prevent the demolition of the Tors inspired a hit Broadway play, it's the views from their peaks that are the real showstoppers, with the Hudson River unfolding directly below and the Catskills and Shawangunks visible far to the northwest. No less enjoyable are the scramble up both summits, over wrinkly volcanic basalt, and the deep-woods flavor of their surroundings.

## DESCRIPTION

Like most hikers, we don't relish chewing the same scenery twice, and as a rule we'll opt for a good loop over an out-and-back trek any day. There are exceptions to every rule, however, and a few linear romps—Fitzgerald Falls, Sterling Ridge, and Sandy Hook come readily to mind—are quite exceptional indeed. The jaunt to High Tor and Low Tor belongs in this category of out-and-back hikes that are so memorable, and memorably rewarding, that we simply can't exclude them from this volume.

And yet if it had been left to the New York Trap Rock Company, there would be little to say about the Tors. That's because back

------------------------------------------

*Directions* ⟶

**Follow I-95 across the George Washington Bridge to Exit 74, and merge onto the Palisades Interstate Parkway North. Drive to Exit 10 and turn right on Germonds Road. After 0.7 mile turn left on NY 304/South Main Street. Proceed 3.8 miles and make a left on Ridge Road. Continue 0.8 mile and veer right on Haverstraw Road. Park on the left shoulder in about 250 feet, right by the trailhead. The main park entrance and office are 2 miles west from here, on the right.**

### i  KEY AT-A-GLANCE INFORMATION

**LENGTH:** 5.8 miles

**ELEVATION GAIN:** 1,751 feet

**CONFIGURATION:** Out-and-back

**DIFFICULTY:** Moderate

**SCENERY:** Woodsy ascent to two eroded, basaltic summits, with expansive views of the Hudson River and Haverstraw

**EXPOSURE:** Mostly dense canopy in summer, sun-struck on bald summits

**TRAFFIC:** Fairly light weekdays, heavy weekend visitation

**TRAIL SURFACE:** Largely rocky, some packed dirt

**HIKING TIME:** 3 hours

**DRIVING DISTANCE:** 28 miles

**SEASON:** Year-round, sunrise–sunset

**ACCESS:** Free; foot traffic only, pets on leash not exceeding 6 feet

**MAPS:** At park office; USGS *Haverstraw*

**FACILITIES:** No toilets, public phone, or water at trailhead, but all may be found, along with a swimming pool, by the park's main entrance.

**COMMENTS:** In icy or snowy conditions, the tricky rock scramble descent off the north side of High Tor, leading to Low Tor, may be extremely hazardous. For further information, call 845-634-8074 or visit nysparks .com/parks/78/details.aspx.

## GPS COORDINATES

N41° 10.609'  W73° 57.616'

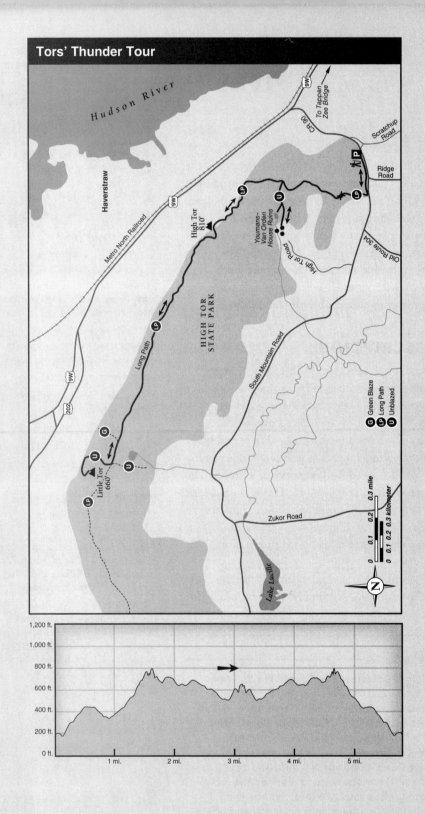

# Tors' Thunder Tour

in the 1930s, Trap Rock planned to "develop" the land into a quarry, reducing High Tor's crest, which today towers 832 feet above the Hudson River, into gravel and sand for paving roads. That we hikers can still enjoy a 360-degree, kick-you-in-the-seat-of-the-pants panorama from that peak says a great deal about the determination of conservationists of that era, as well as Elmer Van Orden, who owned a large section of the summit and resisted New York Trap Rock's efforts to buy it. Van Orden's neighbor, Maxwell Anderson, memorialized that struggle in *High Tor,* a play he wrote in 1937 that was performed on Broadway and won the New York Drama Critics Circle Award. (It was later rewritten as a TV movie starring Bing Crosby and Julie Andrews.) After Van Orden's death six years later, 23 acres of his property were donated to the Palisades Interstate Park, with an additional 470 acres being given by Archer Huntington, a railroad magnate, from his private estate. High Tor State Park now totals more than 600 acres, with a community pool and picnic grounds among its amenities.

On exiting your automobile, step around the abundant roadside litter and walk west, away from the Hudson River, sticking to the right shoulder of the road. After the fourth telephone pole, the aqua blazes of the Long Path (LP) jag to the right, by a large tree, into the forest. The trail, passing among myriad oaks, black birches, and beeches, as well as wild violets and garlic mustard, is rocky to start with, as it bumps over duckboard planks and begins to gain elevation. The mild ascent continues through secondary growth, including a smattering of cedars, before leveling off, in about 10 minutes (and a slight gain of 150 feet of elevation), amid a rumpled, corrugated landscape where wild turkeys often roam. An unblazed spur to the left, indicated by a large sign, leads in less than a quarter-mile to the site of the Youmans–Van Orden House and a former winery. Little more than a tiled floor area remains, but the adjacent pond is attractive and lends the short detour some extra value.

Once back on the main trail, the uphill slog resumes for another 3 to 5 minutes before you reach the shoulder of High Tor, with a filtered view of the Hudson straight ahead. The LP then lunges left, over terrain that is reminiscent of the Timp, at neighboring Bear Mountain, for the intimidating amount of rocky scree piled up at the base of the peak. As at the Timp, the LP skirts the worst of that obstacle, looping to the left of the rocks, at the same time giving you an opportunity to observe chipmunks at play in and around the chinks and crevasses of the moraine heap. After working around that rough, beautifully formed outcropping of traprock, with lichen settled over it like a blanket of oxidized copper, the LP moves on to another node, then a third, higher one, before cresting atop High Tor. This loge-level vantage point of the Shawangunk range to the north, and to the east, the Hudson River, was used by colonial troops as a signal post during the Revolutionary War to alert people to the comings and goings of the British army. Today it is favored as a local party spot, with a distressing amount of graffiti smeared across the wrinkled texture of the volcanic substrate under your feet, but we find the vultures flying by at eye level (as well as blue azures and mourning

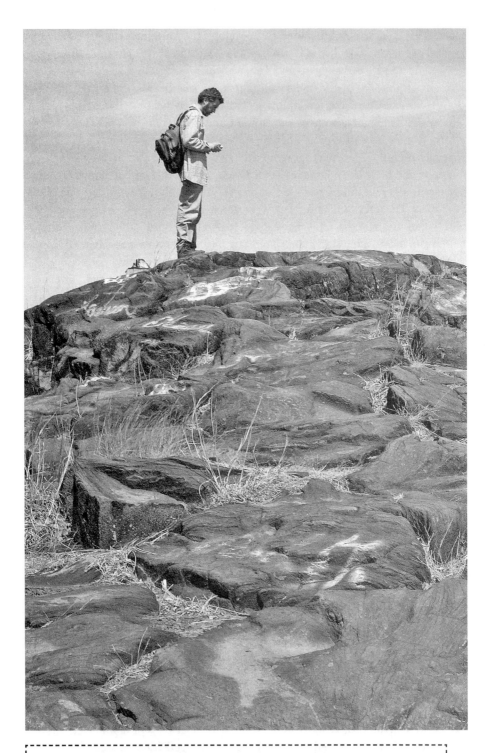

How high *is* High Tor's bald summit? Our GPS indicates 801 feet and the topo map shows 810 feet, while other sources list it as high as 832 feet.

cloak butterflies in warm weather) a more thrilling distraction. That rock quarry far below you to the southeast, by the way, is a stark reminder of what might have happened to the ground you're hiking through if not for Van Orden and the labors of conservationists.

The trek continues on the north side of this dome, where the scramble down can be seriously challenging when there's snow or ice on the path. Once off High Tor's peak, the LP veers to the right, eastward, then to the northeast, along a former forest road. This wide and easy stretch lasts for 20 minutes, with a green-blazed spur materializing to the right about the time the surface of the lane turns to gravel. Ignore that turn, persisting on the LP until just after it dips by a swamp stream and then rises to a diagonal intersection, the latter notable for the presence of a large graffiti-marred erratic. Skim to the right there on the unblazed forest road, which curves uphill, edging gradually toward the north, culminating in an easy ascent to Low Tor. This lesser Tor, which is also scarred by graffiti and too much broken glass, abuts a similar knob, which, given its comparatively clean surface, is our preferred choice of sandwich spot. Views atop Low Tor, while marginally less pronounced than those of its big brother, are still rather breathtaking, with the Hudson Highlands beckoning from across the river. When you tire of the setting, or as sunset deepens to darkness, retrace your steps back to the trailhead.

## NEARBY ACTIVITIES

Stellar views and prime, private picnic spots don't come any easier than the short, level walk at nearby **Tallman Mountain State Park.** The breezy 2-mile loop there leads to an overlook high above the Hudson River, where birding and boat-watching are extra attractions. If you're bounding with energy, you can connect this trail with an extended campaign along a piece of the Long Path. For further information, call 845-359-0544 or visit **nysparks.com/parks/119/details.aspx.**

High Tor is not the only landmark in the vicinity to play a role in the American Revolution. **Stony Point,** on the Hudson, was of strategic importance to the British, who fortified it with a garrison and used it to control the river. In a risk-all gambit, colonial troops, commanded by Brigadier General Anthony Wayne, launched a midnight raid on July 15, 1779, reportedly armed solely with bayonets. Astonishingly, it took them a mere half-hour of skirmishing to take the fort, effectively ending the Crown's presence on the Hudson. The story of this amazing victory, as well as that of the Stony Point Lighthouse (one of the few remaining such beacons still lining the river), is on full display at Little Stony Point Battlefield State Historic Site, in Stony Point. For further details, call 845-786-2521 or visit **nysparks.com/historic-sites/8/details.aspx.**

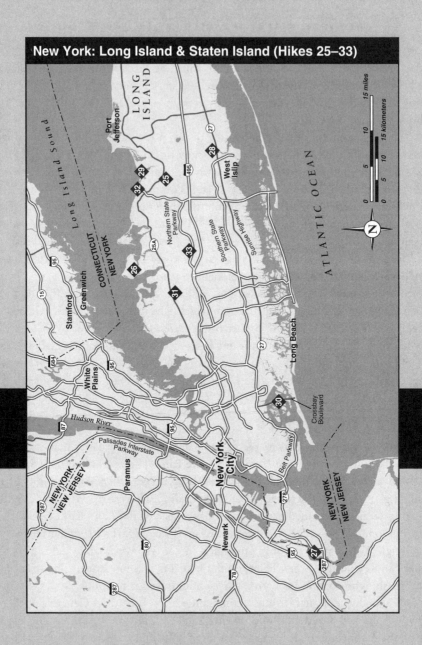

## New York: Long Island & Staten Island (Hikes 25–33)

# NEW YORK:
## LONG ISLAND AND STATEN ISLAND

# 25 CALEB SMITH FULL CIRCUIT

## KEY AT-A-GLANCE INFORMATION

**LENGTH:** 2.9 miles

**ELEVATION GAIN:** 222 feet

**CONFIGURATION:** Double loop

**DIFFICULTY:** Easy

**SCENERY:** Surprisingly secluded park contains fields, streams, and ponds; wetlands and upland forests; and a gorgeous Colonial-style nature museum.

**EXPOSURE:** Mostly shady

**TRAFFIC:** Light to moderate

**TRAIL SURFACE:** Sandy with root network

**HIKING TIME:** 1.5 hours

**DRIVING DISTANCE:** 46 miles

**SEASON:** Year-round, Wednesday–Sunday, 8 a.m.–4 p.m.

**ACCESS:** $8 parking fee; no dogs, no bicycles

**MAPS:** At park office and posted at entrance kiosk; USGS *Central Islip*

**FACILITIES:** Restrooms, water, and public phone at park office

**COMMENTS:** The preserve is a popular winter venue for cross-country skiers and a great spot for fly-fishers. For further information, call 631-265-1054 or visit nysparks.com /parks/124/details.aspx.

## GPS COORDINATES

N40° 51.107'  W73° 13.526'

## IN BRIEF

You don't have to be a big fan of the Colonial era to enjoy Caleb Smith State Park Preserve—but it doesn't hurt. Wander beyond its historic house and first-rate nature center, though, and you'll be on your own—on a really fun hike, that is, through successional fields, pine barrens, swampy hollows freckled with wildflowers and skunk cabbage, with birds all around. Caleb Smith is a tranquil oasis in the heart of suburbia, with trails suitable for even the littlest Bigfoot in your tribe.

## DESCRIPTION

To stop by Caleb Smith State Park Preserve is to ingest a good-size bite of Long Island history. The Colonial house that now serves as a nature museum, with a rat snake in an aquarium and various child-friendly exhibits, was built by Daniel Smith in 1752. Smith's grandfather, Richard "Bull" Smythe, was a founding father of neighboring Smithtown, while his son, Caleb, became a thorn in the side of the British troops when they occupied Long Island during the Revolutionary War. Because Caleb, a graduate of Yale who was elected to the state assembly and also became a judge of common pleas, refused to take an oath of loyalty to King George, "he was shot at, roused from

## Directions

Follow the Long Island Expressway/I-495 East to Exit 42 and merge onto the Northern Parkway East. Continue to Exit 45 and take the Sunken Meadow Parkway North. Proceed 1.9 miles to the junction with the Jericho Turnpike/NY 25 East at Exit SM3E. Drive 3.1 miles and turn left into the preserve. Make another quick left into the parking lot.

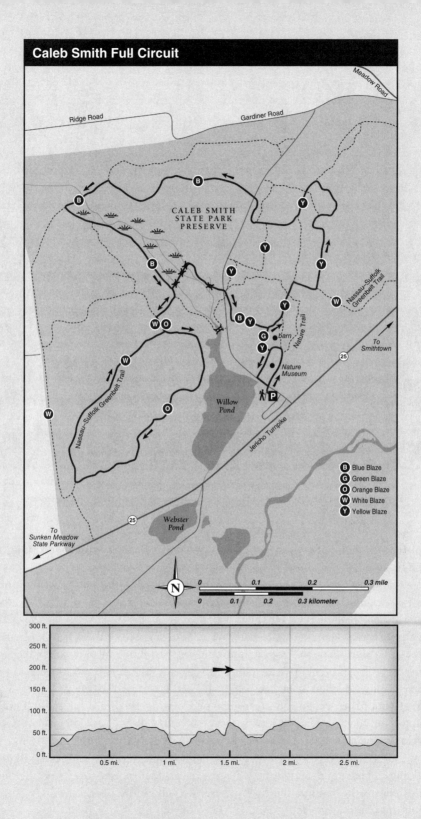

# Caleb Smith Full Circuit

Meadow Road

Ridge Road

Gardiner Road

CALEB SMITH
STATE PARK
PRESERVE

Nassau–Suffolk
Greenbelt Trail

barn

Nature Trail

Nature
Museum

To
Smithtown

25

Willow
Pond

Jericho Turnpike

Nassau–Suffolk Greenbelt Trail

To
Sunken Meadow
State Parkway

25

Webster
Pond

**B** Blue Blaze
**G** Green Blaze
**O** Orange Blaze
**W** White Blaze
**Y** Yellow Blaze

N

| 0 | 0.1 | 0.2 | 0.3 mile |

| 0 | 0.1 | 0.2 | 0.3 kilometer |

300 ft.

250 ft.

200 ft.

150 ft.

100 ft.

50 ft.

0 ft.

0.5 mi.    1 mi.    1.5 mi.    2 mi.    2.5 mi.

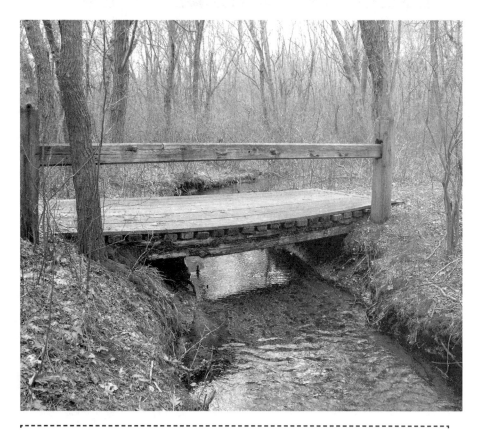

The many small streams of this park feed into secluded swamps, where birds and amphibians nest.

bed, [and] lashed with hickory gads up and down Willow Pond," according to park records.

It shouldn't take hickory gads to get you to saunter up and down the pond these days, or to hike the park's shady circuit of trails, for that matter. Fair weather and a decent pair of walking shoes are all that is required. Many of the paths overlap firebreaks, and most are fairly wide, allowing two or three people to stroll abreast. To start a double loop of approximately 2.8 miles, head from the parking area to the Smith home, passing along the paved road to its right. Once past this green clapboard-sided structure, obey the black arrow that points to the left. Forget about the orange-and-green-diamond blazes—those are for cross-country skiing—and focus instead on staying with the yellow discs inset with black arrows. Circle around to the left of the red barn, beyond the main house, and bear right by the gas pumps, drifting away from burlap-covered wigwams and scattered out-buildings. Hang another right in 30 yards, then go left on the dirt lane.

Keep to the right at the fork, where the yellow discs break away from the green ones, and swing left a moment later on the dirt forest road. Now among dense clusters of chokeberry, oaks, and red maples, many aged and sporting wrinkled, splintery goiters, you may notice a few birdhouses spaced out among the trees. They're intended for wood ducks and owls, which we presume don't cohabitate. Shortly after the forest road crosses over the cinder-surfaced nature trail, it divides, with yellow blazes continuing to the right toward a pocket meadow with scattered conifers at its center. Hug the far right of that open space, and in several strides you will enter a corridor of cedars, at which point you should turn left. (Straight ahead is a white-blazed section of the Suffolk Greenbelt Trail.) The meadow is now on your left, faintly visible through the hedgerow of cedars and a smattering of black birch. Once you reach the north end of that field, jog right onto the narrow, wood chip–surfaced trail, then right again at the slanted four-way crossing. The track passes a couple of white pines as it tapers downhill, then abruptly loops to the right, regaining lost ground. Launch left at a little circle or roundabout, where a branch-and-leaf lean-to has been constructed off the trail; now back on an unpaved service road, strut straight with the yellow discs as the cross-country-ski blazes skip off to the right. Hew to the right in another 60 to 70 paces, leaving the park road, while the dirt trail remains flat and wide.

Blue discs appear at the next intersection, and you continue straight with those as the yellow ones split to the left. Steer right on this peaceful path just before it meets a patch of pavement, no more than 200 yards from the previous junction. The track cuts to the left, crosses the paved park road, and proceeds through a vestigial pine barren of cedars and white pines, imperceptibly losing elevation. Break left at the fork, now walking westward, then left again, shifting toward the south, at the four-point intersection. Remain with the sandy, blue-blazed route as it begins to climb and passes a couple of maverick, unmarked spurs, as well as a pair of disused stairs leading up to the right. Incidentally, on hearing a rustling among the oak leaves covering the ground here, you may con-clude that an industrious squirrel is intently gathering acorns. Take a closer look: more likely what your ears have caught is the sound of a rufous-sided towhee scavenging for a smaller scale of seed. This is one of the more appealing parts of the park, where a lowland swamp, decorated with ferns and skunk cabbage, colors the left side of the trail, and the ground, shaded by a mature mix of hardwoods, rises sharply to your right.

In a little while, the Blue Trail (BT) breaks left, hopping over a serpentine swamp stream via a little bridge. You will take that path later, heaving right for now with the orange-and-white blazes—the latter path, incidentally, being a continua-tion of the Suffolk Greenbelt Trail (SGT). Ascend the erosion-control steps—nearly hidden under a heap of bark and mulch—and scoot left at the triangular T, still adhering to the orange-and-white markings. When the two colors diverge in 30 seconds of ambling, go with the orange blazes to the left. You are now in an upland forest populated by cedars, many types of oaks, and a fair number of white pines—not to mention dense clusters of catbrier. As you mosey along over roots and moss, the rather sizable Willow Pond comes into view down to the left, with the orange circuit all too soon rejoining the SGT at a T. Cruise right, and in 5 minutes pull to

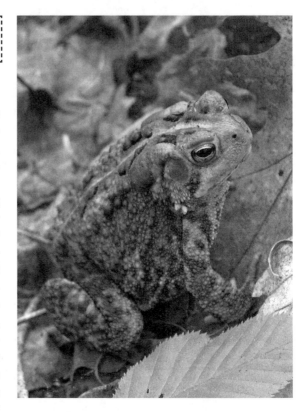

Go ahead and give him a kiss: this plump American toad may turn out to be your Prince Charming.

the left, bounding by the spot where this mini-loop diverged awhile earlier. Traipse down the steps to return to the BT.

Once more following the blue blazes, walk over the small bridge and, a few seconds later, another couple of such spans. The level track, flanked by ferns, garlic mustard, and skunk cabbage, soon jags to the right, where a fourth bridge appears. Turn right just after crossing the park road, as yellow discs now unite with blue, and stick with yellow as they lead you back to the open field, just above the wigwams. The Caleb Smith House and trailhead lie to the right, a couple of minutes away.

## NEARBY ACTIVITIES

If you can't bear being on Long Island without catching a glimpse of the coast, **Heckscher State Park** is the place to be. Never mind the 1 million annual visitors, the Great South Bay is roomy enough for a cool dip, and there's a swimming pool as well. To camp or picnic, hike or bike, plan your visit at **nysparks.com/parks/136 /details.aspx,** or call 631-581-2100 to find out more.

# CAUMSETT NECK LOOP

## IN BRIEF

It's all downhill once you get past Caumsett State Historic Park Preserve's most obvious landmarks, a dairy farm and brick manor house. *Literally,* as the extensive trail system meanders among open fields and mature stands of hardwoods, reaching a physical low point by a series of bluffs abutting Long Island Sound. Abundant wildlife—including gray foxes—and a wealth of birds endow every step in this beautiful park with the possibility of surprise or discovery. Springtime, when blossoms color the trees and wildflowers carpet the ground, is our favorite time to visit.

## DESCRIPTION

Have you ever wondered what it would be like to have a few million dollars burning a hole in your pocket? To be as rich as Croesus, sitting on top of a golden heap? Well, stop wondering and get yourself over to Caumsett State Historic Park Preserve. A trip to this peninsula—1,500 acres of meadows, marshes, forests, and farmland that extend dramatically into Long Island Sound—won't magically make you a millionaire, but it may help to visualize what a boatload of money can buy.

------------------------------------------

## *Directions* ———————————→

Follow the Long Island Expressway/I-495 East to Exit 39. Make a left on Glen Cove Road, drive 2 miles, and go right on Northern Boulevard/NY 25A East. Continue 11 miles and make a left on Goose Hill Road. After 0.8 mile turn right on Huntingdon Road. Proceed 0.5 mile and swing left on West Neck Road, which becomes Lloyd Harbor Road. Continue for 3.8 miles to the park entrance, on the left; the parking lot is 0.2 mile ahead.

### KEY AT-A-GLANCE INFORMATION

**LENGTH:** 7.3 miles

**ELEVATION GAIN:** 423 feet

**CONFIGURATION:** Loop

**DIFFICULTY:** Easy

**SCENERY:** Peaceful peninsula harbors woodlands and grasslands, salt marsh and rocky shoreline, freshwater pond, and an old dairy farm.

**EXPOSURE:** Very open in meadows and beach areas, some shady trails

**TRAFFIC:** Light to moderate, but sunny days attract many outdoors fans.

**TRAIL SURFACE:** Grass, sand, and dirt

**HIKING TIME:** 3.5 hours

**DRIVING DISTANCE:** 40 miles

**SEASON:** Year-round, sunrise–sunset

**ACCESS:** $8 parking fee April–November; no pets. Some paved trails are wheelchair-accessible.

**MAPS:** At entrance booth; USGS *Lloyd Harbor*

**FACILITIES:** Restrooms, telephone, and water at dairy-farm complex

**COMMENTS:** Beautiful setting and gentle terrain encourage people with strollers to take advantage of expansive domain, which also accommodates equestrians, cyclists, and joggers. Call 631-423-1770 or visit nysparks.com/parks/23/details.aspx.

## GPS COORDINATES

N40° 55.050'  W73° 28.372'

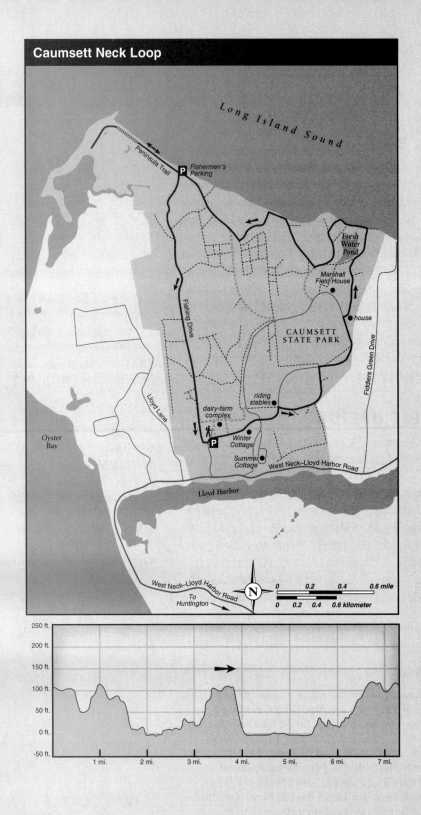

# Caumsett Neck Loop

Long Island Sound

Fishermen's Parking

Peninsula Trail

Fresh Water Pond

Marshall Field House

house

Fishing Drive

CAUMSETT STATE PARK

Fiddlers Green Drive

riding stables

Lloyd Lane

dairy-farm complex

Winter Cottage

Summer Cottage

West Neck–Lloyd Harbor Road

Oyster Bay

Lloyd Harbor

West Neck–Lloyd Harbor Road

To Huntington →

N

| 0 | 0.2 | 0.4 | 0.6 mile |
| 0 | 0.2 | 0.4 | 0.6 kilometer |

250 ft.
200 ft.
150 ft.
100 ft.
50 ft.
0 ft.
-50 ft.

1 mi.   2 mi.   3 mi.   4 mi.   5 mi.   6 mi.   7 mi.

When Marshall Field III, grandson of the founder of Chicago's renowned department store, bought this spit of soil in 1921, he didn't have hiking in mind. With a fortune in his billfold and the collaboration of architect John Russell Pope, he created a self-sufficient community centered on a dairy farm, complete with 80 head of award-winning cattle and a magnificent manor house modeled on those of 19th-century Europe. True to the British tradition, visitors to the estate could indulge in hunting, skeet shooting, swimming, fishing, polo, boating, tennis (both outdoors and in), and, of course, riding.

It is still possible to ride horses at Caumsett, which was acquired by the Empire State in 1961, but the egalitarian pursuit of hiking allows one to see the grounds under more serene circumstances. *Caumsett,* incidentally, means "place by sharp rocks," a name given to the property by Field in honor of the Matinecock Indians who used to live here. From the parking area and entrance booth, proceed along the maple-flanked paved road in an easterly direction, keeping the dairy-farm complex to your left. The Winter Cottage, a stone construction on the right that is a "cottage" only by the standards of a Vanderbilt or Field, appears just before a four-way intersection. Walk straight through the junction, passing the sprawling brick riding stables on your left. Remain with the paved road as it bends to the left, all the while showcasing the surrounding landscape, with mature plantings running the gamut from white pines, yews, and cedars to dogwood, forsythia, and honeysuckle.

The flora grows considerably wilder when you turn off the drive onto the unpaved lane to the right, opposite the horse corral (GPS: N40° 55.231' W73° 27.914'). This easy, pebble-strewn track descends slightly for 100 yards or so before tapering to the left, with garlic mustard, chokeberry, briar, and black birch springing up along the grassy margins. Skip the two spurs to the right, with the first leading to an open field, the second toward a low animal pen in that same lush sward, maintaining instead a straight direction. Then swing left at the T, by a vine-draped chain-link fence. The abundance of scrub growth provides great ground cover for birds, and to judge by the melodious jabbering that reaches one's ears, a number of sundry species take advantage of it.

After the sudden surge uphill, hang a right, back on the main road. Remain with this as it swoops to the left and then straightens out. When you see a cinder drive, by a cluster of rhododendrons, steer right on it. This seems at first to lead to a private dwelling, but as the driveway edges toward the house, on the right, the trail branches off to the left. (Pay no attention to that turn to the trace that diverges to the right.) We have seen a gray fox treading stealthily among the wild violets and laurel here, as well as a great horned owl hooting above the magnolia trees (which blossom beautifully in early spring). On bearing left at the Y, this untamed setting segues to an open expanse of lawn (where ospreys are known to nest atop a tall snag), punctuated periodically by a few mature maples. As you approach the freshwater fishing pond, hew to its right side, following the unpaved lane.

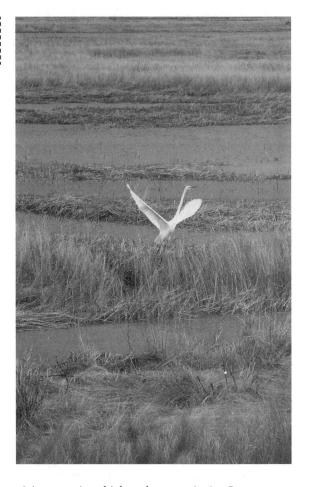

A tidal salt marsh is the favorite hunting ground of elegant white egrets.

Moseying counter-clockwise around the pond, look for birds among the cedars, black birches, maples, and briar that ring its shore. At its north end, where auburn-colored phragmites rises above the water, the picturesque panorama encompasses not only the pond but also Long Island Sound and the rocky shoreline below the trail. Stay with the sandy track as it parallels the Sound, yielding meanwhile a view to the left of the stately brick Marshall Field house, high atop the grassy hill. In a couple of minutes, the path comes to a low bluff over the shore, with large-bodied oaks adding the allure of shade to an enticing area in which to laze or picnic. Cormorants often roost on the rocks that jut above the water, and you may observe seagulls dropping shellfish on the stones in an attempt to open them.

From this enchanting spot, the trail veers sharply left and inland along a pebble-and-sand-surfaced lane, fertile ground that flourishes with daffodils, vinca, and wild forsythia in spring. Stick with this wide track as it arcs to the right and passes a small dam at the west end of the pond. Stride right 2 minutes later onto the dirt-and-grass path and persevere all the way back to the bluffs. The grass-topped overlook here is a mere 15 feet above the beach, the rocks farther out crusted with seaweed. Stroll left along the bluff, cutting away from the water view in 150 yards, moving inland toward the knoll's grassy recess. The pebbly path resumes once you're by the large maple, winding southward uphill. On entering this small maze of trails, keep hard to the right at the first fork, and right again at the top of the slope. In about a minute this grassy lane merges with a sandy one, beside a superannuated dogwood tree. Amble to the right and continue along this route for roughly half a mile, all the way to the Fishermen's Parking Lot. Don't put away your birding specs, as we've spied a green-breasted warbler, blue jays, catbirds, a wood thrush, a nuthatch, red-winged blackbirds, and even an ever-elusive pileated woodpecker in this portion of the park.

Having reached the parking lot, march dead ahead to the hard, sandy track that marks the start of the Peninsula Trail, a half-hour side trip. Here, fully exposed to the sun, you can enjoy great views of the Sound on one side (with a few intriguing erratics decorating the shore like the odd flotsam of a shipwreck), while on the other is a salt marsh where great and snowy egrets frequently fish. In a few paces, the firm surface of the path evolves to soft sand, and then board-walk, succeeded by soft sand again, with any number of wildflowers and—sur-prisingly—prickly pear cacti springing up among the surrounding bayberry, cedar, and chokeberry. Although you may choose to wander along the shore to the end of the cove, the spur ends at the rotting wooden platform—the remains of docks used by Marshall Field III to land *Coursande,* his steam-powered yacht.

On returning to the Fishermen's Parking Lot, turn right on the dirt road. Remain with this route, which is known as Fishing Drive, for the next 2 miles, all the way back to the dairy farm. When the road has drawn within 200 yards of the farm and breaks to the left toward it, continue straight on the slightly rutted track, with open fields on either side of you. The trailhead parking lies a couple of minutes ahead.

## NEARBY ACTIVITIES

A guided tour through Theodore Roosevelt's home in Oyster Bay provides a fas-cinating portrait of how one of our country's great presidents lived. **Sagamore Hill,** as he called it, is a typical dark Victorian mansion, enlivened by TR's per-sonal belongings and collections. For details, visit **nps.gov/sahi.**

# 27   CLAY PIT PONDS CONNECTOR

## KEY AT-A-GLANCE INFORMATION

**LENGTH:** 1.7 miles

**ELEVATION GAIN:** 148 feet

**CONFIGURATION:** Double balloon

**DIFFICULTY:** Very easy

**SCENERY:** Gaping clay-mining pits and ponds, hidden in wetlands and woodlands, surrounded by sandy barrens

**EXPOSURE:** Mostly dense canopy

**TRAFFIC:** Generally light

**TRAIL SURFACE:** Dirt, sand, roots, and wood chips

**HIKING TIME:** 1 hour

**DRIVING DISTANCE:** 35 miles

**SEASON:** Year-round, sunrise–sunset

**ACCESS:** Free; no bicycles, no pets

**MAPS:** At visitor center; download from tinyurl.com/claypitpondsmap; USGS *Arthur Kill*

**FACILITIES:** Fully accessible interpretive center, restrooms

**COMMENTS:** Hikers are not permitted on the horse trails that run through the preserve, and vice versa. For further information, call 718-967-1976 or visit nysparks.com /parks/166/details.aspx.

## GPS COORDINATES

N40° 32.348'  W74° 13.932'

## IN BRIEF

It may be hard to believe, but many of Manhattan's buildings and sidewalks were once made from the clay drawn from the ground of this pocket-size park. The 19th-century brick plant is long gone, replaced now by a fun series of lilting trails that loop by idyllic swamps and peaceful ponds, which serve as a backdrop for a colorful variety of birds and wildflowers.

## DESCRIPTION

Recent history notwithstanding, one of the most horrific events in New York's past occurred the evening of December 16, 1835, when a fire broke out in a downtown dry-goods store. It was a bitingly cold night, and at a time when most structures were made of wood, gale-force winds whipped the flames into an inferno, rapidly spreading the fire from block to block. With temperatures well below freezing, cisterns and wells were iced over, and what water the fire department could obtain quickly froze in their hoses. Only by dynamiting a broad break through the city was the blaze brought under control, after it had raged for 15 hours and destroyed nearly

--------------------------------------------

### *Directions*

Follow I-95 over the George Washington Bridge, and drive south to Exit 13. Merge onto I-278 East and continue to Exit 5 to merge onto NY 440 South. Drive 5.9 miles to Exit 3 (Bloomingdale Road). Proceed straight onto Veterans Road West and make a quick left on Bloomingdale Road, followed by a right, after 0.8 mile, on Sharrotts Road, and a final right, also after 0.8 mile, on Carlin Street. Proceed straight to the park entrance and parking lot, 0.1 mile ahead.

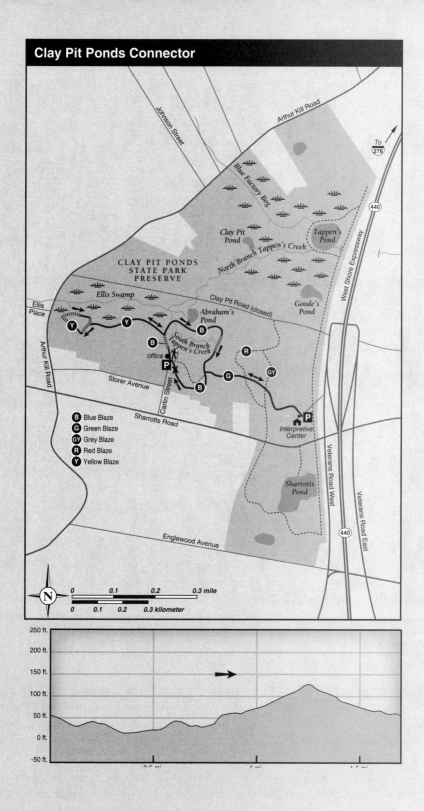

# Clay Pit Ponds Connector

Johnson Street

Arthur Kill Road

To 278

440

Blue Factory Bog

Clay Pit Pond

Tappen's Pond

North Branch Tappen's Creek

CLAY PIT PONDS STATE PARK PRESERVE

West Shore Expressway

Ellis Swamp

Clay Pit Road (closed)

Goode's Pond

Ellis Place

Y

Y

Abraham's Pond

B

South Branch Tappen's Creek

B

office

P

B

R

G

GY

Arthur Kill Road

Storer Avenue

Carlin Street

Sharrotts Road

B Blue Blaze
G Green Blaze
GY Grey Blaze
R Red Blaze
Y Yellow Blaze

P

Interpretive Center

Sharrotts Pond

Veterans Road West

Veterans Road East

440

Englewood Avenue

N

| 0 | 0.1 | 0.2 | 0.3 mile |
| 0 | 0.1 | 0.2 | 0.3 kilometer |

250 ft.

200 ft.

150 ft.

100 ft.

50 ft.

0 ft.

-50 ft.

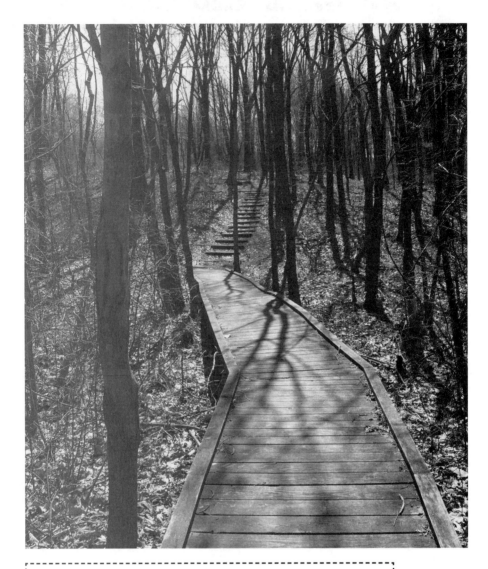

Trails meander through wetlands and pine barrens while showcasing rare wildflowers and scores of birds.

700 buildings, including the post office, the Merchants' Exchange, and most of the financial district. In the aftermath of this disaster, the city restructured the fire department to reduce chaotic competition among volunteer outfits and implemented more-stringent building codes to encourage the use of fire-resistant construction materials.

Enter German immigrant Balthasar Kreischer. Arriving at the Big Apple following the Great Fire (as it has come to be known), Kreischer made his fortune from a wheelbarrow full of bricks, you might say. With wood out of favor, brick (along with iron and stone) became the material of choice for rebuilding the city, and Kreischer's flame-resistant variety was considered to be among the best. What, you might ask, does all this have to do with Staten Island's Clay Pit Ponds State Park Preserve? Much of the clay for Kreischer's bricks was mined here, and by 1854 his gargantuan Staten Island brick factory stood on 700 acres of land. Near the end of the 19th century, more than 300 people worked at that plant, churning out 3.5 million bricks annually at its peak. Clay mining was largely finished by 1927, but it was not until 1976 that this 260-acre property was developed into a state preserve. You can still see vestiges of clay mining on this short, easy hike, which passes through a delightful mixture of habitats, ranging from wetlands and spring-fed streams to sandy barrens and open fields.

The trailhead is behind the park office, a shingle-and-clapboard-sided house with wisteria growing by its side. Pick up the yellow-and-blue blazes to the left of the picnic pavilion, on the bark-covered path. From initially overlooking a swamp, with a small stream beside you, the trail soon descends through oaks, maples, sycamores, briar, birches, beeches, and an occasional azalea, to a boardwalk, where skunk cabbage reigns. Shortly after that, the yellow-and-blue discs diverge; continue straight with yellow.

There is a fun lilt to the moss-sided track as it gently ascends and falls through this swamp. Bypass the spur to the right—that's where this mini-loop comes to a close—and note the corrugated texture to the land around you, the lingering effects of clay mining. Any squealing of seagulls you may hear overhead is a reminder that the park, on the southwest side of the island, lies very close to the water. The ensuing boardwalk, shaped like an upside-down U, runs for 100 feet and passes beneath sweet gum trees, maples, and oaks. Midway along that span is a short spur to the left that leads, in a few paces, to a phragmites-enclosed cluster of swamp ponds; look for frogs and turtles cooling themselves in the water. As you continue on the main path, dirt and moss alternate with a couple more segments of boardwalk, as it rises to the right to reconnect with the outgoing route. A step or two before that is an appealing nook, to the left, where a bench is set under pin oaks, in front of a modest cascade.

Persevere along the yellow-blazed trail, swinging left at the close of the loop, and return to where the blue discs earlier branched off. Canter left there and cross the 20-foot-long span, beneath which creeps a slowly moving stream. The track bends abruptly to the right, paralleling that arroyo, with a bench and a bird-viewing platform on the left, where Abraham's Pond is gradually silting up, becoming more of a marsh with every successive season. If you're lucky, you may observe a muskrat swimming among the cattails and yellow bullhead lilies. Keep straight at the trace, to the left of a large, twin-trunked black birch, and stay to the right in 80 feet at another false junction. The scrub-filled bowl to the right is one more relic of when this locale was extensively mined for clay.

Three brief boardwalks follow, in the dips of the rolling trail, with a pocket meadow succeeding the last of those. Walk directly past the bench there by about 100 feet, stopping short of the tree cover opposite, and turn left on the

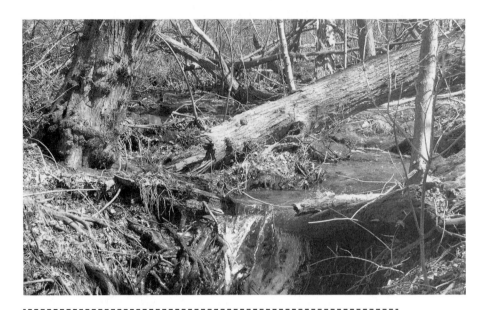

The swamp surrounding Tappen's Creek comes to life in spring, when frogs, toads, and peepers let loose with a lusty chorus.

green-blazed trail (GPS: **N40° 32.341' W74° 13.837'**), an easy-to-miss spur to the park interpretive center. Created late in 2002, this out-and-back route is a bit rough around the edges, as evidenced by sundry debris discarded within the cover of the forest. But the reward for taking it, a spanking-new interpretive center, is well worth enduring the minor eyesores. Having slaked your thirst for knowledge on the center's exhibits, backtrack to the pocket meadow where you jumped off the blue-blazed track, and lunge left on it. In about 100 feet the trail jogs right, by a gate, and descends a touch over erosion-control steps. With a sharp arc to the right, it emerges abruptly by a kiosk at the parking area.

If you have extra time at the conclusion of the hike, plan to cross Sharrotts Road for a stop at Sharrotts Pond. Look for great lobelia around the banks of the water, as well as various types of bladderwort. If you're really lucky, you may also see an Eastern mud turtle, which supposedly is found nowhere else on Staten Island. Herons, snowy egrets, and ring-necked ducks frequent this attractive pond, too.

## NEARBY ACTIVITIES

Time to let your body and spirit relax in the serenity of a Tibetan mountain temple. The **Jacques Marchais Museum of Tibetan Art** exhibits paintings and art objects from Nepal, Mongolia, and Tibet. It features a sculpture garden and a couple of ponds. For information, call 718-987-3500 or visit **tibetanmuseum.org**.

# CONNETQUOT CONTINUUM

## IN BRIEF

Critics carp that this is a long, arid hike without the payoff of vistas or dramatic scenery. They're missing the larger picture, one that starts with a nucleus of historic houses by a placid lake and loops through pretty pine barrens, enticingly lush fields, and swampy streams, achieving a rollicking climax by an active fish hatchery. Much of the time you'll be all on your own, with only birds, butterflies, and white-tailed deer for company.

## DESCRIPTION

Connetquot River State Park Preserve is one of the largest parcels of public land on Long Island, with hiking trails that go on for miles. You don't need to be a descendant of Bigfoot to get the best out of this varied terrain, though. All that is required, some insist, is a fishing rod or an appreciation for Colonial architecture. No doubt about it: angling and area history are as interconnected as the Yankees and the Bronx.

From the Secatogue Indians, who dubbed the river *Connetquot*, meaning "great river," this land passed to William Nicoll sometime around 1684. He dammed a portion of the river and built a gristmill against the edge of

## Directions

Follow the Long Island Expressway/I-495 East to Exit 57 and merge straight with Expressway Drive South, which becomes Express Drive South. Continue 0.5 mile and veer right on Veterans Memorial Highway/NY 454 East. After 4.2 miles make a right on CR 93/Lakeland Avenue. Proceed 1.8 miles and turn right on Sunrise Highway. Drive 0.1 mile and merge onto NY 27 West/Sunrise Highway. The park entrance is 2.9 miles ahead, on the right.

---

### KEY AT-A-GLANCE INFORMATION

**LENGTH:** 8.6 miles

**ELEVATION GAIN:** 157 feet

**CONFIGURATION:** Loop

**DIFFICULTY:** Easy

**SCENERY:** Mostly level with pine barrens, grasslands, streams, fish hatchery, and pond

**EXPOSURE:** Open along fire roads in first half, covered in second half

**TRAFFIC:** The southern part draws the most visitors.

**TRAIL SURFACE:** Mostly sandy, some packed dirt, some grass

**HIKING TIME:** 4.5 hours

**DRIVING DISTANCE:** 55 miles

**SEASON:** Year-round, sunrise–sunset

**ACCESS:** Call ahead for free permit at 631-581-1005; $8 parking fee; no pets

**MAPS:** At entrance booth and visitor center; USGS *Bay Shore East*

**FACILITIES:** Restrooms, water, and public telephone at visitor center; restrooms at fish hatchery; museum

**COMMENTS:** The Connetquot River is highly rated for trout fishing; permit required. Horseback riders share most of the trails. For further information, call 631-581-1005 or visit nysparks.com/parks/8/details.aspx.

### GPS COORDINATES

N40° 44.935'  W73° 9.122'

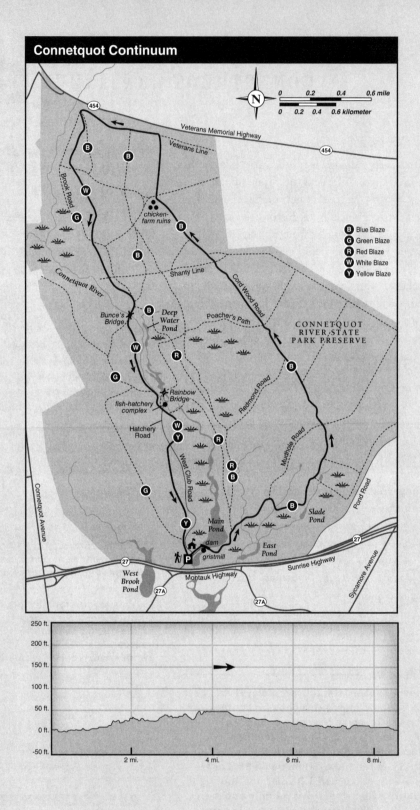

# Connetquot Continuum

**B** Blue Blaze
**G** Green Blaze
**R** Red Blaze
**W** White Blaze
**Y** Yellow Blaze

CONNETQUOT RIVER STATE PARK PRESERVE

Veterans Memorial Highway
Veterans Line
Brook Road
chicken-farm ruins
Shanty Line
Connetquot River
Cord Wood Road
Poacher's Path
Bunce's Bridge
Deep Water Pond
Redmond Road
Rainbow Bridge
fish-hatchery complex
Hatchery Road
West Club Road
Mudhole Road
Pond Road
Slade Pond
Main Pond
dam
gristmill
East Pond
Sunrise Highway
Connetquot Avenue
West Brook Pond
Montauk Highway
Sycamore Avenue

250 ft.
200 ft.
150 ft.
100 ft.
50 ft.
0 ft.
-50 ft.

2 mi.    4 mi.    6 mi.    8 mi.

the resulting pond. Fast-forward to 1820, when Eliphalet "Liff" Snedecor leased a parcel of land abutting the millpond. Liff, who had a good nose for business, erected a tavern there, which soon became an important stagecoach stop. In little more than a decade, as the fishing grew in popularity, affluent sportsmen flocked to the tavern, with the result that it was easier to catch a fish than snag a room at the inn. Eventually, a number of Snedecor's most committed guests bought the tavern, along with 879 acres around it. Their group, incorporated in 1866 as the South Side Sportsmen's Club of Long Island, built a trout hatchery on the estate and continued to acquire land until their holdings totaled 3,473 acres. New York State purchased the property from the club in 1963 and opened it to the public 10 years later. The pond, river, and affiliated streams are still considered among the top trout-fishing destinations in the Northeast.

When you've finished fishing (or poking around Snedecor's Tavern), proceed up the lane to the millpond. Keep to the left of the Oakdale Grist Mill, which was constructed around 1750, and walk over the dam. This hike rates an "easy" because it follows level trails, but for those people who might find its relatively long mileage taxing, shorter excursions are possible via an abundance of side tracks. Initially, the utility road sports both red and blue blazes. Stay to the left at the fork, walking between the old pillars. Outflow from the nearby pond results in swampy conditions on both sides of the track, with low reeds, skunk cabbage, and white flowering anemones thriving by the feet of chestnut oaks.

Turn right at the ensuing fork (leaving the blue blazes for now), shortly after a viewpoint by the edge of the pond. Minks, ferrets, star-nosed moles, and even flying squirrels are among the mammals making their homes here, though you are more likely to see horses, judging by the "apples" that punctuate the sandy surface of the trail. At the next major intersection, steer to the right, as pitch pines begin to grow in number. This wide, exposed forest lane is called Cord Wood Road (CWR, haphazardly marked with blue blazes), which you follow for an hour or so. It bends to the left at the Y, in about 5 minutes, and left again in a similar amount of time, then continues straight at the four-way crossing in an additional handful of minutes. Notice how the surroundings, cloaked in oaks and pines, have grown more arid as the CWR pulls away from the pond. Boggy hollows still spring up on the left from time to time, depending on the meanderings of various streams, and in early spring you may see wild violets and an occasional daffodil.

Ignore the side spurs, first to the right, then to the left, and hang with the wide CWR as it slips through a couple of four-way junctions (the first of these leads in the direction of a red-fox den, where the young are especially active in mid-May). Skip also the grassy lane that appears to the left, just after a rather large, parklike expanse (but keep your eyes open for deer, which often graze near the edge of the woods). The succeeding intersection, in less than a quarter-mile, marks the site of the old chicken farm. The ruin—concrete debris, basically—lies several hundred feet to the left (GPS: **N40° 46.996' W73° 9.439'**). Your route, though, is to the right, toward the grassy, pine-dotted plain. March straight ahead

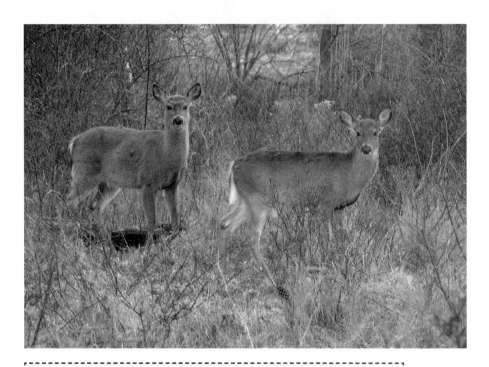

White-tailed deer are no longer hunted in Long Island's largest park, allowing this pretty duo to roam undisturbed.

and, within 8 or 9 minutes, cars should be visible ahead of you, zipping along the road beyond the tree line. That signals the end of the CWT; veer left at the T, following the elusive blue blazes onto Veterans Line (VL).

In 10 minutes, the VL starts to arc left, with the spur to the right leading to a gate by the road. As you swing around on the VL, the blue blazes break sharply left, while your direction is the middle path (more of a soft left). Leave that in 35 to 40 paces, seizing the narrow trace to the left. This shaded route, which bears the white blazes of the Suffolk Greenbelt Trail (SGT), runs through a wedge of pitch pines and scrub oaks sandwiched between a pair of wide, sandy, sun-struck trails. It is a pleasantly wild-looking stretch that fords, in roughly 7 minutes, one of those sandy lanes. As you saunter along this flat turf, scan the overgrown understory for deer and such butterflies as lavender-colored blue azures and yellow tiger and black spicebush swallowtails.

The trail merges to the left briefly with a wide, loamy track and, in about 60 strides, breaks right, back under the cover of the forest. It intersects that sand trap once more, then merges with it. Remain with the sandy lane as you pass the blue-blazed connector to the left. Pursue the white blazes a few steps beyond that, branching to the right and crossing Bunce's Bridge. The SGT then moseys through a swampy area, where fishing spurs are grooved into the moss, and scoots to the left, snaking through a jungle of head-high sheep laurel and a handful of black birch. On skirting a picturesque bog, the path arrives at a fork, with the white blazes cruising left.

Stay with the SGT as it draws you by the bog and approaches Rainbow Bridge. Shift to the right, then jog left onto the park road. Keep strolling straight toward the parking area as the road tapers to the right, just beyond the latrine. Yellow blazes join the white ones here and together parallel the road. Before continuing, though, make a side trip left to the fish hatchery, a small complex built in 1890 that still turns out a variety of trout in much the manner it did a century ago. The water here so often churns with flopping, hyperactive fish, you may be inclined to run for your tackle box. Birding specs might make an even better choice, however, as we've seen ospreys, yellow-crowned night herons, great egrets, blue herons, titmice, Canada geese, and guinea fowl in the vicinity.

On leaving the hatchery, the trail hugs the left side of West Club Road. In a few minutes, though, it hops to the other side of the pavement and slips behind a thin curtain of oaks. Remain with this wide track as it brushes by the periphery of a series of open fields—developed by the Sportsmen's Club to attract game birds—all the way back to the parking area.

## NEARBY ACTIVITIES

From March through October, there is always something blooming at **Bayard Cutting Arboretum**. Visit **bayardcuttingarboretum.com** for a list of activities. An elegant lunch and tea are served in the former Cutting Manor; for reservations, contact the park directly at 631-581-1002.

Liff Snedecor's tavern ceased serving long ago, but that doesn't mean you'll be left with pond water to slake your thirst at the conclusion of this hike. The **Southampton Publick House**, at 40 Bowden Square, has a variety of delectable brews on tap. To learn what's *hop*pening, telephone 631-283-2800 or visit **publick.com**.

# 29 DAVID WELD SANCTUARY TOUR

## KEY AT-A-GLANCE INFORMATION

**LENGTH: 3.2 miles**

**ELEVATION GAIN: 354 feet**

**CONFIGURATION: 3 connected loops**

**DIFFICULTY: Very easy**

**SCENERY: Splendid variety of habitats includes fields, swamp, deciduous forest, beach frontage, and kettle holes.**

**EXPOSURE: Open at outset, followed by shady canopy (except for some bluff viewpoints), and open at finish**

**TRAFFIC: Usually light but popular on weekend afternoons**

**TRAIL SURFACE: Grassy, packed dirt, and roots**

**HIKING TIME: 1.5 hours**

**DRIVING DISTANCE: 52 miles**

**SEASON: Year-round, sunrise–sunset**

**ACCESS: Free; no pets, foot traffic only**

**MAPS: Posted and handouts at kiosk; tinyurl.com/weldmap; USGS *Central Islip***

**FACILITIES: None**

**COMMENTS: Glacial erratics are rare on Long Island, but this charming preserve has several sizable specimens. For further information, visit tinyurl.com/davidweldsanctuary. For a self-guided science walk, download details from tinyurl.com /weldsciencewalk.**

## GPS COORDINATES

N40° 54.318' W73° 12.522'

## IN BRIEF

Talk about bang for the buck: at the David Weld Sanctuary, you get blufftop vistas of Long Island Sound, flowering fruit trees, a hardwood forest highlighted by colossal tulip trees, colorful swamps, a remote group of kettle-hole depressions, and even a few glacial erratics. All that and more, without being nicked for an admission fee!

## DESCRIPTION

David Weld, and in later years his widow, donated much of this turf to The Nature Conservancy, which explains why it bears his name. History buffs might argue, though, that the preserve could just as well be called the Richard "Bull" Smythe Sanctuary. Smythe, after all, was one of the property's earliest owners, back in the 1600s. In truth, he held title to most of the acreage in these parts, including what is known today as Smithtown. Legend has it that a local Indian chief, grateful to Smythe for having rescued his kidnapped daughter, gave him claim to all the land he could ride a bull around in one day. Waiting for the summer solstice, the longest day of the year, Smythe hopped on the back of Whisper,

------------------------------------------

### Directions ⟶

Follow the Long Island Expressway/I-495 East to Exit 56 onto NY 111 North. Drive for about 4 miles to the junction with NY 25 and NY 25A. Go straight across NY 25, following NY 25A East briefly, then bear quickly left on (Nissequogue) River Road. Continue for 3.4 miles and turn left onto Moriches Road (which becomes Horse Race Lane). After 0.5 mile, make a left on Short Beach Road and proceed for 0.1 mile to the preserve entrance and parking area, on the right.

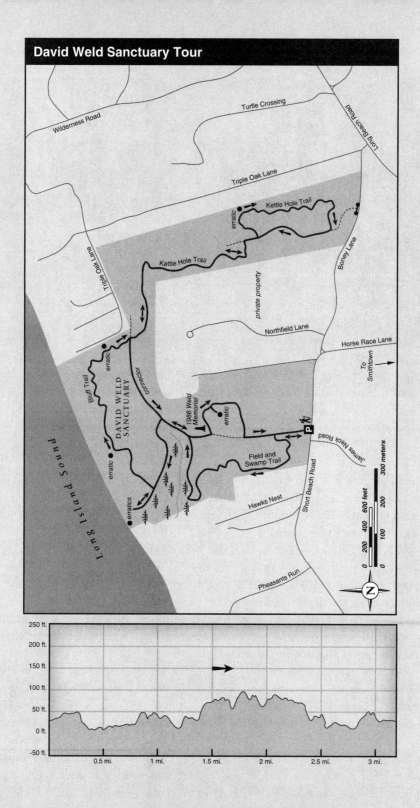

# David Weld Sanctuary Tour

Wilderness Road

Turtle Crossing

Long Beach Road

Triple Oak Lane

Kettle Hole Trail

erratic

Kettle Hole Trail

Boney Lane

Triple Oak Lane

private property

Northfield Lane

Horse Race Lane

erratic

To Smithtown

Bluff Trail

erratic

DAVID WELD SANCTUARY

connector

1986 Weld Memorial

erratic

P

N

Long Island Sound

erratic

Field and Swamp Trail

James Neck Road

Short Beach Road

300 meters

erratics

Hawks Nest

0   200   400   600 feet

0      100      200

Pheasants Run

N

250 ft.

200 ft.

150 ft.

100 ft.

50 ft.

0 ft.

-50 ft.

0.5 mi.        1 mi.        1.5 mi.        2 mi.        2.5 mi.        3 mi.

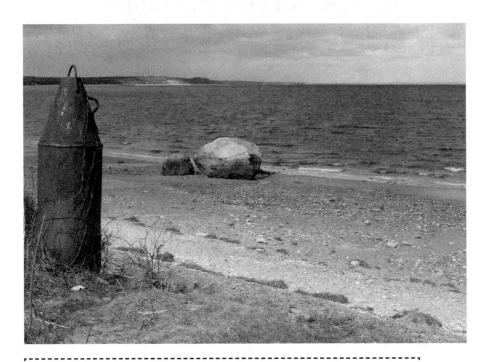

This pocket-size preserve abutting Long Island Sound displays a handful of sizable erratics.

his pet bull, and galloped from sunup to sunset, stopping only briefly on what is now called Bread and Cheese Hollow Road for a simple lunch of—what else?—bread and cheese. By nightfall, Smythe possessed a 35-mile swath of prime real estate, as well as a new nickname.

Whether the story is bull or not, the fact is that the David Weld Sanctuary is a diamond in the rough, packing shorefront bluffs, successional fields, wetlands, glacial kettle holes and erratics, and a hardwood forest into a modest 125 acres. From scattered stands of pines and red cedars to one of the tallest tulip trees on Long Island, from bluffs that rise 50 feet above the Sound to vestigial farms, this easy hike offers something for just about everyone over terrain that as recently as 1920 was largely a clear-cut pasture.

With the elevation all of 30 feet at the five-to-six-car-capacity parking area, the highest you can expect to reach is about the century mark, found at the well-forested farthest end of this horseshoe-shaped preserve. To get to that spot (which is near the kettle-hole formations) while seeing the most that David Weld has to offer, walk straight in for about 70 yards to the kiosk, where a trail map is posted. Hang a left directly beyond the information board onto the Field and Swamp Trail, where Eastern red cedars, sumac, and an assortment of fruit trees (blossoming beautifully in early May) contribute some texture—but not much shade—to the grassy meadow. Cottontail rabbits love to cavort here, in turn attracting an occasional coyote, to judge by telltale trailside spoors.

In a few strides, the field undergoes a transition as dogwood, chokeberry, briar, wintergreen, and other scrub interweave like a thick hedge maze around the path, while many species of birds twitter from the shady shelter of their branches. Soon maples and oaks are among the mix, and then, suddenly, you are in a hardwood forest. Those greens, by the way, with the long, tender leaves growing amid the Canada mayflowers are ramps—a kind of cross between wild leek and scallion that tastes wonderful when sautéed with butter and garlic. (Of course, gathering plants is a no-no in a nature preserve.) The scenery evolves still further when you turn right at the Y, still on the Field and Swamp Trail. Skunk cabbage and marsh reeds line the fairly wide track, which is scarred by a fair share of roots, while a slow-moving stream putters along on the left.

This swampy swale continues even as you dart to the left at the T. The rising ground to the right, though, is more densely forested, with a smattering of conifers outnumbered by beech, black birch, and oak trees. That lasts for all of a minute, until the next fork, where a left puts you squarely in the middle of a colorful swamp that is anything but dismal. Along the way, you may notice some tulip trees to the left that are truly gargantuan in scale, with the tallest, at 106 feet, being one of the largest on Long Island.

You may also notice the scent of brine increasing with every step you take. That's because this track, now called the Bluff Trail, is edging closer to—you guessed it!—a row of bluffs overhanging Long Island Sound. A spur to the left, just as the main route bends right, leads out to a grassy overlook of the water, as well as the beach below, where a couple of glacial erratics serve as dark pedestals for sunbathers. Within this triangular patch of grass is a fragment of a foundation stone, all that remains of a rustic retreat that former resident Cornelia Otis Skinner once occupied. Skinner, a thespian and playwright, reportedly used the bungalow, which burned to the ground in 1987, to rehearse her monologues.

There is a scattering of a few more erratics in addition to some knobby oak, as you stroll east along the Bluff Trail. If the weather is clear, you can see Connecticut from a bench a couple of minutes down the path. Be careful by the railing there, though, as the ground just beyond it is eroding away. Moving along, the serpentine path winds through a tangle of briar and barberry, past yew trees, holly, and an enormous oak before finally drifting inland among cedars, maples, and, at ground level, jack-in-the-pulpits. Continue straight across the four-way intersection, shortly after a huge erratic, on what is now the Kettle Hole Link.

From an elevation of 20 feet at that junction, the trail makes an abrupt rush uphill, gaining in scant seconds 40 additional feet of altitude. Just shy of the crest, it scoots to the left, skirting the perimeter of a dilapidated farm where generations of debris have spilled onto the path behind a red barn, amounting to an agricultural archeologist's dream dig. After the track jumps right, onto a grooved surface, Kettle Hole Link ends at a fork, with the Kettle Hole Trail running both straight and left. We like to go left here, but it doesn't really matter which direction you take on this mini-loop. Leftward, the route wends down a bit by a minor erratic,

> Immature red-tailed hawks have not yet developed adult behavior, making them highly trainable hunting assistants for falconers.

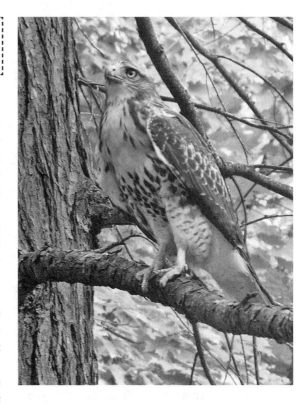

passing through the depression of a glacial kettle hole. (Unlike the ones at Westmoreland Sanctuary in Westchester County [Hike 15], the kettle holes here contain no water.)

The moss-sided path wanders over a corrugated landscape that is appealingly forested with silver-barked beeches, black birches, and oaks. It arcs to the right a couple of times before hitting a T, where it then continues to the right. In a few minutes, the loop is closed and you swing left at the earlier dogleg, back on Kettle Hole Link. Backtrack on that all the way to the four-way intersection at the bottom of the hill, where you should launch to the left. There may be a few rotting trees down across this leg, but you'll have little trouble navigating through. In 5 minutes, this wide, smooth track meets a forest road, with a left returning you to the trailhead.

On the way there, though, make the short detour to the left, just after the David and Molly Weld monument stone. From swampy terrain limned with skunk cabbage and jack-in-the-pulpits, you are now entering a largely open, grassy area, so keep an ear up for cottontails. The landmark along this spur, listed on the map as a "huge erratic," lies to the right, tucked under some trees. A slanted, sedimented slab of slate-colored granite that protrudes some 5 to 7 feet off the soil, the otherwise-photogenic rock suffers, it seems, from a case of elevated expectations. At the conclusion of this side trip, swing left onto the grassy forest road. The parking area is dead ahead.

## NEARBY ACTIVITIES

An art museum and a carriage museum house very different collections in **The Long Island Museum.** The displays include American paintings, antique hunting decoys, and horse-drawn vehicles, but the changing shows are no less spectacular. Call 631-751-0066 for current activities, or visit **longislandmuseum.org.**

# JAMAICA BAY WEST POND TRAIL  30

## IN BRIEF

This hike is for the birds—and for those who love to observe them in all their curious shapes, plumages, and idiosyncrasies. The richest sightings are during the spring and fall migrations, when the ponds and surrounding marshlands teem with waterfowl, but this is a refuge of calm worth visiting throughout the year. Among its huge array of exotic plants is an abundance of colorful wildflowers that bloom from spring through early autumn.

## DESCRIPTION

On the surface of a New York–area map, it is easy to overlook Jamaica Bay Wildlife Refuge. In spite of its prime position east of Brooklyn and south of Queens, Jamaica Bay's close proximity to JFK Airport evokes images of ambling with one's ears stoppered against sonic boom as the sandy soil constantly quakes from crisscrossing jet traffic. Who would willingly walk in such cacophonous conditions?

Well, serious birders, for one. The fact of the matter is that the flyovers are not as frequent—or as nasty—as you might think, with many more birds soaring through the air than 747s. The refuge was established in 1951 by the New York City Parks Department, which promptly created two freshwater ponds and

### *Directions*

Follow I-678 South to Exit 1W. Keep right onto North Conduit Avenue/NY 27 West, then merge onto the Belt Parkway West. Drive 1.9 miles and take the Cross Bay Boulevard via Exit 17 South. Drive 3.6 miles, over the North Channel Bridge, to the signposted refuge entrance on the right. Access the trail through the visitor center.

### i KEY AT-A-GLANCE INFORMATION

**LENGTH: 2 miles**

**ELEVATION GAIN: 45 feet**

**CONFIGURATION: Loop**

**DIFFICULTY: Very easy**

**SCENERY: Coastal marshes, city views, exotic plants, a brackish pond**

**EXPOSURE: Mostly open; some shade in North and South Gardens**

**TRAFFIC: Very popular on weekends**

**TRAIL SURFACE: Packed dirt, gravel**

**HIKING TIME: 1 hour, more for serious birders**

**DRIVING DISTANCE: 24 miles**

**SEASON: Year-round, sunrise–sunset**

**ACCESS: Free, but you must obtain a permit at the visitor center; no bikes, no smoking, no pets. Trails are partially wheelchair-accessible.**

**MAPS: At visitor center; USGS *Far Rockaway***

**FACILITIES: Restrooms and water at visitor center; water fountain by bird blind near South Garden**

**COMMENTS: Sunsets can be gorgeous, but beware of breezy winter winds. Bring good binoculars or a spotting scope to watch abundant and fascinating birdlife. East Pond, across the road, is accessible when the tide is low. For additional information, call 718-318-4340 or visit nps.gov/gate and nyharborparks.org /visit/jaba.html.**

## GPS COORDINATES

N40° 37.011'  W73° 49.511'

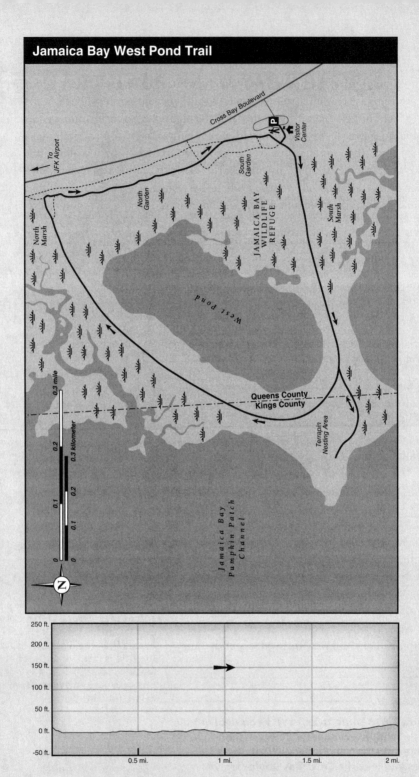

# Jamaica Bay West Pond Trail

transformed what was then barren land into a veritable garden. In 1972, the National Park Service assumed management of the 9,155-acre refuge, under the umbrella of the Gateway National Recreation Area, which has two other units within the metropolitan region. Since then, more than 325 species of birds have been identified in the park.

The West Pond is the more accessible of the two principal bird-watching zones, with a 1.8-mile gravel path circling it. Throughout the year, feathered creatures of all stripes, shapes, and colors can be seen by its shore and in its water, as well as on the surrounding marshlands. But if you are one of those who knows a booby from a bunting and a grackle from a grosbeak, you should consider timing a visit to coincide with major avian activity. The park service notes that evenings in late March are ideal for observing the mating behavior of American woodcocks; a multitude of southbound migrators starts appearing in mid-August; and autumn months are ripe for seeing songbirds, raptors, and warblers.

Once through with the obligatory registering at the sleek visitor center, which was christened in August 2006, pick up the start of the West Pond Loop behind the building. Right away you'll arrive at turnoffs to the Upland Nature Trail and the South Garden Trail. If you choose to travel counterclockwise, start with the South Garden Trail. It flows in a meandering fashion first into Upland and then the North Garden Trail before emerging at the northeast corner of the West Pond circuit. A left at that point completes the tour around the pond and marshes.

We prefer to roam in a clockwise manner, initially bypassing those two side spurs. The path is wide and level, with viewpoints spaced out between thriving stands of winged sumac and a wondrous array of wildflowers, including the yellowish-orange gaillardia, purple loosestrife, blue vervain, purple gerardia, evening primrose, salt marsh fleabane, goldenrod, rose mallow, and—perhaps the biggest botanical surprises—prickly pear cactus and flowering yucca. Clearly, this preserve is as much fun for amateur botanists as it is for birders.

Look left toward the South Marsh and you may see such salt-loving waterfowl as snowy and great egrets, yellow-crowned night herons, and possibly an osprey up on the nesting stand. Gil Hodges Memorial Bridge is also visible off in the distance. In a few dozen yards, the vegetation cloaking the trail opens up more, offering greater views of the phragmites-flanked West Pond. So many birds are drawn to its brackish water that you might more easily count the leaves on a tree as put a number on them. The Terrapin Nesting Area spur is farther on to the left (closed during the diamondback terrapin's breeding season—typically mid-summer–mid-September); it dead-ends in about 750 feet at an unobstructed view of Manhattan across the bay. Continuing along the loop, the North Garden appears on the right, notable for its invitingly grassy grove of mature willow oaks, cedars, and sweet gum trees.

By all means explore the North Garden trails, since landscaping along the main path becomes less attractive as it parallels the noisy Cross Bay Boulevard back to the parking lot. The North Garden, on the other hand, while offering no further

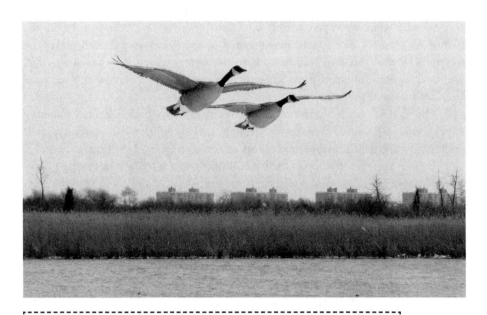

West Pond makes a soft landing, for Canada geese as well as scores of other waterfowl.

views of the West Pond or saltwater marshes, is a peaceful, less-trammeled oasis. Many of its trees (as well as those in the South Garden), including white birches, cottonwoods, American hollies, white pines, and trees of heaven, were planted by the refuge's first supervisor, Herbert Johnson, back in the 1950s and early 1960s.

Now somewhat overgrown, a small warren of trails threads in and out of the thicket, leading eventually to a tiny bird pond, complete with a viewing blind. This is a fun area of the park to wander around while listening attentively to all sorts of little critters crackling noisily in the underbrush. And because the North Garden, Upland Trail, and South Garden are interconnected, with the West Pond on one side of you and the main path on the other, there's no real chance of getting lost. Just keep moving southward, and soon enough you'll be back by the visitor center.

## NEARBY ACTIVITIES

Fort Tilden and Jacob Riis Park have bathing, beaching, and golfing facilities. Breezy Point is another birders' paradise. All three locations are to the southwest of Jamaica Bay. For further information, call 718-338-3799 or visit nps.gov/gate /planyourvisit/thingstodojamaicabay.htm.

# MUTTONTOWN MYSTERY TRAIL  31

## IN BRIEF

You don't have to be a fan of murder mysteries or obscure Albanian history to enjoy wandering the woods of Muttontown, not with such an appealing variety of habitats tucked into the domain. A vast network of trails and old estate lanes weaves through swampy swales, miniature savannas, a rhododendron jungle (that transforms in July into a fairyland of pale-pink blossoms), some glacial deposits, and even a few ghostly ruins. Of course, if you do have a thing for unsolved mysteries, so much the better.

## DESCRIPTION

Thumb through the brochures at Muttontown's nature center, and you will learn that the 550-acre preserve runs the gamut of habitats, from open fields and lowland swamps to rolling hills, kettle ponds, and upland forests. One pamphlet talks about the variety of animals in Muttontown, with raccoons, red foxes, star-nosed moles, and masked shrews among its denizens. Another brochure boasts of the birds that nest here, including flickers, rose-breasted grosbeaks, bobwhites, and bobolinks. There is even a brief account of how the preserve came

### KEY AT-A-GLANCE INFORMATION

**LENGTH:** 3.3 miles

**ELEVATION GAIN:** 237 feet

**CONFIGURATION:** Double loop

**DIFFICULTY:** Very easy

**SCENERY:** Six different habitats, including wet woodlands, rolling fields, kettle ponds, and upland forests, as well as mysterious ruins

**EXPOSURE:** Sheltered at start, then exposed in fields, followed by more tree cover

**TRAFFIC:** Light to moderate, except when school groups are exploring the grounds

**TRAIL SURFACE:** Grass, sand, roots, pebbles, and plenty of mud in spring

**HIKING TIME:** 1.5 hours

**DRIVING DISTANCE:** 30 miles

**SEASON:** Year-round, 9 a.m.–5 p.m.

**ACCESS:** Free; no pets, no bicycles

**MAPS:** At nature center; USGS *Hicksville*

**FACILITIES:** Restrooms and water behind nature center

**COMMENTS:** Bridle paths and cross-country skiing trails wind through the preserve. For further information, call 516-571-8500 or visit tinyurl .com/muttontownpreserve.

## *Directions* →

Follow the Long Island Expressway/I-495 East to Exit 40E. Turn left on NY 25 East/Jericho Turnpike and drive 1 mile. Merge onto NY 107 North/NY 106 North and, after 0.3 mile, veer right to continue on NY 106. Proceed for 3.5 miles to the intersection with NY 25A West/Northern Boulevard. Go left and, after 0.1 mile, turn left again onto Muttontown Lane. Drive 0.2 mile—through two stop signs—to the preserve entrance on the right, and veer left at the fork to the parking area.

## GPS COORDINATES

N40° 50.289'  W73° 32.073'

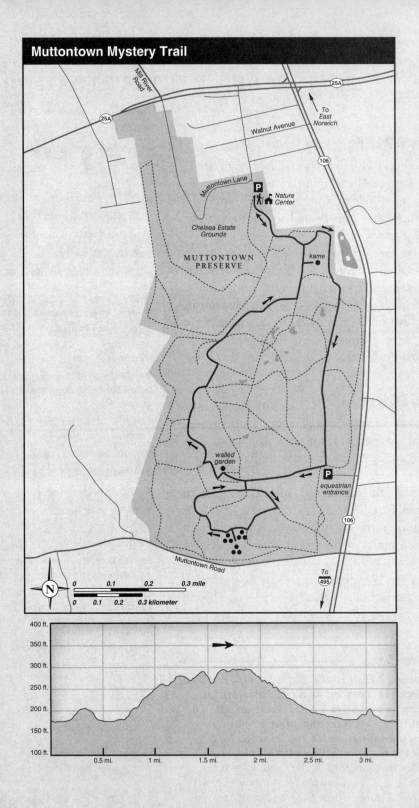

# Muttontown Mystery Trail

Mill River Road

25A

To East Norwich

Walnut Avenue

106

Muttontown Lane

P — Nature Center

Chelsea Estate Grounds

MUTTONTOWN PRESERVE

kame

walled garden

P — equestrian entrance

106

Muttontown Road

To 495

N

| 0 | 0.1 | 0.2 | 0.3 mile |
| 0 | 0.1 | 0.2 | 0.3 kilometer |

400 ft.
350 ft.
300 ft.
250 ft.
200 ft.
150 ft.
100 ft.

0.5 mi.   1 mi.   1.5 mi.   2 mi.   2.5 mi.   3 mi.

into being, with 400 acres purchased from the estate of Lansdell Christie, 100 acres donated by Alexandra McKay, and a 20-acre lot given by Mrs. Paul Hammond. What you won't find is any mention of the ruins of Knollwood, the international intrigue surrounding King Zog, rumors of hidden treasure, and a murder mystery that is still unsolved.

To call Knollwood an estate would be to injure it through understatement. Built in 1907 by Charles Hudson, a venture capitalist, Knollwood was a 60-room granite palace that combined such myriad architectural flourishes as Italian Renaissance, Greek Revival, and Spanish Churrigueresque. Lying at the center of what is now the Muttontown Preserve, Knollwood was purchased in 1951 by Ahmed Bej Zogu, better known as King Zog of Albania. Zog, who had a penchant for poker and perfumed cigarettes (reportedly smoking an average of 150 a day), became president of Albania in 1925 and proclaimed himself king three years later. Not all of his subjects were delighted by this turn of events, so to consolidate power, Zog put each of his four sisters in command of an army division, while his mother ran the royal kitchen—just to make sure his food wasn't tampered with. Still, Zog was almost gunned down by two assassins in 1931, and by 1939, after Italy invaded Albania and defeated its army in two days, he "retired" to England, bringing with him a fair balance of his country's bullion. It was during a visit to the United States in 1951 that King Zog saw Knollwood and purchased it with—so it was rumored at the time—"a bucket of rubies and diamonds," to the tune of $102,800. Such tales can take on a life of their own, and although Zog reportedly never lived at Knollwood, treasure hunters, convinced that his booty was hidden within the domain, climbed over the walls and vandalized the establishment beyond repair. In 1955, the estate was sold to Lansdell Christie, a mining tycoon, who four years later razed the mansion to the ground.

More recently, in November 2001, six men were practicing orienteering in Muttontown when one saw a glint of sunlight shining beneath a tree. That reflective matter turned out to be bone—part of a human skeleton curled in a fetal position below a light layer of leaves. The authorities were summoned, and after an extensive forensic examination, the corpse was determined to be that of a woman of approximately 35 years, 5'1" to 5'3" in height. The victim—she had been murdered, the police concluded—was missing a top front tooth, as well as the metal or plastic denture that would have filled the gap. With few clues to go on, the case remains open.

You won't require a deerstalker cap and a pal named Watson to follow the scent in this beautiful sanctuary—sturdy-soled walking shoes and the park map should more than suffice. Pick the latter off the rack on the back porch of the nature center abutting the parking area. Turn around there and face the woods: the trail to the right is the shorter interpretive path, while left—your direction— leads into the larger part of the park. In spring, the trails may be a bit soft— downright muddy in spots—but that inconvenience is more than balanced by a colorful collage of wildflowers, including grape hyacinth, blue penstemon,

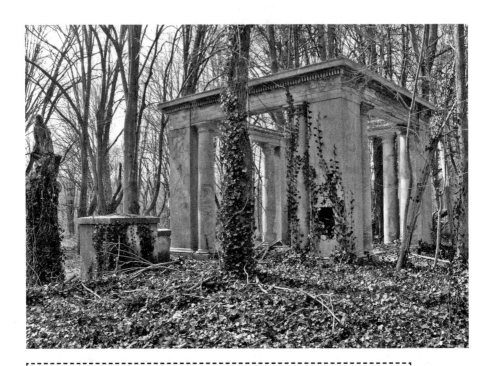

The man who would be king: this is all that's left of Zog's palace-in-exile, in Muttontown.

mayapple, periwinkle, wild violet, and anemone, that sparkle on the ground like precious jewels.

The trail bends to the left, initially following the contours of a chain-link fence. Bear left in a few seconds at the wide fork, then right at the next junction, exchanging the dirt track for a grassy path. Ignore the trace to the right as you cruise higher through a cluster of white and black birch trees, maples, cedars, and pines on the way to a T. Hang a right there, then take another hard right in a dozen steps, when you reach the boundary fence. On swinging left at the ensuing intersection, in 200 yards, you will find yourself in an area of flowering dog-woods, oaks, and an occasional fruit tree. Not for long, though. Steer right at the Y, marked by a rare trail blaze, and after striding 150 feet, go right at the subsequent fork, now moving toward an open field. Keep to the left at the next turn, marching along the west side of the meadow, and proceed through the following junction, in about 30 yards.

As you strut forward, look sharply for bluebirds flitting about the field. Remain with this open stretch for several minutes, eventually passing a couple of horse corrals. Turn right directly after the kiosk by the equestrian parking area, onto the broad dirt lane, and bypass the spur to the right that appears almost immediately. The easy walking along this maple-shaded carriage road lasts for several minutes, until it begins to bend toward the north, whereupon you glide left on a narrower path. This route enters a labyrinth of trails where much of the fun derives from exploring off the beaten track. Saunter left at the four-way intersection, and then—in a couple of minutes—right at the fork. From an overgrown estate road overhung with aged apple trees, you are now on a narrower track sided by rhododendrons and ivy. The forest grows wilder as you break to the right at the next fork, with yews dwarfed by a handful of cyclopean pines and beech trees.

And then—suddenly—you are standing among the ruins of Knollwood, with two raised, columnar temples flanking a low, rising stair (GPS: N40° 49.530' W73° 32.141'). As you stroll first south of the stairs to the overgrown bunker, then retrace your steps and head north between the two temples, try to imagine what this looked like more than half a century ago when it was lavishly landscaped with reflecting pools and formal gardens, marble fountains, Greco-Roman statues, and ivy-filled urns. Stick with the trace that extends north above the stairs; it leads to an imposing wall. A baroque gargoyle fountain leers from its center, with symmetrical staircases—now collapsed—rising on either side. This is all that remains of the mansion itself. The trail resumes to the left as you face this crumbling edifice, swooping around its far side. Dart left at the T with the asphalt-covered lane, reentering a forest of rhododendrons. Stay with this until the four-way intersection (you met this same crossing from the opposite direction on the way to the ruins), where you venture left and, in 75 feet, left again at the T. Take the middle of three choices at the upcoming junction; it brings you to the front of what is listed on the map as a walled garden. This is yet another remnant of the Knollwood era, an imposingly large enclosure with a stucco-covered wall that measures about 8 feet high and a football field long.

To continue, cut left of the garden wall; when the trail breaks toward the west, bear right, or northward. Then take the second option to the left, avoiding the open expanse, and go left at the post, followed by yet another left, once more skirting the field. As you near a chain-link fence, roll right (or, if you have extra time on your hands, pass through the gap in that barrier to enjoy a quiet stroll in the neighboring preserve). Bypass the subsequent right and instead launch left at the meadow. Once through that, turn left at the T and left again at the Y that follows. Take the moderately steep spur to the right that occurs a minute or two later; this side trip ends atop a kame, or glacial deposit, sitting at an elevation of 220 feet. Return to the main track and jump left at the succeeding fork; you are now on familiar turf, backtracking along the first leg of the hike.

## NEARBY ACTIVITIES

**Planting Fields Arboretum State Historic Park,** at 1395 Planting Fields Rd., Oyster Bay, was landscaped by the Olmsted brothers of Massachusetts, whose father designed Central Park. It includes impressive greenhouses, stately gardens, woodlands, and lawns, as well as Coe Hall, a Tudor Revival mansion open to the public. To learn more, call 516-922-9200 or visit **plantingfields.org.**

# 32 SUNKEN MEADOW TO NISSEQUOGUE RIVER TRAIL

## KEY AT-A-GLANCE INFORMATION

**LENGTH: 5.1 miles**

**ELEVATION GAIN: 596 feet**

**CONFIGURATION: Out-and-back**

**DIFFICULTY: Easy to moderate**

**SCENERY: Views of the Sound and Nissequogue River; tidal flats and rolling hardwood forests**

**EXPOSURE: Shady, except for boardwalk section at start and end**

**TRAFFIC: Intense weekends**

**TRAIL SURFACE: Sandy, dirt, roots**

**HIKING TIME: 3 hours; more if birding or exploring Kings Park**

**DRIVING DISTANCE: 49 miles**

**SEASON: Year-round, sunrise–sunset**

**ACCESS: $8–$10 parking fee, free in winter; dogs allowed only in undeveloped areas and on leash not exceeding 6 feet. Boardwalk start of the hike is wheelchair-accessible.**

**MAPS: At visitor center; Long Island Greenbelt Trail Conference; USGS *Northport***

**FACILITIES: Restrooms, water, and public phone at visitor center**

**COMMENTS: Bring binoculars for birding or for views, and a swimsuit for a dip in Long Island Sound. Call 631-269-4333 or visit nysparks.com/parks/37/details.aspx. Part of the walk includes the grounds of the former Kings Park Psychiatric Center— a defunct mental institution. Most buildings remain closed to the public.**

## GPS COORDINATES

N40° 54.633'  W73° 15.399'

## IN BRIEF

Birds and bees, beaches and trees, from boardwalks to blufftops, Sunken Meadow packs a rich range of nature into a short stretch of trail. This serene, scenic hike offers extended contact with Long Island Sound and the Nissequogue River, passes fleetingly through an isolated upland forest, and culminates at a spooky old lunatic asylum, where the palatial grounds are landscaped with flowering fruit trees, dogwoods, and daffodils.

## DESCRIPTION

The official title of the domain from which this hike begins is Governor Alfred E. Smith/Sunken Meadow State Park. Like the cumbersome nature of that *nom d'état,* the initial impression you may have on arriving here in summer is of one vast ocean of cars, of a parking lot without end. Scratch beneath the surface of that paved expanse, though, and what you will find— beyond fabulous views of Long Island Sound— is a great hike that offers some of the best birding in the region and a pastel palette of wildflowers in spring. From sandy bluffs overlooking the Nissequogue River to an eerie amble through the grounds of a defunct veterans' hospital, this out-and-back jaunt, while neither strenuous nor overly long, is nonetheless the sort that leaves a lasting impression.

------------------------------------------------

## *Directions* ⟶

**Follow the Long Island Expressway/I-495 East to Exit 53 and—via the Sagtikos State Parkway—merge onto the Sunken Meadow State Parkway North. Proceed 7.3 miles to the park tollbooths, then continue for 1.2 miles to the visitor center and the parking lot, straight ahead.**

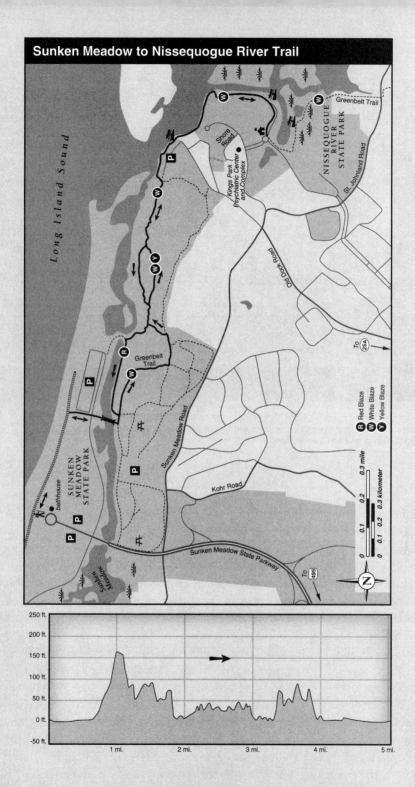

# Sunken Meadow to Nissequogue River Trail

Long Island Sound

Greenbelt Trail

NISSEQUOGUE RIVER STATE PARK

St. Johnland Road

Shore Road

Kings Park Psychiatric Center and Complex

Old Dock Road

To 25A

Greenbelt Trail

SUNKEN MEADOW STATE PARK

bathhouse

Sunken Meadow Road

Kohr Road

Sunken Meadow State Parkway

To 495

Sunken Meadow

**R** Red Blaze
**W** White Blaze
**Y** Yellow Blaze

0   0.1   0.2   0.3 mile
0   0.1   0.2   0.3 kilometer

250 ft.
200 ft.
150 ft.
100 ft.
50 ft.
0 ft.
-50 ft.

1 mi.   2 mi.   3 mi.   4 mi.   5 mi.

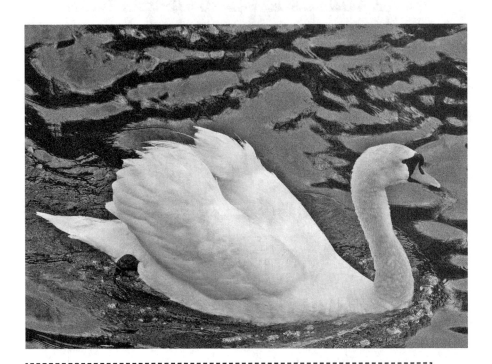

Careful! A graceful mute swan will become very aggressive when defending its nest: it will hiss, smack its wings, and bite any intruder.

To start, stroll from the main parking area (lots 1 and 2) through the bathhouse pavilion, and turn right onto the boardwalk. With the gentle waves of Long Island Sound lapping at the sand to your left, stick with the wide wooden boardwalk for 5 minutes, until you reach a paved path branching off from the second opening in the railing on the right. Take that conduit and, in 200 yards, after passing parking lot 3 and shuffling over a bridge (great white and snowy egrets, loons, cormorants, and Canada geese often skim across the reed-rimmed water below), hang a left at the T, where you meet the picnic grounds. Still on macadam, you may notice the white blazes of the Suffolk County Greenbelt Trail (SGT) underfoot. Although the SGT connects Sunken Meadow to the Atlantic Ocean and Heckscher State Park 36 miles to the south, this particular trek runs only 3.1 miles before returning.

The track shifts to the right in a couple of minutes, moving uphill and away from a cedar-lined fence. It proceeds more steeply after encountering a pair of concrete benches, with the pavement being replaced by bark as it passes through a gap in the fence. For the next mile or so, the SGT is intersected by a dizzying number of social trails, but if you hew to the white blazes, you should do fine. Try to follow those markings through the narrow passage of catbrier to a four-way intersection, where they branch left. If you succeed in sticking with them, you should find yourself atop a sandy bluff, ringed by pitch pines, with the far end of parking lot 3 visible to the left, a few brackish ponds down below, and a great view of the Sound beyond the latter. Bear to the right as the sandy track scuttles along the bluff, where oaks, cedars, pines, and catbrier do little to obstruct the fine water vistas. For a brief spell, yellow and white blazes run concurrently, and as the white tags continue along the rise you may also notice red ones diving off to the left, downhill in the direction of the water. The Atlantic Flyway overlaps the area, and this lovely, untamed spot is often alive with the chirping and twittering of an abundant assortment of birds.

The SGT soon spurts right, away from the yellow trail, once more clawing through thorny catbrier before looping back to the bluff, where it again connects with yellow blazes and traipses to the right. Additional views of the Sound and those salt-marsh ponds below ensue, and then, after a marina parking lot materializes to the left, the white blazes veer inland and dive into a tangle of thorny plants. Dart left at the fork that occurs a minute later, and go left again in a yard and a half, descending over a set of steps to the marina's parking area. Cut directly toward Long Island Sound to the far side of the lot, then swerve to the right along the sidewalk. Beeline across the boat launch, cruising to the left of the Old Dock Inn (note the white blaze on the telephone pole there). A dogleg left—and right— around the rail fence delivers you to the sandy beach, where the Nissequogue River converges on the Sound and a bevy of boats often shuttle around. Continue on this colorful strip of shore for about 300 yards, until the white blazes signal a break to the right, up a sandy mound and a piling-supported staircase (GPS: N40° 54.193' W73° 13.718').

Oaks and birches shade a bench up on this high ground, and with a commanding panorama of the Nissequogue and the marina, you could do a lot worse for a lunch spot. The SGT exits to the left of the bench, holding mostly to the edge of the bluff as it snakes by orange lilies, periwinkles, grape hyacinth, fruit trees, cedars, dogwoods, and daffodils. You may also see a number of slender, vertical bat houses mounted on an occasional maple. When the path, which features more curves and clefts than a Victoria's Secret catalog, hits a T, dog it to the left, then step to the right at the next fork.

Not long after that, a handful of boarded-up brick buildings appears through the trees to the right. At first glance, these spooky structures look vaguely like a decommissioned military installation, or maybe an old school. Close, but no cigar. What you are moseying by was once the Kings Park Psychiatric Center, better known to county residents as the local loony bin. Established more than a century ago to aid shell-shocked veterans of the Spanish-American War (and later expanded to accommodate World War I GIs), Kings Park held 9,300 inmates, er, *patients*, at its peak in 1954, and consisted of 150 buildings. The number of residents dwindled in later years, and in 1996 the hospital was finally shuttered. Happily, much of the compound and surrounding land have been preserved as Nissequogue River State Park, which came into being in 1999.

The SGT skirts the property for 5 minutes, until it descends gradually toward a duff-colored concrete building, its windows covered with green boards, and then heaves to the right. The park visitor center lies straight ahead, with exhibits inside on native plants and animals, in addition to a history of Kings Park. This is the turnaround stage of the hike, the point at which you backtrack to Sunken Meadow. But before making your return, consider lingering here for a walking tour of the former institution. It is hard not to be impressed by the sheer scale of this sprawling complex, and by the vaguely spectral nature of all the decaying, moldering edifices.

Once back on the bluff, beyond the Old Dock Inn and above the marina parking lot, you might try a change of pace with the yellow blazes as they diverge to the right from the SGT. Ignore the many ruts that have been burned into the soil by mountain bikers, and in a couple of minutes the yellow trail reconnects with the white. Then, in a matter of several strides, go with the red blazes as they surge right. This initiates a steady descent from the bluff, drawing you under pitch pines, by a few ponds (swans brood in the adjacent marsh during the spring), back toward parking lot 3. Instead of marching off in that direction, though, remain straight with the level trail as it hugs the left side of the canal. Enjoy the birding here, but remember to fly right at the bridge, where you reunite with the white blazes.

With the boardwalk once again underfoot, you are nearing the end of the hike. As rich as its earlier portions were for birds, the beach area is prime people-watching turf. And given the right temperature, the water ain't so bad for swimming, either.

## NEARBY ACTIVITIES

What would Long Island be without a Vanderbilt mansion? This Spanish Revival–style building in Centerport, called **Eagle's Nest,** houses the Vanderbilt Museum and is furnished with original period pieces, paintings, family photos, and eccentric collections. For guided tours and information, call 631-854-5579 or visit **vanderbiltmuseum.org.**

# WALT WHITMAN SAMPLER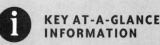

## IN BRIEF

The seaside vistas are overgrown from when Walt Whitman roamed this historic woodland, but the densely forested hills still provide a poetic setting for a short hike. A labyrinth of trails snakes by a picturesque pond amid laurels, white pines, and rhododendrons—as well as a full complement of hardwoods—on the way to Jayne's Hill, the highest point on Long Island.

## DESCRIPTION

"West Hills is a romantic and beautiful spot. It is the most hilly and elevated part of Long Island . . . afford[ing] an extensive and pleasant view," Walt Whitman wrote in 1850 of the hills that rise above his boyhood home. In Whitman's day it was possible to view the Connecticut shore from atop the highest peak, Jayne's Hill, and watch schooners sailing by Fire Island to the south. Those vistas are gone now—overgrown by mountain laurel, beech, and birch trees—but this remains a delightful place, no less hilly and inspiring today than it once was to one of our country's great poets.

In 1825, when Silas Wood, an early historian of Long Island, had "High Hill" surveyed, its top crested at 354 feet of elevation. While paltry by Western standards, that was

## KEY AT-A-GLANCE INFORMATION

**LENGTH:** 3.6 miles

**ELEVATION GAIN:** 473 feet

**CONFIGURATION:** Loop

**DIFFICULTY:** Easy

**SCENERY:** Rolling, mixed deciduous forest hiding a quiet pond, gnarly laurel thickets, and Long Island's highest point

**EXPOSURE:** Lush canopy protection

**TRAFFIC:** Light on weekdays; can get really busy on weekends

**TRAIL SURFACE:** Dirt, roots, and pebbles

**HIKING TIME:** 2 hours

**DRIVING DISTANCE:** 35 miles

**SEASON:** Year-round, sunrise–sunset

**ACCESS:** $6 parking fee for Suffolk County residents Memorial Day–Labor Day ($13 for nonresidents), free rest of year; no bicycles on most trails, pets on leash

**MAPS:** At Walt Whitman Birthplace; USGS *Huntington*

**FACILITIES:** Restrooms, water, and public phone at picnic area

**COMMENTS:** Horse riders share most trails. For further information, call the park office at 631-854-4423 or visit tinyurl.com/westhillspark.

## Directions

Follow the Long Island Expressway/I-495 East and take Exit 42, merging onto the Northern State Parkway East. Drive to Exit 40 and merge onto Walt Whitman Road/NY 110 South. After 0.3 mile, turn right on Old Country Road and continue 0.4 mile, then go right again on Sweet Hollow Road. Proceed 0.5 mile to the parking lot and picnic area on the right.

## GPS COORDINATES

N40° 48.100'  W73° 25.278'

# Walt Whitman Sampler

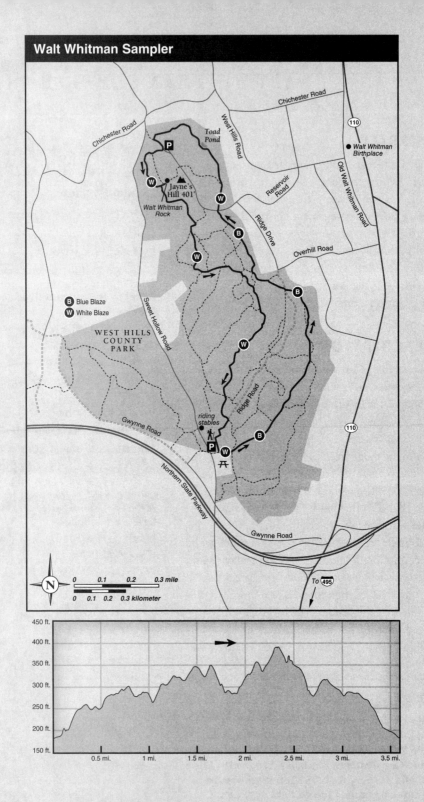

Chichester Road

Chichester Road

West Hills Road

110

Walt Whitman
Birthplace

Toad
Pond

P

W

Jayne's
Hill 401'

Walt Whitman
Rock

Reservoir Road

Old Walt Whitman Road

Ridge Drive

B

W

Overhill Road

B

B  Blue Blaze
W  White Blaze

W

WEST HILLS
COUNTY
PARK

Sweet Hollow Road

W

B

110

Ridge Road

riding
stables

Gwynne Road

P
W

Northern State Parkway

Gwynne Road

To 495

N

| 0 | 0.1 | 0.2 | 0.3 mile |

| 0 | 0.1 | 0.2 | 0.3 kilometer |

| | | | | | | |
|---|---|---|---|---|---|---|
| 450 ft. | | | | | | |
| 400 ft. | | | | | | |
| 350 ft. | | | | | | |
| 300 ft. | | | | | | |
| 250 ft. | | | | | | |
| 200 ft. | | | | | | |
| 150 ft. | | | | | | |
| | 0.5 mi. | 1 mi. | 1.5 mi. | 2 mi. | 2.5 mi. | 3 mi. | 3.5 mi. |

enough to rank this mount as highest on the island. Its name was later changed to Jayne's Hill, after the family that lived here, and having been resurveyed a number of times since, it now officially tops out at 400.9 feet above sea level. This meandering hike circles through the colorful forests of the West Hills, crossing the top of Jayne's Hill about halfway out. Many maverick bike and bridle trails intersect your route, but the main path is well blazed and fairly easy to follow.

The trail begins at the far side of the picnic grounds, by the edge of the woods. Keep to the right, walking toward the fenced field, looking for white blazes on a few of the oak trees. Stay with those as the markings glide to the left (or wooded) side of the sports field–cum–dog walking area. Just past the corner of the fence is a path to the left, blazed with blue paint. Turn there and then left again on the sandy bridle path. Stick with the blue blazes as they veer right at the Y, and right another time in an additional 10 steps. Now drifting among birches, oaks, and an occasional dogwood—to say nothing of scads of mountain laurel—the well-indicated, pebbly track shifts left at a T. It then passes a number of spurs as it ascends steadily to higher ground, swinging left in 3 minutes at the T-junction with a bridle trail. For hikers with a good sense of orientation, the many side trails in this forest offer great bushwhacking possibilities.

In due time, the clearly blazed trail loops to the left of a gray house. About a minute later, it meets a wide crossing with another bridle path, where it continues straight ahead, single-file, until it merges with a horse track, where you pivot left. Bear left once more at the next broad fork, steering away from the private dwellings. With laurels now the dominant plant, the blue blazes swerve sharply right off the main route in 150 feet, adhering closely to the line of a ridge. Vault to the right when you hit the T with still another bridle path and, a couple of minutes after passing a horse stable to the right, just beyond the park boundary, you will come to a set of erosion-control piling steps.

The access lane to Jayne's Hill is at the top of that staircase. Instead of following the road, though, stroll across the pavement, picking up the white blazes on its opposite side near a chain-link fence. With that barrier to the right and white pines towering overhead, you have now started the more enjoyable half of the hike. On reaching a small rise, the path descends sharply away from the majestic conifers, moving swiftly into a beech-and-birch-shaded gully. The trail levels off briefly, trots right at a Y, goes right at the ensuing crossing, then dives downhill again among a green carpet of false lilies of the valley. The white blazes hop left at the succeeding fork and in a few paces guide you to Toad Pond. Though marred by a metal fence stretched over its right end, this is an attractive (albeit gradually silting up) body of water, shaped like a crooked, elongated smile.

Ignore the steps that lead away from the pond and proceed along its boggy bank. A few strides later, the white blazes branch to the left, with the path fording a small stream in another moment or two via a log corduroy. With the track running beside a bog, the next several yards can be quite wet in spring, but soon enough the ground grows steadily steeper, plugging upward toward Jayne's Hill.

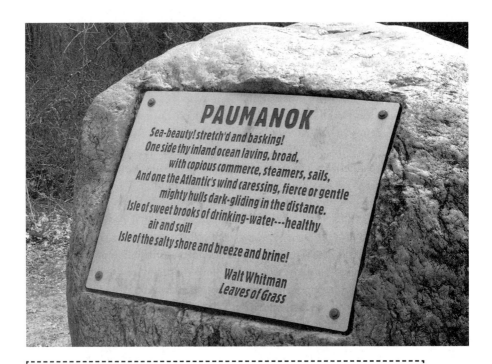

PAUMANOK

Sea-beauty! stretch'd and basking!
One side thy inland ocean laving, broad,
with copious commerce, steamers, sails,
And one the Atlantic's wind caressing, fierce or gentle
mighty hulls dark-gliding in the distance.
Isle of sweet brooks of drinking-water---healthy
air and soil!
Isle of the salty shore and breeze and brine!

Walt Whitman
Leaves of Grass

Jayne's Hill was a favorite inspiration point for a young Walt Whitman, who grew up nearby.

(There were a number of trees down the last time we passed through, with one low-hanging trunk requiring a limbolike effort to continue.) It only takes a minute to get by the most precipitous part of that climb—one breathtaking, heart-pounding minute. From there the elevation gain is more gradual, almost imperceptible. Heave to the left on the bridle path, and in a few dozen strides the trail spits you out at the Jayne's Hill parking lot.

Hug the right side of the lot, rounding a pine tree and hewing hard to the right when a swing set and dilapidated latrine come into view. Stick with this wide, white-blazed track, which is lined with lavender-flowering myrtle, dog-woods, and oaks, as it cruises to the right at the subsequent fork and left at the one after that. The terrain grows more lush with every step you take, as mountain laurels, white pines, and black birches creep back into the forested mix. The top of Jayne's Hill lies just ahead, a site marked by two benches, a rock (sadly stained with graffiti) with a plaque on it, and a pale-blue water tower. Second-growth trees now block out the view that Whitman enjoyed from this, the highest ground on Long Island, but you may still derive pleasure from the tranquility of the spot, as well as the Whitman quote that adorns the plaque.

The trail continues to the right of the rock, down several steps through an overgrown tangle of briar, chokeberry, and poison ivy. It levels off in a minute among ferns and oaks, then rolls with the undulating texture of the hillside. This pleasantly secluded, moss-sided track ends at a split-rail fence, where you scoot right onto a bridle path. In 45 yards, the white-blazed foot trail scuttles to the left at a four-way crossing, descends through briar, maples, birches, and cedars, and then crosses another four-way intersection. From a leveling off, the path rises negligibly, culminating in a left turn at a T. Pull to the left at the ensuing fork, and with the white blazes clearly visible, hang a right at the next major turn, in about 25 feet. Some 100 yards later, the track diverges to the right—then left in 30 paces—and, having descended briefly, darts through a narrow livestock barrier.

You remain on this ridge for a while, slightly above the trees of the surrounding hills, as rhododendrons make a surprise appearance, blanketing the sides of the slope. A further descent over log steps leads to a second livestock barrier. Once through that, the white blazes shift to the left, crossing the bridle path and slipping through a rail fence (look for spotted wintergreen in springtime). In a few minutes of walking, you should see the roof of the riding stables to the right. A short descent follows, delivering you to yet another set of rails. The horse trails here trot left, right, and straight ahead, with your route running between the right and straight options. A few furlongs more and the path ends, dropping you off by the picnic grounds, with the parking lot directly beyond.

## NEARBY ACTIVITIES

What better place to start (or unwind from) this hike than the **Walt Whitman Birthplace State Historic Site**? Displays in this recently renovated early-19th-century farmhouse, at 246 Old Walt Whitman Rd., include portraits of Whitman, his poetry, letters, a tape recording of his voice, and more. Call 631-427-5240 for details, or visit **waltwhitman.org**.

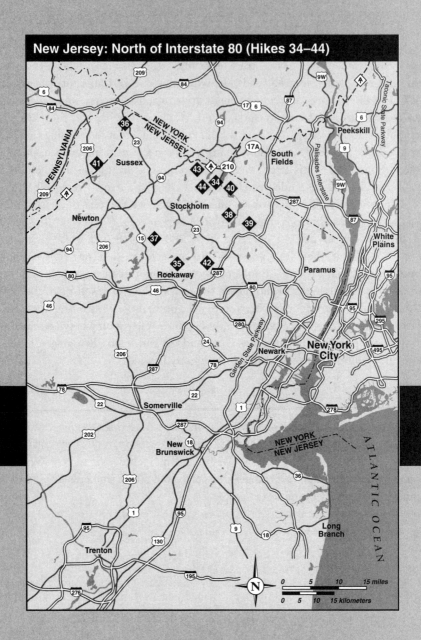

# New Jersey: North of Interstate 80 (Hikes 34–44)

# NEW JERSEY:
## NORTH OF INTERSTATE 80

# 34 ABRAM HEWITT'S BEARFORT RIDGE

## KEY AT-A-GLANCE INFORMATION

**LENGTH:** 8.3 miles

**ELEVATION GAIN:** 1,651 feet

**CONFIGURATION:** Loop

**DIFFICULTY:** Moderate to strenuous

**SCENERY:** Puddingstone ridge, partially covered by pitch pines and scrub oaks, with access to upland swamps, a lake, a pond, and views of distant hills and lakes

**EXPOSURE:** Large stretches of open sun on extended plateaus

**TRAFFIC:** Hardly anyone on weekdays; very light most weekends

**TRAIL SURFACE:** Largely rock and rubble, some stretches padded with pine needles

**HIKING TIME:** 4.5 hours

**DRIVING DISTANCE:** 36 miles

**SEASON:** Year-round, sunrise–sunset

**ACCESS:** Free; pets on leash, no bicycles, no motorized vehicles

**MAPS:** At Wawayanda State Park office; USGS *Greenwood Lake*

**FACILITIES:** None

**COMMENTS:** Hunting allowed. Keep an eye out for rattlesnakes in warm weather and black bears in early autumn. For further information, call 973-853-4462 or visit tinyurl.com /abramhewitt.

## GPS COORDINATES

N41° 9.343'  W74° 21.768'

## IN BRIEF

After a few hours of rolling along the rocky ridges of Hewitt, you'll swear you've been magically airlifted to the middle of Maine. A big reason for that is the stark, natural beauty of your surroundings, which range from bubbly puddingstone plateaus to an abundance of pitch pines, laurels, and scrub oaks, to the extended views of lakes in several directions, to near-total solitude. The only things missing for a truly authentic Down East experience are incessant swarms of mosquitoes.

## DESCRIPTION

In taking to the hills of Hewitt, you really have to love rocks. Not simply a glacial erratic here, a fin of granite there, but great, towering bluffs of the stuff: big boulders, colossal cliffs, and fractured highways of rocky rubble and seismic schist. This is a hike that draws you through a series of upland swamps, over several streams, to a couple of pristine bodies of water; with so few people venturing into these woods, you're more likely to encounter five-lined skinks—if it's warm weather—than other hikers. Beyond all that, though, the dominant quality of this 8-mile circuit is the

---

## Directions

Follow I-95 over the George Washington Bridge and take Exit 72A onto NJ 4 West. Drive 8.3 miles, then stay straight and follow NJ 208 North for 10.2 miles before merging onto I-287. Take Exit 57 onto Skyline Drive and proceed 4.9 miles, bearing right onto the Greenwood Lake Turnpike. Continue for 8.1 miles and stay straight onto CR 513/Union Valley Road. After 0.3 mile, bear right on the Warwick Turnpike. The small trailhead parking is 0.4 mile ahead, on the right.

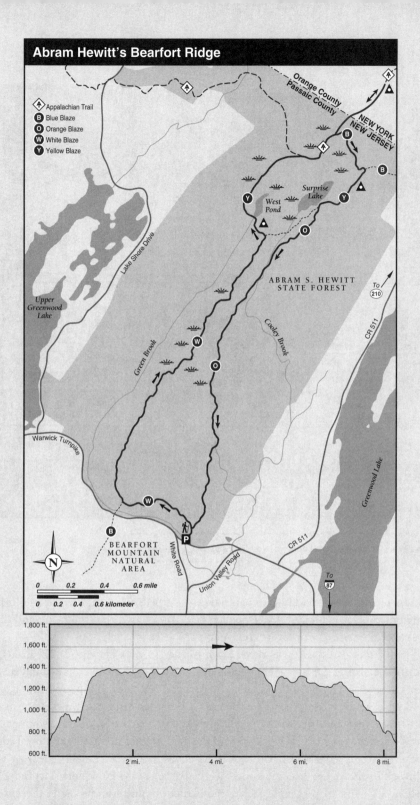

# Abram Hewitt's Bearfort Ridge

Orange County
Passaic County

NEW YORK
NEW JERSEY

Ⓐ Appalachian Trail
Ⓑ Blue Blaze
Ⓞ Orange Blaze
Ⓦ White Blaze
Ⓨ Yellow Blaze

Lake Shore Drive

Surprise Lake

West Pond

ABRAM S. HEWITT
STATE FOREST

To 210

CR 511

Upper Greenwood Lake

Green Brook

Cooley Brook

Greenwood Lake

Warwick Turnpike

CR 511

BEARFORT MOUNTAIN NATURAL AREA

White Road

P

Union Valley Road

To 87

N

0    0.2    0.4    0.6 mile

0    0.2    0.4    0.6 kilometer

1,800 ft.
1,600 ft.
1,400 ft.
1,200 ft.
1,000 ft.
800 ft.
600 ft.

2 mi.    4 mi.    6 mi.    8 mi.

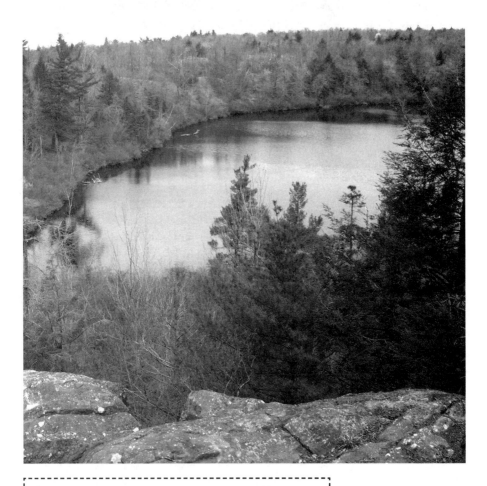

This peaceful mirage is West Pond, viewed from a puddingstone ledge.

prolonged plateau of puddingstone it navigates, a bedrock composed of a colorful conglomerate larded with egglike nuggets of milky quartz, the trail rising and dipping over the corrugation of its contours.

This state forest takes its name from Abram Stevens Hewitt (1822–1903), a man of English and French Huguenot descent who, in all likelihood, never set foot in the domain. Hewitt was born in Haverstraw, New York, and graduated from Columbia College, where he then taught mathematics. Such was the prosaic start of a rather colorful life, in which Hewitt survived a transatlantic shipwreck, was elected mayor of New York City (defeating, among other candidates, Teddy Roosevelt), helped establish Cooper Union, was a founder (and trustee) of the Carnegie Institute, and became known as the Father of the New York City Subway System, after his creative approach to construction and funding made the enterprise possible. The Cooper-Hewitt National Design Museum was later created by his three daughters.

There is no subway stop anywhere near this hike, but you'll find a curbside parking area, which is spacious enough for about four vehicles, just 20 steps to the west of the trailhead, along the north shoulder of the road. The fun begins by the brown sign that reads JEREMY GLICK TRAIL. Go left there, away from the metal gate barring the end of the forest road, and you'll soon spy the white blazes of the Bearfort Ridge Trail (BRT), which spears directly uphill. The greatest physical demands of this hike occur over the ensuing 20 to 30 minutes, as you scale the south side of the Bearfort Ridge without the benefit of any switchbacks. Which is not to say that it's a continuous slog upward, barren of any level patches of path upon which to catch your breath. On the contrary, in 60 seconds or so of maneuvering through rhododendrons and mountain laurels, and after passing a crackling stream, you swing left on a wide track, breaking left again in 30 paces, when the white tags dive once more into the thick of the forest. (The orange-blazed Quail Trail to the right is your return leg.) The BRT then meanders among a mix of oaks and birches while hopping over a rock-filled streambed, providing, meanwhile, a great view of an impressive escarpment straight ahead of you. (Be alert here for wild turkeys, which are attracted to the water source.) The trail circles around this rugged bulwark to the west rather than scaling it head-on, losing a touch of elevation in the process, before meeting a blue-blazed spur on the left, just above a rhododendron-filled ravine. Remain with the white blazes, straight onward, as the BRT resumes the uphill trend.

A great pausing point during this steep climb is approximately three-quarters of the way to the ridgeline, by a lichen-encrusted rock outcropping. Better yet is the minor scramble onto an angular knob of puddingstone, near the top, which lies to the left of the trail. From that pitch pine–dappled outpost, take a gander to the south of the ridge's extension across the Warwick Turnpike. That blue spur you skipped over a short while earlier leads there, into Wawayanda State Park's Bearfort Mountain Natural Area, amounting to a marvelous marathon hike. Oh, and on a clear day you can see the Manhattan skyline to the southeast. On pulling away from this beautiful spot, ignore the old, faded red markings that lead into the hemlock forest (and then peter out); the BRT breaks to the right, over a rocky fin of the ridge, continuing higher as it navigates around several protruding knuckles of puddingstone.

And then, in just a few seconds, you're at the crest, cruising by hemlocks, pitch pines, and laurels, in a fun scramble from one rocky node to the next. The second moss-and-lichen-coated rise features a filtered view of Greenwood Lake through the pitch pines. There's a wonderfully wild look to the trail here as it hugs the glacially fractured puddingstone, drops into a slight gully, then surmounts a parallel fin. As you look for the blazes, many of which are painted on bedrock, scan the understory for Dutchman's breeches, tiny violets, Canada mayflowers, even pink lady's slipper orchids. All part of the pleasure of hiking in this rock-pocked forestland.

One of the highlights of this stretch surfaces a few minutes later, as the path edges from the cover of hemlocks to a perch, 15 feet above a transitional swamp, where massive slabs of puddingstone have broken off vertically from the main body of the ridge. Additional eye candy follows, even after the BRT ends, in roughly an hour and a half of hiking, and you turn left onto the yellow-blazed Ernest Walters Trail (EWT) (GPS: N41° 10.916', W74° 21.166'). This is an easy junction to miss as you tread along in thrall to the beauty of the setting and far-reaching views, because the blazes, painted on bedrock, are readily overlooked. The EWT drops off this arm of the ridge, ascends the neighboring appendage, and then does the same with it, climbing over a third hump, before steeply—if briefly—descending yet again. At the base of the rocks, the yellow markings direct you both left and right, with the hike continuing to the left. Before proceeding, however, take the detour to the right, which leads, in 60 paces, to a splendid vista point above West Pond. This puddingstone crow's nest, well shaded by pitch pines, makes for a splendidly secluded spot in which to enjoy one's lunch.

Back on the main circuit, carefully scramble through the rock declivity and jump over the narrow stream, the latter being runoff from West Pond. From initially coursing west-northwest, the EWT finally bends north, delivering, meanwhile, filtered views of West Pond through a tangle of laurels, oaks, and pines. When the path eventually drops off the ridge, the yellow blazes end at a junction with the Appalachian Trail (AT, long white markings). Roll right, as the track returns you to the ridge crest for a fleeting glimpse of Surprise Lake through trees, then pulls to the left and once more leaves the high ground. The AT surges north at the subsequent intersection, while the continuation of the loop cuts right, or east, on the State Line Trail (STL, blue blazes). Those who know these woods well, however, recommend sticking with the AT for a further half-mile to an extended plateau, where you can enjoy outstanding views not just of Greenwood Lake but also of Sterling Ridge to the east (note the fire tower at its apex), the Catskills and Shawangunks to the north, and, down south, the Manhattan skyline. While there, look for the buttery yellow blossoms of trout lily, too, in spring.

Back at the STL turnoff, swing left, momentarily moving downhill, and then, on the ensuing upward swing, bear left at the unblazed fork. Two more ridgelines follow before the rubbly track, which has devolved into an eroded streambed, begins to descend in earnest. Keep a sharp lookout as you shuffle through this groove for the yellow blazes of the EWT, to the right, or the red-shale heap of a cairn that marks this turnoff (GPS: N41° 11.270' W74° 20.439'). All that elevation you lost on the way down the STL you'll now regain as you crawl back to the ridge. Take the time, though, as you suck air on the way up, to look for wildflowers: pretty pink and white trailing arbutus often carpet the ground here. Yet more views await once you reach the ridgetop, with the panorama of Greenwood Lake stretching from the islands dotting its jadelike surface to the south, clear up to its heavily forested north end. (It's in looking down off the opposite side of this

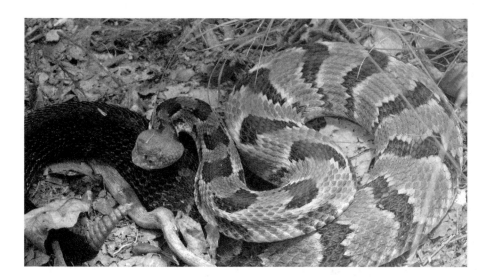

Watch your step! The venomous timber rattler is rather docile but will strike if harassed.

monolith, at the massive slabs of puddingstone that have splintered apart and fallen into a heap below, that one's knees might turn to Jell-O.)

The EWT hugs this plateau for a few minutes, and then, just like that, darts to the southwest and delivers you to the bank of Surprise Lake, where the waterside setting is gorgeous despite suffering the sullying effects of local partiers. Look closely here, not at the trash that litters the ground, but for the orange blazes of the Quail Trail (QT), which join with the yellow markings briefly before splitting off to the left. The QT is far from Hewitt's best trail, and if you're not wearing your sturdiest hiking boots, its hard, uneven surface, which has been degraded in places by illegal ATV usage, may feel as if it's pounding your soles into hamburger. But it also happens to pass through one of the more appealing parts of the preserve, showcasing an attractively dense forest and a delightful boulder field to the right of the path, where a seasonal stream crackles merrily over the rocks. The steep descent ends, in 10 minutes, by an intersection with a forest road. Bear right, and in a couple hundred yards pivot right again, back on the white-tagged BRT. The trailhead is just ahead.

## NEARBY ACTIVITIES

If you're an über-hiker, you might consider trekking across the Warwick Turnpike into part of **Wawayanda State Park** (Hike 44). Remember the blue trail that forked left, about 0.6 mile into the hike? In 2 miles it will bring you to lovely Terrace Pond. The connecting white trail—1.5 miles in length—goes completely around the water. Just retrace your steps on blue to return to your car.

# 35 FARNY HIGHLANDS HIKE

### KEY AT-A-GLANCE INFORMATION

**LENGTH:** 8.5 miles

**ELEVATION GAIN:** 1,806 feet

**CONFIGURATION:** Triple loop

**DIFFICULTY:** Moderately strenuous

**SCENERY:** Mixed-oak forest, several stream crossings, historic iron-forge ruins, a hawk watch, and an impressive dammed reservoir

**EXPOSURE:** Well shaded throughout, except for hawk watch and dam area

**TRAFFIC:** Fairly light, but people flock to the hawk watch and the dam.

**TRAIL SURFACE:** Dirt, rocks, and leaves

**HIKING TIME:** 4.5 hours

**DRIVING DISTANCE:** 39 miles

**SEASON:** Year-round, sunrise–sunset

**ACCESS:** Free; pets on leash, no bicycles, no motorized vehicles

**MAPS:** wcrhawkwatch.com/kiosk.html; USGS *Boonton*

**FACILITIES:** None

**COMMENTS:** From spring through early summer, this rock-filled forest teems with insects, so wear repellent. Hunting is allowed in some areas. For further information, call 973-962-7031 or visit njparksandforests.org /parks/farny.html and mtnlakes.org /Environment/farny.htm.

## GPS COORDINATES

N40° 56.692'  W74° 29.575'

## IN BRIEF

You might justifiably expect a hilly hike with "Highlands" a part of its name, but Farny's near-continuous up–down contours are just the start of what this outstanding circuit delivers. A high elevation ledge that's great for birding, a historic iron forge, several stream crossings (including one that may leave you wet to the knees), a remote cemetery, and even an eerie bat cave are just a handful of the highlights you'll encounter on this lively tour through a hilly hardwood forest.

## DESCRIPTION

If you've never heard of the Farny Highlands, you're not alone. Situated in the heart of New Jersey's lakes district, Farny tends to be overlooked in deference to such nearby hiking icons as Ramapo Mountain, Norvin Green State Forest, Bearfort Ridge, and High Mountain. This works in Farny's favor—and yours—in the near-total absence of hikers traversing the 35,000 acres that make up this wilderness area, a domain that boasts some 907 species of animals and plants, including 71 that have been designated threatened or endangered (the red-shouldered hawk and barred owl among them). The following 8.4-mile trek through Farny's Wildcat Ridge Wildlife Management Area showcases the beauty of its rolling hills,

- - - - - - - - - - - - - - - - - - - - - - - - - - - - - - - - - - - -

*Directions* ─────────────────────────➤

**Follow I-95 across the George Washington Bridge and take Exit 69 to merge onto I-80 West. Take Exit 37 (for Hibernia/Rockaway) and drive north on NJ 513/Green Pond Road for 2.8 miles, then turn right on Sunnyside Road/Lower Hibernia Road. Make an immediate left into the parking lot.**

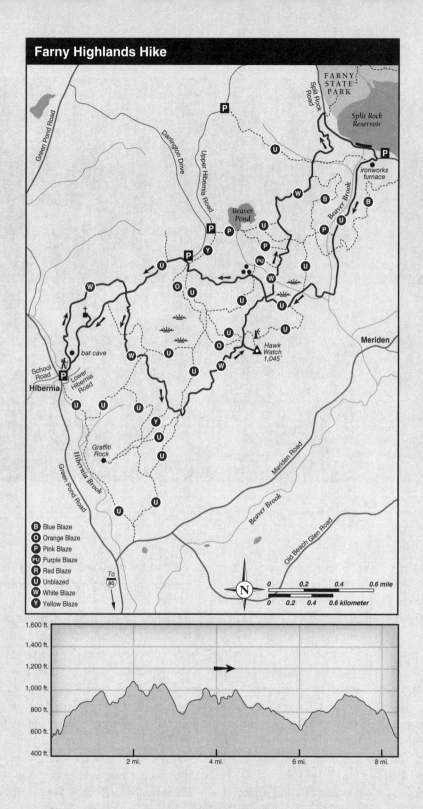

# Farny Highlands Hike

Blue Blaze
Orange Blaze
Pink Blaze
Purple Blaze
Red Blaze
Unblazed
White Blaze
Yellow Blaze

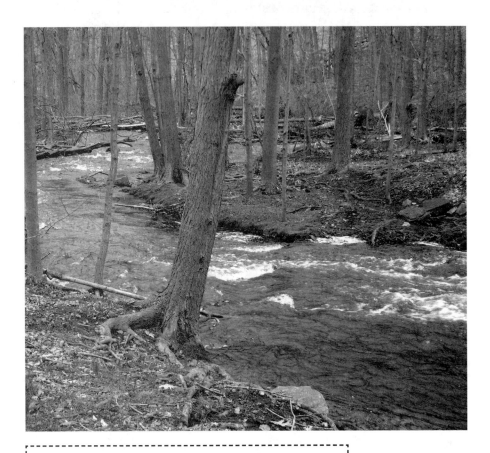

In early spring, tumultuous Beaver Brook makes for a challenging crossing.

glacier-wracked rockscapes, densely foliated lowland swamps, and numerous rivulets. Along the way, you'll also encounter the ruins of an ironworks, a couple of ancient blast furnaces, even a spooky bat cave.

This outing begins inauspiciously, in a well-settled residential neighborhood, but rapidly puts the sounds of civilization behind it by plunging deeply into a second-growth forest. Pick up the white blazes at the trailhead, on the concrete barrier in the parking area (where you will also see the orange and blue ones of other trails), and plan to stick with those for the entire first half of this hike, all the way to Split Rock Reservoir. Initially, the white-blazed Four Birds Trail (FBT) brushes against the ruins of an old ironworks, where it bears right, even as the orange markings of the Hibernia Brook Trail (HBT) cut left. In a few short strides, the FBT hits a T. Swing left, and bear left again in a few moments as an old forest road breaks right. A few derelict slag heaps color the setting here, among a mix of oaks and the occasional wild violet. The grass-surfaced FBT then hops across a junction with the HBT as it gradually climbs higher, past some impressive rock outcroppings. From the appealing setting of the laurel-rimmed ridge, continue by the small stream, where trout lily and Canada mayflower flourish, then head east, paralleling the groove in the ground that marks the old trail. In the course of a couple of miles your route is traversed by a number of unmarked paths, first from the left, then the right, and so on, but the white blazes remain easy to follow.

Shortly after crossing a narrow forest road, the WT crests on a higher hill, this one lush with long grass, and then hops over yet another woods road, now moving south among white birches, beeches, and chestnut oaks. From a southward angle, the path zigs north and zags east, crisscrossing the hillside as it descends to a seasonal stream, where the water cascades colorfully against a broad, slanted rock face. Eventually you'll rock-hop over that trickle, along with the skunk cabbage, scarlet gilia, and false hellebore that grow by its muddy edges, as the white markings lead you upward again, now among a thrilling array of granite outcroppings. These formations rank high in pulchritude, so take your time as you amble through the oversize rocks and boulders. At the summit is a junction with an orange-blazed track, a short and worthwhile detour to a cliff edge where an unobstructed view of Torne Mountain to the south serves as a hawk watch for amateur ornithologists, who also search the open sky for warblers, kestrels, and other birds.

Back on the FBT, a steady descent commences, attaining its perigee, after roughly 15 minutes, by a narrow stream. Use the rocks to leap across, keeping your eyes open meanwhile for wild turkeys, which frequent this area. Bear right at the next junction as the path again begins to gain ground, and do the same at the ensuing intersection, near the crest, where a red-blazed track leading to Beaver Pond forks off to the left. Ignore the subsequent traces as you stretch your legs over a couple more streams and gingerly work your way through a boulder-speckled mud field. A second patch of boulders follows, this one highlighted by several sizable erratics; ignore the blue-blazed Split Rock Loop, which materializes to the right at the crest of that outcropping. One more stream fording ensues, just after you cross a yellow-tagged path: at periods of high water, this water flow can be a challenging 10 to 15 feet wide. That bit of up-and-down concluded, it's back uphill, steaming toward an imposing granite ridge. The white-blazed trail skirts the highest part of that promontory and crosses a power-line cut, and if the trees are leafless, you may be able to glimpse Split Rock Reservoir through their upper branches.

Turn right at the base of this slope onto the unpaved Split Rock Road, walking toward the reservoir dam. The scene to your left, where swallows often fly low over the water, is magnificent, but pay attention, as well, to the inland setting, down beyond the spillway. That giant stone behemoth, which rises 32 feet high and measures 22 feet across at its base, is Split Rock Furnace, which was built in 1862 to forge iron for Union troops in the Civil War. (A similar structure, a short distance downstream, was used as a lime kiln.) Once across the dam, stay with the dirt road until it begins to bend to the left (about 100 feet), and then trot to the right down the rutted and rubbly path toward the water. Bear right at the fork and stick with the trail as it veers left by the streambed. (Take a few minutes, though, for an up-close examination of the colossal ruins before moving on.)

Adhering to the correct route is more of a challenge over the return leg of this hike. Don't worry that few of the paths are marked, though, as much of the time you'll be taking the more dominant track. A fork soon appears as you tread downstream on the left side of the flow, with red blazes leading across the river at a point that can be rather daunting during times of snowmelt and spring showers. Ignore that junction, persisting straight on the wide, hard-packed forest road, and in less than a minute a blue-tagged trail crosses the river (look for the blue paint on a large rock by the right side of the trail). Although the stream is wider here, and punctuated with an extended series of small cascades, the presence of numerous rocks and moss-crusted trees growing out of the water makes this an easier fording place. Nonetheless, your crossing point lies 5 minutes farther downriver, where a wide, unblazed trace forks right by a sizable erratic, aiming directly over the river (GPS: N40° 57.099' W74° 27.821'). (You've gone too far if you reach a very prominent Y-intersection.) Dutchman's breeches abound in the mossy turf on the far side of the water, with the trail moving uphill from there. Stay with the grooved track for maybe 3 to 5 minutes (meanwhile easing your way by a few fallen trees), to a junction with another trail, then break left. As the path arcs toward the west, it hops over a small stream and comes to a fork, where you should roll right onto the more defined track. Now plowing uphill in a northerly direction, you'll quickly come to an intersection with, and cross, the FBT. A brick ruin lies off to the right at the subsequent intersection, and beyond that is a scenic pond. Your return route is straight ahead, however, gradually gaining ground until it ultimately tops out under a power line.

Ignore the yellow-blazed trail that joins the path just before the power line, and turn right, away from the yellow gate, when you hit the forest road. Vault left as the road forks, and hang with the forest road for the next mile, until you reach the turnoff to the bat cave. Along the way you should see a fair number of slag heaps and other remnants of ore mining, in addition to a smattering of detritus left by latter-day litterers.

After a short while you will once more cross the FBT; then, in something like a minute, the wide, rocky track enters the cover of trees and meets a trail emerging from the left. Continue straight, descending gradually, and in a further few seconds the path merges left into a wider track, once more under open sky. At the next divergence steer to the right (the left-hand trail is blazed orange), venturing slightly downhill on rockier ground for a short visit to St. Patrick's Cemetery. Once there, you may spook a lonesome deer grazing among the little white crosses that indicate where, up until 1869, many of Hibernia's mine workers were buried.

Backtrack from that picturesque spot to the previous intersection and bolt to the right, taking the level orange-blazed route. Keep to the main track as the descent resumes and grows steeper, and the orange tags disappear, and skip the spur to the left that leads to private homes. The trailhead is to the left at the subsequent three-way junction, but a brief side trip, to the right, will bring you to the old Hibernia Mine, its entrance blocked off with sturdy iron bars. If you're lucky,

Just below the dam of Split Rock Reservoir this iron furnace, which dates to 1862, still proudly stands.

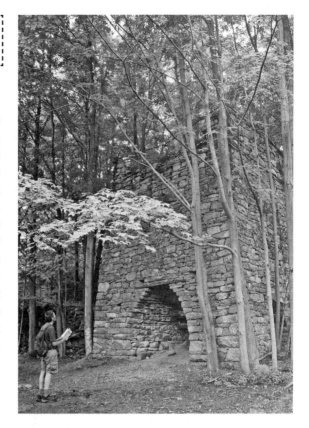

or you've planned your hike well, and it's sunset when you reach this spot, you'll probably find people on the wooden viewing platform opposite the dark aperture. Join them and wait for the spectacular flight of nearly 30,000 bats as they soar up from a shaft 2,500 feet beneath the ground and exit the cavern. Among those dark-brown critters are a number of endangered Indiana bats.

## NEARBY ACTIVITIES

Just up the road, in Kinnelon, is the 1,000-acre **Silas Condict County Park.** Its pristine lake is ideal for fishing, and there are miles of hiking trails, too, if you haven't had enough of *that.* The park is also a popular spot for picnics, and its "Casino" is famous not for gambling but for the historic murals that adorn its interior. For further information, call 973-326 7600 or visit **morrisparks.net/asp parks/silasmain.asp.**

# 36   HIGH POINT DUET

### KEY AT-A-GLANCE INFORMATION

**LENGTH:** 9.8 miles

**ELEVATION GAIN:** 1,416 feet

**CONFIGURATION:** Figure-eight

**DIFFICULTY:** Moderately strenuous

**SCENERY:** Rocky ridges leading to scenic views of surrounding mountains, valleys, fields, and lakes

**EXPOSURE:** Partially shaded at best

**TRAFFIC:** Popular on sunny weekends, light traffic on weekdays

**TRAIL SURFACE:** Pointy rock upheavals, grass, dirt, a few rooty stretches

**HIKING TIME:** 5 hours

**DRIVING DISTANCE:** 62 miles

**SEASON:** Year-round, 8 a.m.–8 p.m.

**ACCESS:** Entrance fee is charged Memorial Day weekend–Labor Day. Residents: $5 weekdays, $10 weekends; double that for nonresidents. Dogs on leash.

**MAPS:** At park office; USGS *Port Jervis South*

**FACILITIES:** Restrooms, water, and public phone at park office

**COMMENTS:** In winter, the Cross-Country Ski Center at Lake Marcia welcomes skiers with all things warm: soup, food, a fire, and a smile. In summer, the water belongs to swimmers. Even campers are pampered with secluded sites along the pretty lake. For more information, call 973-875-4800 or visit njparksandforests .org/parks/highpoint.html.

## GPS COORDINATES

N41° 18.274'  W74° 40.233'

## IN BRIEF

High Point State Park lies in the heart of black-bear country. Don't fret too much about that, though, as you are far more likely to encounter birds and butterflies on this rough-cut loop than any ill-tempered Smokey. There are also views galore from along the Appalachian Trail, access to a secluded lake on the back half of the hike, and a profusion of wildflowers throughout the spring.

## DESCRIPTION

Have you ever thought about getting high—*really* high? Just say yes, and slip your bunions into boots for a rousing hike in High Point State Park. The aptly named park achieves an elevation of 1,803 feet atop High Point Monument, making it the Garden State's tallest peak. The 360-degree panorama there extends to the Delaware River and the hills of Pennsylvania, the Catskill Mountains, and the fertile farmlands of northwestern Jersey. Our suggested hike does not summit High Point Monument, though you should save time for a side trip there. Which is not to imply that the following jaunt is devoid of views—far from it. More than half of the 10 miles of this trek overlap the Appalachian Trail (AT), with a number of fine vistas occurring en route. That's just for starters: the AT clings to a series

-------------------------------------------

### *Directions* ⟶

**Follow I-95 across the George Washington Bridge and take Exit 69 to merge onto I-80 West. Take Exit 53 onto NJ 23 North. Continue approximately 43 miles to the visitor center, on the left. The trailhead parking is 0.1 mile earlier, also on the left side, by the maintenance building.**

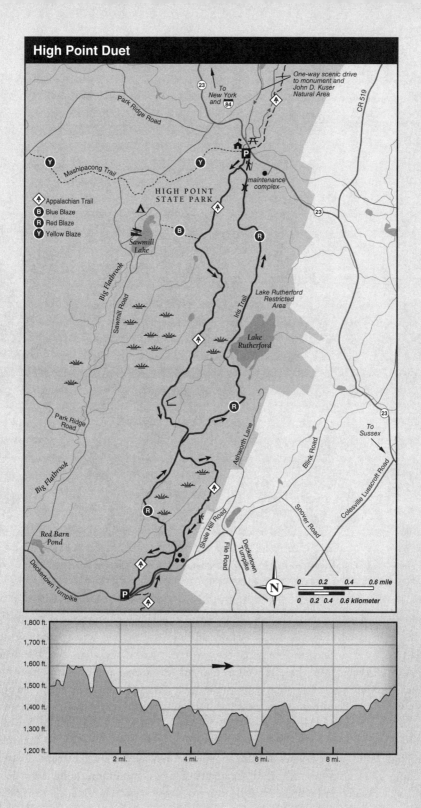

# High Point Duet

Appalachian Trail
B Blue Blaze
R Red Blaze
Y Yellow Blaze

HIGH POINT
STATE PARK

Park Ridge Road

To
New York
and 84

23

One-way scenic drive
to monument and
John D. Kuser
Natural Area

CR 519

Mashipacong Trail

Big Flatbrook

Sawmill Road

Sawmill
Lake

Iris Trail

Lake Rutherford
Restricted
Area

Lake
Rutherford

maintenance
complex

Park Ridge
Road

Big Flatbrook

Ashworth Lane

Blink Road

To Sussex

23

Snover Road

Colesville Lusscroft Road

Red Barn
Pond

Shale Hill Road

File Road

Deckertown
Turnpike

Deckertown Turnpike

N

0   0.2   0.4   0.6 mile
0   0.2  0.4   0.6 kilometer

1,800 ft.
1,700 ft.
1,600 ft.
1,500 ft.
1,400 ft.
1,300 ft.
1,200 ft.

2 mi.        4 mi.        6 mi.        8 mi.

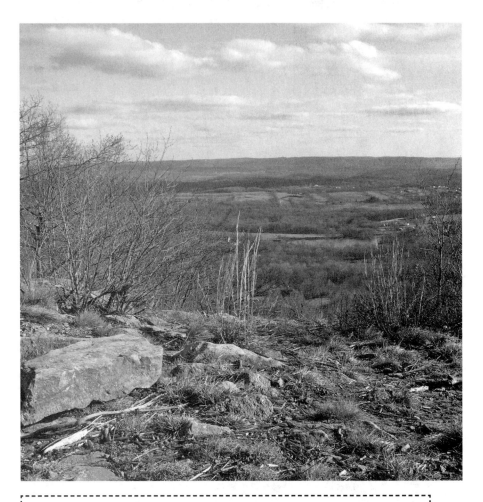

Splendid views of rural New Jersey await along the Kittatinny Mountain Ridge section of the AT.

of bluffs and rugged rock formations along the spine of Kittatinny Mountain Ridge, where wildflowers and wildlife sightings are all but guaranteed. White-tailed deer are among the more common of the woodland denizens, but black bears roam these parts, too, as well as bobcats, raccoons, and possums. You may even hear the exotic chirruping of the elusive pileated and red-breasted wood-peckers and, in the lower swampy areas, the hooting of barred owls.

Time for a bit of history, though, before you set off. In 1888, Charles St. John built a vacation resort, the High Point Inn, on the edge of Lake Marcia, thus pinning the High Point name to this locale. When St. John later went bankrupt, Colonel Anthony Kuser and John Kuser, descendants of Swiss immigrants, bought the property. By 1911, High Point Inn had been refashioned into "The Lodge," to serve as Anthony Kuser's summer retreat. The Colonel had already consolidated all of the power companies in and around Trenton and was president of Southern Jersey Gas and Electric. He was so flush with cash that he ponied up $200,000 in seed money for the establishment of what later became 20th Century–Fox, as well as $60,000 to finance a 17-month expedition to the Far East to study and draw pheasants. High Point became a state park in 1923, after the land was donated to New Jersey by the Colonel and his wife, Susie Dryden Kuser (whose father, U.S. Senator John Dryden, founded Prudential Life). Park officials later hired the Olmsted brothers of Boston—landscape architects and the sons of Frederick Law Olmsted, designer of New York City's Central Park—to beautify the preserve's grounds.

The influence of the Olmsteds is omnipresent as you drive the park roads, most obviously in the wide, swooping lawns that wrap around mature stands of trees. The responsibility for what you see on the trail, on the other hand, rests securely on the shoulders of Mother Nature. The trailhead is at an altitude of 1,400 feet, and your later elevations will vary from that by little more than a couple hundred feet. Thus, the greatest challenge you are likely to face is from the hard, chunky rubble that covers great passages of the AT. The trail at the kiosk, where a map is posted, is blazed with both red and yellow markings. When it hits the T, in 20 feet, turn left, joining the Appalachian Trail (long white blazes). In 150 yards, the yellow markings break to the right, with the red tags shifting left just after that, while you continue straight on the AT, with black birches, maples, various oaks, and a handful of shagbark hickory trees shading the area.

The AT is level for a spell, gliding over an old stone wall and paralleling a rocky bluff rising 40 feet high to the right. Soon, though, the trail ascends that ridge, a 3-minute effort that culminates in a steep, lung-sucking scramble to the top. As is typical of these AT ridge walks, a dip ensues, succeeded by another rise, then a dip, and so on. In a little less than a mile, the path brushes by a blue-blazed spur to the right, a connector to Sawmill Lake. Keep strolling on the AT, and in about a minute it rubs up against a broad bench of fractured granite, from which Sawmill Lake and the adjacent campground are visible. Approach this spot quietly and, while you probably won't encounter any pheasants, you may see a vulture or raptor perched on the rocks.

The AT tapers rapidly downhill, doglegging around a mound of glacial debris and slithering through a rock-limned gully between parallel ridges. The rocky upheaval underfoot resembles a cobblestone street in a war zone, but it improves when the track levels off and begins to climb. After an elevation gain of 150 feet, the AT passes among white birch and white pine on its way to a viewpoint looking out to the west. The path then jogs to the east side of the ridge, providing a glimpse of Lake Rutherford, a reservoir, a couple hundred feet below. The ghostly series of snags you see, by the way, are American chestnuts, killed off by a fungal blight that arrived in the US a century ago.

Forget the trace that slices left to a view of the lake; there's a better vantage point dead ahead, on top of a rocky knob. For the next several minutes, the AT flanks an attractive shelf of granite that extends south from that node, a plateau that is enticingly easy to scramble up for more views of Lake Rutherford, or to just laze in the sun awhile. On passing the sign for the Rutherford Shelter, a backpack-ers' lean-to, the track skirts to the right of the stony ledge and drops downward over chunky ground. The Iris Trail (IT, red blazes) then merges from the left, overlapping the AT for a minute. Steer left on the AT when the two diverge, as the path descends to a swamp where white anemones, violets, and jack-in-the-pulpits preside in spring. More bog pots follow, with the track finally rising through blueberry bushes and pitch pines to a break carved into the forest for an underground pipeline. The AT continues directly across that opening, but first amble left to enjoy the rocky bird's-eye view, with what seems like all of rural Sussex County unfolding below.

Back within the shade of the trees, the path cruises right at a fork in roughly 100 feet and meets a staggered four-way intersection just beyond a trail register. Remain with the white blazes as they steam directly across, passing over the IT yet again. (If you're feeling winded, you can tumble right on the red-blazed route and begin your return.) After a gradual loss of elevation, the track emerges from the forest by a small parking area. Swing left, then left again in a few steps, departing the AT where it crosses the road. Hug the left shoulder for the ensuing 5 to 8 minutes of brisk walking (about a third of a mile), until you come to a cinder drive, also on the left (GPS: **N41° 15.327' W74° 40.986'**), where you pick up the IT and commence your return trip. Unlike the AT, which is restricted to foot traf-fic, Iris is a multipurpose track, shared by hikers, bikers, equestrians, skiers, snow-mobiles, perhaps even people on pogo sticks, so a heads-up vigilance is called for.

After passing the ruins of an old cabin, on the right, the path descends for about 4 minutes before bottoming out at a low swamp. Skunk cabbage lines the grass-sided trace here, along with Indian strawberry and violets. In June, you may stumble upon pink flowering lady's slipper orchids, too, and frogs croon from the muddy depths for most of the summer. Naturally, when it comes to hiking, what goes down must surge up again, and in a short time the trail rises to drier ground, where a network of mortarless walls serves as a reminder that most of this was once open farmland. At the pipe break, Iris doglegs right over buttercups and anemones for 10 steps before swinging left, once more into the forest. (Several hundred yards to the east is the ridge you walked over earlier.) It then briefly reunites with the AT; remember to trot right in a few minutes with the IT when the routes split.

A loss of elevation follows, with Iris, well below the high bluff, meandering through a swamp. There among the ferns and other wetland vegetation, where tiger and spicebush swallowtail butterflies frequently flutter about, you may notice a few purple-flowering irises, justifying the trail's moniker. Shortly after, the red blazes jump left at a T with a forest road, and then lunge right in 150 feet at a Y. This wide, level track draws enticingly close to Lake Rutherford, arcing away to the left before you reach the water. On navigating an S-curve around a mound of angular boulders and a bridge crossing, the lake comes back into view. The IT then rises to a two-tiered granite platform that overlooks the water by 40 feet. As shore-side spots go, this one ranks among the more picturesque. Proceeding from there, Iris

High Point's stretch of the AT is particularly rocky, and tough on the feet.

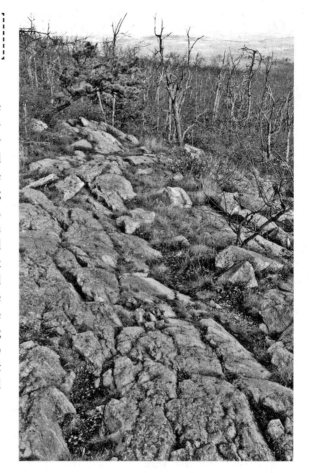

hugs the contours of the reservoir for a spell, eventually gliding into a blueberry heath. Additional dips and climbs ensue, with the undulating terrain boasting a number of glacial erratics, many painted green with lichen. Once you've cruised over a small bridge—look for trout lily, trillium, and jack-in-the-pulpit in the spring—the IT arrives at the staggered four-way crossing where you first picked up the AT. Cut to the right with the red blazes, and return to the trailhead.

## NEARBY ACTIVITIES

Tucked into the northern part of the park is a scenic interpretive trail in an attractive sanctuary. The **Dryden Kuser Natural Area** encompasses a high-elevation cedar swamp, a variety of conifers, rhododendrons, and some endangered plant and animal species. For more details, call 973-875-4800 or visit **njparksandforests.org/parks/highpoint.html.**

Rest your feet in nearby Port Jervis, at the **Gillinder Glass Store,** on Liberty Street, where you can admire the amazing art of glass-blowing. Call 845-856-5375 or visit **gillinderglassstore.com** for more information.

# 37 MAHLON DICKERSON DISCOVERY TRAIL

## KEY AT-A-GLANCE INFORMATION

**LENGTH:** 10.2 miles

**ELEVATION GAIN:** 1,558 feet

**CONFIGURATION:** Figure-eight

**DIFFICULTY:** Moderate

**SCENERY:** Glacially formed bluffs, ridges, and oblong erratics, with many stream crossings, a dynamic cascade, and an active beaver area by a scenic pond

**EXPOSURE:** Mostly tree-shaded

**TRAFFIC:** Fairly light, except for fishers and picnickers at Saffin Pond

**TRAIL SURFACE:** Dirt, moss, and mud, with extended stretches of gravel

**HIKING TIME:** 5 hours

**DRIVING DISTANCE:** 48 miles

**SEASON:** Year-round, sunrise–sunset

**ACCESS:** Free; pets on leash not exceeding 6 feet

**MAPS:** At the park office, at 995 Weldon Rd.; download from morris parks.net/aspparks/mahlontr.asp; USGS *Franklin*

**FACILITIES:** Vault toilets in campground and by picnic area on Weldon Road

**COMMENTS:** Hike may be split into two shorter loops of about 5 miles each; swarms of gnats are a springtime nuisance; park offers excellent camping facilities. Call 973-326-7631 or visit morrisparks.net/aspparks/mahlonmain.asp.

## GPS COORDINATES

N41° 0.675' W74° 34.261'

## IN BRIEF

Don't be thrown by the fact that this double loop brushes by a campground, a picnic area, and a sports field. That's just an iota of the habitat diversity, from a pretty beaver pond to a densely forested pine swamp, that has to be experienced to truly be believed. Better still, for most of the way you'll be out on your own, deep in a rugged wilderness environment of craggy ridges, boggy streams, rolling hills—including the county's highest point—and far-reaching views.

## DESCRIPTION

Yet another fine park within Morris County, this one owes its unusual moniker to native son Mahlon Dickerson (1770–1853). Dickerson's life is a study in contrasts. A self-made man, he was also educated by hired tutors. Although admitted to the bar in 1793, he was awarded the lowly rank of private in the militia during the Whiskey Rebellion. From a position as state commissioner of bankruptcy, in Pennsylvania, he graduated to adjutant general, only to succeed that post with the relatively minor one of city recorder in Philadelphia. After a term in New Jersey's General Assembly, he became a law reporter for the state supreme court, then followed that up as a justice on the same bench. In 1815, Dickerson was elected governor but

---

### *Directions*  ⟶

**Follow I-95 across the George Washington Bridge and take Exit 69 to merge onto I-80 West. Take Exit 34B onto NJ 15 North and drive about 5 miles to the Weldon Road exit. Proceed east for approximately 3.8 miles to the entrance of the tent-camping area, on the right. Park by the kiosk.**

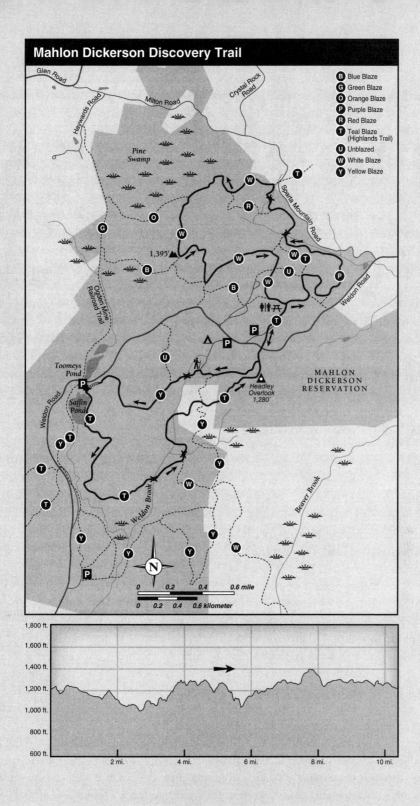

# Mahlon Dickerson Discovery Trail

Glen Road
Haywards Road
Milton Road
Crystal Rock Road

Pine Swamp

Sparta Mountain Road

**B** Blue Blaze
**G** Green Blaze
**O** Orange Blaze
**P** Purple Blaze
**R** Red Blaze
**T** Teal Blaze (Highlands Trail)
**U** Unblazed
**W** White Blaze
**Y** Yellow Blaze

W
R
O
G
W
1,395'
B
W
R
W
T
W
U
T
P
B
Weldon Road

P
P
U
Toomeys Pond
P
Saffin Pond
T
Headley Overlook 1,280'
T

MAHLON DICKERSON RESERVATION

Ogden Mine Railroad Trail
Weldon Road

Y
T
T
Y
T
W
Y
T
Weldon Brook
Y
W
Beaver Brook

T
Y
Y
W
P

**N**

0     0.2     0.4     0.6 mile
0   0.2   0.4   0.6 kilometer

1,800 ft.
1,600 ft.
1,400 ft.
1,200 ft.
1,000 ft.
800 ft.
600 ft.

2 mi.          4 mi.          6 mi.          8 mi.          10 mi.

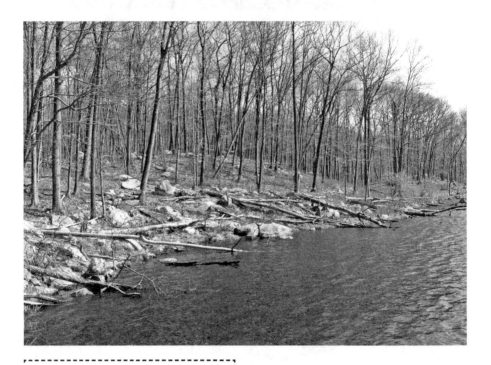

Saffin Pond is home to a zealous beaver colony.

only stuck around for two years, having run for, and won, a seat in the U.S. Senate. He remained a senator until 1833 but spent less than a year in retirement before assuming the mantle of secretary of the navy, serving in the cabinets of both Andrew Jackson and Martin Van Buren. On leaving that post, in 1840, Dickerson was appointed to the U.S. District Court in New Jersey.

Like its namesake political lion, Mahlon Dickerson Reservation is also a study in contrasts, its rich range in topography providing a beautiful backdrop for a memorable hike. To get started, head south from the parking area, by the entrance to the tent campground, to site 8, where the yellow-blazed trail (YT) begins to the left. Keep to the right at the fork, in 15 yards, and in a few seconds more you will arrive at an attractive swamp stream, where the scent of skunk cabbage fills the air. The setting grows wilder once you cross the bridge, as the YT desultorily climbs to an elevation of 1,230 feet, passing not just various oak, beech, and birch trees but also lichen-and-moss-crusted glacial uplift. Ignore the sign indicating Saffin Pond, to the left, and continue right instead, still on the YT. Additional granite outcroppings and large erratics appear as the wide, mossy path slips through a couple of swamp pots and arcs toward the west, then south, bypassing, meanwhile, a short spur on the right that leads to the road. A 25-foot-long boardwalk helps skirt a fertile swamp, rife with peepers in spring, and in no time at all the YT emerges at the northeast corner of Saffin Pond. Switch here to the Highlands Trail (HT, black dot on teal diamonds for now, plain teal diamonds away from the pond), heading left instead of straight, and make your way clockwise along the shore. You'll remain with the HT for the next 3.75 miles, clear across Weldon Road.

While traipsing by the waterside, be sure to note all the pointed tree stumps in the vicinity. No, those aren't the work of some overactive Paul Bunyan wannabe; they're evidence of active beavers living nearby. On reaching the picnic tables, to the left of the dam, the HT leaves the lakeside, lunging back into the woods. Follow it uphill, breaking right with the teal diamonds at the T. A gradual, if prolonged, descent ensues, one that involves fording a seasonal stream, which cascades musically during periods of wet weather. Are you wearing waterproof boots? Let's hope so, as the path tends to be downright muddy as it bends to the east. The spur to the right leads to Weldon Brook, which you've been flanking, but the HT proceeds leftward, to the east-northeast. Five minutes later it comes to another stream, crossing it by means of a spiffy wooden bridge. Check out the enormous erratic at the top of the next hill, with its wig of ferns and moss, and then bolt left, still with the HT, when it meets the Beaver Brook Trail (white blazes).

And so commences what is possibly the sweetest part of the hike. From the leap across the broad, rocky Weldon Brook, in which the churning, cascading water roils noisily beneath you; to a wide circumnavigation of a moss-covered, granite escarpment; to an encounter with a chockablock rock field, sizzling with many little cataracts, and a challengingly primitive log span to get over the water; to an eye-poppingly awesome, fractured boulder scene of great busted-up blocks of glacial erratics, speckled green like oxidized bronze—the raw, natural beauty seems to go on and on. Shortly after hopping over a tributary of Weldon Brook, while still wading through a picturesque field of boulders, the HT rises to a beautiful resting spot on a pocket plateau, where you may observe five-lined skinks soaking up the sun. Beyond that stone shelf, the trail continues to gain elevation, leveling off by a wide intersection with a different stem of the YT. Leap over that interloper (unless you want to call it quits, in which case swing left, then left again, for a swift return to the trailhead), moving uphill once more with the teal markings. The short spur that soon arises provides access to a protruding ledge, yielding an unobstructed view of Lake Hepatcong, the Delaware Water Gap, and the hills to the south. For an even grander vista point, however, persist on the HT as it hugs this granite lip, with far-reaching views along much of it. In something like a hundred yards, you'll arrive at the spur to the Headley Overlook, a laurel-decked, pitch pine–shaded knob, with a long enough row of sizable rocks to satisfy the derrieres of a dozen or two hikers.

On departing this enchanting picture-spot, return to the main trail and turn right. Now scuttling north, the HT breaks right at the fork and shoots across the paved Weldon Road, bound for the Pine Swamp Loop. Steer to the right, moments later, on reaching the parking lot, walk by the kiosk (first making use of the vault toilet, if necessary), slice to the right at the fork in the macadam, and keep to the pavement through the picnic grounds. Once you're past the horseshoe pits and ball field, the teal diamonds usher you back into forest, and in a matter of moments the path hits a junction with the Pine Swamp Loop (PSL, white blazes). Remain with the HT, to the right, as it overlaps the PSL for a part of the latter's circumference. The path, now sporting both white blazes and teal diamonds, passes spurs to the right and then left (the latter leading to the RV campground) before coming to yet another trace, again to the right. Take this unblazed option, which is the Cascades Trail (CT), and stick with it as it curves toward the left, or east, merging with a trace (that first spur you skipped) from the right. In 2 minutes of plodding, you'll reach an overlook, within a spitball's range of Jefferson High and Middle Schools, far below.

You probably won't feel inclined to linger here, on account of how the surrounding rocks and trees have been horribly disfigured with yellow, blue, purple, and teal paint. Happily, the situation improves remarkably in just a few long strides, as the CT descends toward the lower runoff of the Wallkill River. Long before you obtain a view of that flow, your ears should detect the roiling, rollicking symphony of the water as it crashes downhill in one long cascade, pouring over an extended series of stone steps. The CT dips and rises in drawing nearer that flow, which becomes swampier the higher you go upstream. After passing a disused forest road (which forges directly through the water), the CT ends at a convoluted intersection; rejoin the HT (and PSL) here, bolting to the right. The HT immediately crosses the swamp stream (the source of that extended cascade) and then glides left at the well-blazed fork. This is a colorful area, one in which the trail clings to the right side of an oversize bog, shielded by laurels, shaded by hardwoods, with mossy rocks leavening the soggy soil. If it's been rainy of late, you'll need to stretch and leap at various stages where the path is subsumed by mud. All part of the joys of playing explorer. Heave to the left at the slanted T with a forest road, then plug to the right, less than 100 yards later, at the subsequent fork. The massive field of stones you'll soon approach looks like the remains of a ruined city, with the HT skirting its east side, meanwhile vaulting you over the meandering stream by means of a wooden bridge–cum–boardwalk. Only when the trail nears Sparta Mountain Road will you finally say goodbye to the HT, which jags to the right there and leaves the park; the continuation of your circuit lies with the PST, toward the left.

Plug onward with the white-blazed main drag even as two options emerge from the left: first an unblazed forest road, then an orange-marked maverick path that descends into the swamp. The PSL gains ground on circling toward the south, encountering en route a connector trail, on the right, which leads to the well-graded rails-to-trails Ogden Mine Railroad Bed. Eventually, the PSL crests at 1,395 feet, the highest point in Morris County, though the achievement is anticlimactic given the absence of views. Coming down off the summit, you pass an unblazed spur on the right, even as your own gravel-surfaced route shifts hard to the left before grinding to a halt at a T. Pivot left there, staying with the white blazes, and left again in 10 steps. (A right turn will deliver you to the RV campground.) There are some fair-size erratics in this subtly pretty area, with a fair amount of sunlight filtering through the young hardwood forest. Five minutes from that last intersection, you'll come to a green-tagged trace on the left; keep right, and right again in a couple hundred yards, when the PSL reaches another T. Don't grow too complacent on this woods road, though, as that turn is only the first part of a delayed dogleg, which is completed in 30 paces with a lurch to the left, following the sign to the picnic area. (The RV campground is indicated as straight ahead.) Skip the next turnoff to the right, and in 170 strides the loop comes to a close as you rejoin the Highlands Trail. Vault right, back on familiar turf, and retrace your earlier route through the picnic grounds and back across Weldon Road. Switch to the yellow-blazed trail, on the right, as you continue by the Headley Overlook. Bear right onto the gravel-covered track at the fork, and in a few moments you'll reconnect with the stem leading to the tent campground.

## NEARBY ACTIVITIES

**Hopatcong State Park,** at the southwest corner of the eponymous lake, is a magnet for fishing, boating, and swimming enthusiasts. What most park visitors don't realize, though, is that the focal point of their entertainment—the lake—came into existence in conjunction with the Morris Canal, a 90-mile sluice flowing from Newark to Philipsburg. During its peak, in 1866, more than 880,000 tons of iron, coal, and zinc were transported along the canal, which relied on Lake Hopatcong as its primary source of water. The development of railroads ultimately doomed the canal, but its vibrant history lives on in the park's Morris Canal Locktender's House, which also features exhibits on the local indigenous people. For further information, call 973-398-7010 or visit **njparksandforests.org /parks/hopatcong.html.**

Why not treat yourself to a restoring experience at the lively **Krogh's Restaurant & Brew Pub,** at 23 White Deer Plaza, in Sparta? Menu, directions, and events are posted at **kroghs.com,** or call 973-729-8428 for details.

# 38  NORVIN GREEN'S HEART AND SOUL

## KEY AT-A-GLANCE INFORMATION

**LENGTH:** 11.5 miles

**ELEVATION GAIN:** 2,683 feet

**CONFIGURATION:** Loop

**DIFFICULTY:** Strenuous

**SCENERY:** Abandoned mines, waterfalls and cascades, gnarly laurel forest, and stellar 360-degree panoramas revealing New York City skyline

**EXPOSURE:** Very shady, except on bald peaks

**TRAFFIC:** Often light, but good weather brings out students and nature-lovers.

**TRAIL SURFACE:** Rubble, loose rocks, rock-filled dirt, some grassy and rooty stretches, bedrock on summits

**HIKING TIME:** 7 hours

**DRIVING DISTANCE:** 32 miles

**SEASON:** Year-round, sunrise–sunset

**ACCESS:** Free; dogs on leash, no bicycles, no motorized vehicles

**MAPS:** At kiosk by Weis Ecology Center; USGS *Wanaque*

**FACILITIES:** Nature center, water, restrooms, and public telephone at Weis Ecology Center

**COMMENTS:** Rain-fed streams may make some water crossings tough. Remember to bring a flashlight if you want to go spelunking in the old mines. Hunting allowed. Call 973-962-7031 or visit njparksandforests .org/parks/norvin.html#trails.

## GPS COORDINATES

N41° 4.186'  W74° 19.423'

## IN BRIEF

If you're considering venturing into Norvin Green, you had better dust off your sturdiest hiking boots. This is a challenging hike into an underdeveloped, seriously rugged locale. Your resourcefulness in fording a couple of stream crossings and several steep climbs (along with an even steeper descent) will be rewarded with mountaintop vistas, majestic waterfalls, spectral erratics, and a couple of historic mines, as well as nonstop natural beauty.

## DESCRIPTION

Are you a child at heart? Do you enjoy being out in the rain, walking through puddles without an umbrella? Does wrestling with a dense, tangled overgrowth deep in a backwoods wilderness fill you with joyful thoughts of playing explorer? If the answer to these questions is an unqualified yes, then Norvin Green State Forest is just the place for you. Don't be misled by the fact that many of its trails coincide with old logging roads; this is an underdeveloped park where *rugged* is the byword and raw natural beauty the reward.

## *Directions*

Follow I-95 over the George Washington Bridge and take Exit 72A onto NJ 4 West. Drive 8.3 miles, then stay straight and follow NJ 208 North for 10.2 miles before merging onto I-287. Take Exit 57 onto Skyline Drive (toward Ringwood). Drive 5 miles and turn left on the Greenwood Lake Turnpike, followed by a right—in 1.7 miles—onto Westbrook Road. Continue 2 miles, then veer left at the fork, and turn left on Snake Den Road in another 0.5 mile. Proceed 0.7 mile past the large parking area on the right, and turn left at the fork, by the sign for the Weis Ecology Center. Make an immediate right into the parking lot.

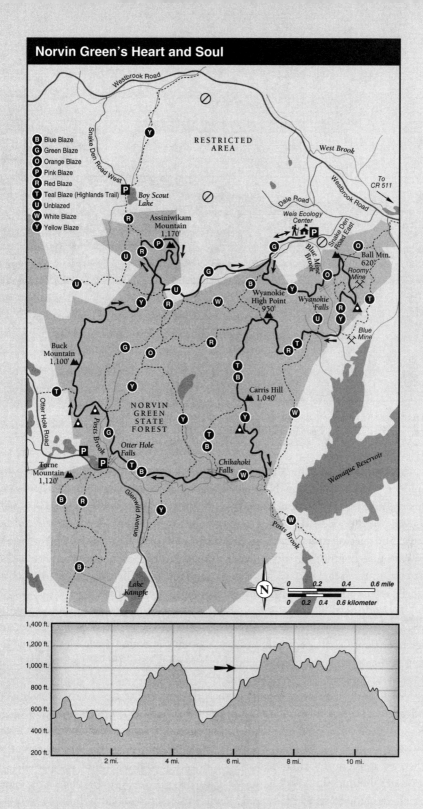

# Norvin Green's Heart and Soul

Ⓑ Blue Blaze
Ⓖ Green Blaze
Ⓞ Orange Blaze
Ⓟ Pink Blaze
Ⓡ Red Blaze
Ⓣ Teal Blaze (Highlands Trail)
Ⓤ Unblazed
Ⓦ White Blaze
Ⓨ Yellow Blaze

Westbrook Road

RESTRICTED AREA

West Brook

Westbrook Road

To CR 511

Dale Road

Snake Den Road West

Boy Scout Lake

Assiniwikam Mountain 1,170'

Weis Ecology Center

Snake Den Road East

Blue Mine Brook

Ball Mtn. 620'

Roomy Mine

Wyanokie High Point 950'

Wyanokie Falls

Blue Mine

Buck Mountain 1,100'

NORVIN GREEN STATE FOREST

Carris Hill 1,040'

Otter Hole Road

Posts Brook

Otter Hole Falls

Chikahoki Falls

Torne Mountain 1,120'

Wanaque Reservoir

Glenwild Avenue

Posts Brook

Lake Kampfe

N

0    0.2    0.4    0.6 mile
0    0.2    0.4    0.6 kilometer

1,400 ft.
1,200 ft.
1,000 ft.
800 ft.
600 ft.
400 ft.
200 ft.

2 mi.    4 mi.    6 mi.    8 mi.    10 mi.

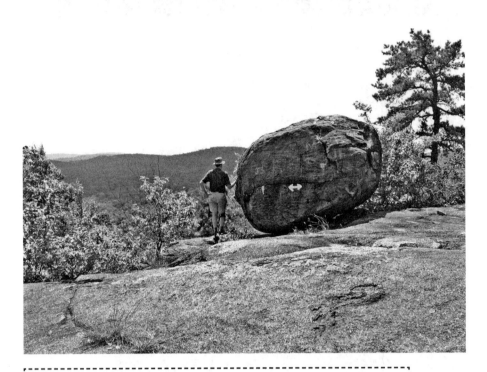

One, two, three, *push*! This giant glacial erratic rests right on the edge of a granite plateau.

So how does parading through puddles relate to the price of pitch pines, you wonder? A typical trek in Norvin Green involves fording numerous seasonal streams, wading on occasion through swift-moving, knee-high water. This thrilling walk on the wild side passes by three delightful waterfalls and involves more than 2,500 feet of cumulative elevation gain, culminating in views of Manhattan from atop a couple of bald domes. Seasoned hikers will enjoy this preserve throughout the year, but we favor visiting in spring, when the forest is freckled with flowers and the challenge of high-flowing water is greatest.

To find the trailhead, cut to the north side of the parking lot and cross the narrow footbridge. Take an immediate left, shy of the concrete picnic tables, and stick with the pine-shaded path, heading west and sporting green blazes. Turn left again at the northwest corner of Highlands Natural Pool (HNP), where the green markings are joined by a couple of others.

Stick with the green blazes as the rock-strewn track crosses a couple of bridges and ascends above the HNP; both the L and W Trails eventually diverge. This circuitous route, which seems to overlap a vestigial streambed under a canopy of black birch, oak, and maple trees, soon arrives at the Richard Warner Kiosk, by a junction with a forest road. Instead of following the green tags to the right, step behind the kiosk and switch to the yellow-dotted white-circle blazes (which overlap with the blue-blazed Hewitt Butler Trail) as the uphill slog resumes.

In a few minutes and an additional gain of 115 feet of elevation, the rubble-rich trail scratches through a laurel patch and reaches a minor crest. Follow the yellow dots as they break left away from Hewitt Butler and, once by a highly scenic series of dramatic uplift and muscular rocky protrusions, swing left again on the orange-blazed Roomy Mine Trail (RM).

The gentle descent that began shortly after that area of colorful boulders gains momentum as you traipse along the RM, until briefly leveling off at the top of Wyanokie Falls. This is a pretty setting, at 550 feet of elevation, where the great cascade tumbles into a jumble of oversize rocks, with a number of flat stones on which to sit and relish the watery atmosphere.

Just as the orange-blazed path encounters a mammoth erratic, it intersects the yellow-on-white blazes of the Mine Trail. Switch to the latter (for now), moving with the yellow markings across the junction and back toward higher ground. It is steep going for a few minutes, but it's worth the effort for the views to come atop an exposed escarpment, Ball Mountain, where chestnut oak, maple, cedar, and a sizable fin of granite bracket the hills to the west. The yellow-dot blazes shift to the right on leaving this extended bedrock, tracing a line south along the rolling contours of the grass-topped hill, re-encountering the orange blazes of the RM along the way. Hang with the main path, now marked by both orange and yellow dots, all the way to its south end, which culminates in a view of the Wanaque Reservoir amid an appealing mix of scrub oaks, cedars, and pitch pines, as well as knee-high grass and lichen-speckled granite.

Descend from here to the base of the headland, where the path splits and the orange-blazed RM leads to the entrance to the Roomy Mine, named after Benjamin Roome (not for the spaciousness of its main entrance), a 19th-century surveyor. Iron ore was excavated here from 1840 to 1857 (and for a short spell in 1890), with the tunnel extending more than 100 feet. Outside of spring, when water often floods it, this shaft can be explored with the aid of a flashlight—and a pair of hip-waders. Note that it is closed from the first of September through the end of April to protect nesting bats.

Having finished exploring the mine, retrace your steps to the previous intersection and bear right, onto the next leg of the yellow-dot route. In due course this path comes to a slanted T with the red-dot blazes of the Wyanokie Circular Trail (WCI): turn left, sticking with both sets of blazes. A minute or so later the trail, now joined by the teal diamonds of the Highlands Trail, bends to the right and crosses a bridge, while the Blue Mine lies toward the left, a few yards beyond the broken-up concrete platform. In spring, the broad Blue Mine Brook flows into the yawning orifice of the mine, as frogs and birds bathe in the eddying current. Water has often inundated the mine, forcing its closure many times since it was initially opened in 1765. Known variously over the years as the London, Whynokie, and Iron Hill mine, this historic operation is now identified by the bluish hue of its iron ore.

Across the wooden span, a steep ascent lifts you from an altitude of 400 feet to a little over 900. Along the way, the WCI encounters a maverick campfire ring and a deteriorating lean-to, where lilies of the valley perfume the air in May. Hold to the left shortly after that, as the yellow blazes finally break away on a spur (stick with yellow if you'd like to bring the trek to a premature end), and then to the right when a white-blazed trace surfaces on the left. We once spooked a grouse in this area that was concealed in the grass by the base of a gargantuan birch; it was only too happy to return the favor, stopping our hearts for a moment with its abrupt flutter of wings.

A field of boulders, succeeded by a stand of dead chestnut trees and, in summer, a broad swath of goldenrod and purple pokeweed, signals the imminent end to this uphill march. To merely say that High Point summit is granite bedrock partly clad in grass, fringed with knee-high ferns, blueberry bushes, and such wildflowers as Indian strawberry and goatsbeard, is to do its beauty an injustice. Even with a cluster of spicebush and pitch pines at the periphery, the view here at 950 feet is spectacular, a 360-degree panorama that takes in I-287 to the south and the New York City skyline beyond that, with the Empire State Building clearly discernible. Your (reluctant) descent from this idyllic dome begins at its northwest side. In about a minute, the Hewitt Butler Trail (HB, blue blazes) merges from the right and for several minutes overlaps the WCI. Continue straight on the HB when the red-dot blazes tack to the right.

Carris Hill, the subsequent summit, though 100 feet above High Point, lacks the latter's dramatic vistas. Nonetheless, it is a highly picturesque plateau, with a foot-wide vein of pegmatite quartz running through it and globular glacial erratics, somewhat like deflated Michelin men, scattered throughout. It requires a brief hand-over-hand scramble up a 35-foot-long slab of granite to reach this knoll, which extends quite some distance to the south. Cruise left at the fork onto the yellow-blazed track, which persists along this delightful, sun-struck shelf for 5 minutes or so before finally losing elevation. A rocky knob partway down the slope faces to the south, providing another opportunity to view the Wanaque Reservoir and the Big Apple from afar. In springtime, fuchsia–yellow penstemon and rare moccasin flowers add a touch of magic to this jagged antediluvian environment. From there, the sharp descent grows more earnest, with the path snaking by one sentinel stone after another, part of a valley of boulders that rolled off the high bluffs eons ago.

Old, faded markings lead over the rocks, but fresh yellow blazes reroute the path westbound, a hair shy of the boulder field and down the moraine-filled, grassy slope. This is an underused segment of trail, and you may have to limbo under some fallen trees and detour around others. A series of seasonal stream crossings coincides with the ongoing elevation loss, with no shortage of rocks to skip over. The yellow blazes end at a slanted T with the Post Brook Trail (PB, white blazes), near a rusty chain-link fence. Slice right, then right again in about 50 yards, at the three-way intersection (GPS: **N41° 2.635' W74° 19.664'**). Rerouting now keeps the path north of Post Brook, a tributary to the Wanaque Reservoir, as it gradually scales a chunky slope of scree and leaps over a couple of minor streams before hitting Chikahoki Falls. Your approach to that explosive waterfall will be heralded by the roar of splashing water and, if you're passing through in early summer (and exceedingly lucky), more examples of the somewhat rare and marvelous moccasin flower, which flourishes in this moist, shady habitat.

Shortly after the dirt path draws to the top of Chikahoki Falls, where a thrilling series of lesser cascades churns Post Brook into a succession of whitewater, the PB ends as blue and teal blazes merge from the right. Stride straight on, using the makeshift bridge of three logs lashed together to ford the following confluence, and continue straight at the subsequent crossing, in 5 minutes, of the Wyanokie Crest Trail (WCR, yellow blazes). Whether you spell it *Wyanokie, Whynokie,* or *Wanaque,* by the way, its root is *winaki,* a local Indian word meaning "land of sassafras." Sassafras does indeed grow throughout the Highlands, but your eyes are more likely to alight upon the endless array of boulders—and the streams that flow by them.

In any case, stick with the blue blazes of the resurgent HB as the trail gains modest elevation and joins an old forest road, churning west. Ignore the two traces to the right that lead toward a stone-studded bluff, steering left instead along the rocky route. Thirty paces beyond the second option, the return leg of your circuit breaks right, on the Otter Hole Trail (OH, green markings). Unless you're feeling tired (or you got soaked back at the falls), though, proceed straight ahead to Otter Hole. We've never seen any otters here, but the picturesque cataclysm of water crashing through the rocks is so appealing that it's easy to understand why they and any number of other animals might be drawn to the site.

When you've had enough of Otter Hole, backtrack to the previous junction and swing left. Now forging northward on the OH, the pebbly track rises gently, then levels off, before striking another leg of the WCR (GPS: N41° 3.086' W74° 21.036'). If you're short on time (or still sloshing along from your spill in the falls), remain with the OH; the trailhead is just 1.6 miles ahead. Otherwise, jump left with the yellow blazes, as the WCR skips across a watery pocket-bog and commences climbing steeply up the rocky slope. After you've brushed by some catbrier and scrambled tooth-and-nail over the lip of an expansive granite plateau (listed on the map as Buck Mountain), your reward is a stellar vista, across the hills of Norvin Green, of far-off Manhattan. Hang with the path as it weaves to the south, over an appealing pine-shaded, rocky knob and then commences coursing back to the north. (Along the way, you will pass a number of unblazed traces, spurs burned into the soft surface of the forest floor by dirt bikers and ATV users who illegally venture into this, a less-trafficked part of the park. Should you encounter any such scofflaws, try to discreetly photograph them and e-mail the images to the New Jersey Department of Parks, which is waging an uphill campaign against this abuse of public land.) Eventually, the WCR doglegs left around a vernal pond, then right

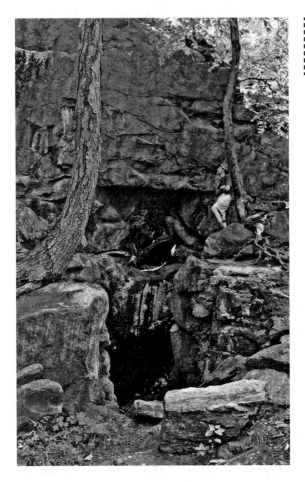

> **Mind the bats! Intrepid hikers have been known to enter Roomy Mine, but only when the water level is low.**

by another such pool, finally departing from this sage-green, lichen-mottled granite ridge.

Having meandered through an attractive rock-spiked swamp, where you may discover artist's conk mushrooms and other polypores attached to the oaks, beeches, black birches, and mountain laurels, the yellow blazes end at a junction with the WCI (red dot on white), the same path you took hours earlier to reach High Point. Ignore the pink blaze of the Will Monroe Loop (WML), directly ahead of you, instead spinning left on the WCI. This route circles to the north-northwest, leading circuitously toward the top of Assiniwikam Mountain. To reach that low peak, jog right onto the far end of the WML (GPS: N41° 4.163' W74° 20.741'), a junction marked with three discreet pink blazes on a slender beech sapling. (Don't worry too much, though, because if you miss it, the Boy Scout Lake parking lot is just ahead on the WCI, and you can easily backtrack from there.) Are you with us now on the pink-blazed trail? Let's hope so, because some stellar scenery lies in wait. First, though, there's a climb to be dealt with, slipping slowly at first by some appealing rock outcroppings, then arcing south and cresting on an extended plateau of granite, where knee-high grass and blueberry bushes provide a colorful contrast to the ubiquitous splashes of sage-green lichen. That's Wanaque Reservoir to the southeast, and Manhattan—again—far beyond it. The WML zigzags over Assiniwikam's cranium, neatly displaying the phrenological beauty of its rounded, multidomed formation before finally jumping off its brow and ending at the junction you passed through a short time earlier, where the yellow-blazed WCR meets the WCI.

Swing left on the WCI (still red-dot blazes) and remain with it as the track winds downhill, toward the southeast, until it comes to a crossing with an unblazed forest road. Turn left onto the latter and proceed downhill on this heavily eroded old logging road to its end, at the green-blazed OH. Take another left and stick with the green blazes, rock-hopping past the washed-out bridge, all the way back to the Richard Warner Kiosk. Break left there and retrace your earlier steps along the OH until you arrive in the parking lot.

## NEARBY ACTIVITIES

True rock-hounds should sniff out a side trip to Franklin's **Mineral Museum,** where mines, minerals, ores, and fossils are featured. For information, call 973-827-3481 or visit **franklinmineralmuseum.com.**

# 39   RAMAPO-RINGWOOD RALLY

## KEY AT-A-GLANCE INFORMATION

**LENGTH:** 13.1 miles

**ELEVATION GAIN:** 2,638 feet

**CONFIGURATION:** Loop

**DIFFICULTY:** Very strenuous

**SCENERY:** Lush forests, babbling brooks, placid lakes, humid swamps, many rock outcroppings and ledges yielding splendid views

**EXPOSURE:** Mostly dense canopy

**TRAFFIC:** Largely light to moderate

**TRAIL SURFACE:** Dirt, grass, stones

**HIKING TIME:** 8 hours

**DRIVING DISTANCE:** 24 miles

**SEASON:** Year-round, 8 a.m.–6 p.m., Eastern standard time; 8 a.m.–8 pm., daylight saving time

**ACCESS:** Free; dogs on leash, no motorized vehicles

**MAPS:** At the Ringwood State Park Office (see below); USGS *Wanaque*

**FACILITIES:** None, but parking lot 1 mile south has posted map, public phone, and portable toilet.

**COMMENTS:** Hunting is allowed. Nearby Campgaw Mountain Reservation and Ramapo Valley County Reservation offer great camping. Permits can be obtained at Darlington County Park in Mahwah: tinyurl.com/darlingtonpark. For further information, call the Ringwood State Park office at 973-962-7031 or visit njparksandforests.org/parks/ramapo.html.

## GPS COORDINATES

N41° 2.852'  W74° 15.083'

## IN BRIEF

You know those Western hikes in which miles go by with only the cacti or an occasional butte lending variety to a uniform landscape? This trek is cut from different cloth, with so much diversity spilling out of it you'll hardly feel the hours slip away. In addition to five scenic lakes, towering bluffs, no end of streams, glacial erratics by the truckload, and a number of memorable ruins, these woods are inundated with wildlife (including black bears), birds beyond count, and a spring flower display any horticulturalist would envy.

## DESCRIPTION

As with numerous other hikes in the Highlands of New Jersey, there are so many trails tattooed into the hills of the Ramapo Mountains, it is sometimes hard to know where to begin. Many of these are logging roads that date back to the previous century, when steel was mined extensively from Ringwood Manor to the north, Ramapo Lake to the south, and west beyond Norvin Green State Forest. During that era, this heavily forested country was denuded of trees, and the smelting forges, where oak, maple, and pine trees were reduced to ash, belched streams of smoke into the

- - - - - - - - - - - - - - - - - - - - - - - - - - - - - - - - - - - -

## *Directions* ⟶

**Follow I-95 over the George Washington Bridge and take Exit 72A onto NJ 4 West. Drive 8.3 miles, then stay straight and follow NJ 208 North for 10.2 miles before merging onto I-287. Take Exit 57 onto Skyline Drive (toward Ringwood). After 0.1 mile, the first parking lot appears on the left. Proceed another mile to the second parking lot on the left, across from the CAMP TAMARACK sign.**

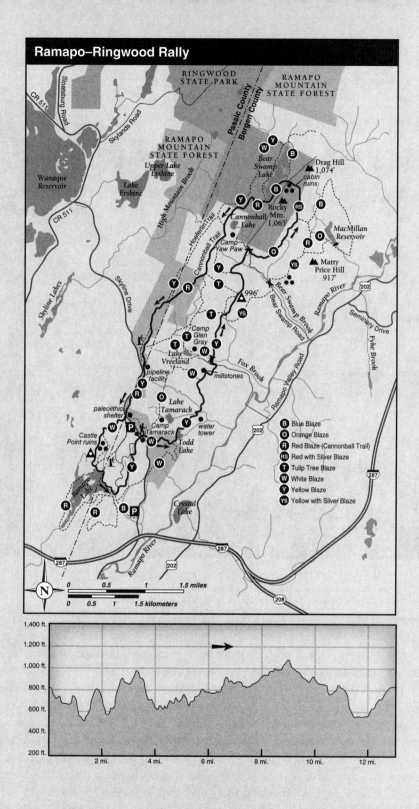

# Ramapo–Ringwood Rally

RINGWOOD STATE PARK

RAMAPO MOUNTAIN STATE FOREST

RAMAPO MOUNTAIN STATE FOREST

Passaic County / Bergen County

CR 511

Sloatsburg Road

Skylands Road

Wanaque Reservoir

Upper Lake Erskine

Lake Erskine

CR 511

High Mountain Brook

Hoeferlin Trail

Cannonball Trail

Skyline Drive

Skyline Lakes

Bear Swamp Lake

Drag Hill 1,074'

cabin ruins

Rocky Mtn. 1,065'

Cannonball Lake

MacMillan Reservoir

Camp Yaw Paw

Matty Price Hill 917'

Bear Swamp Brook

Ramapo River

202

Seminary Drive

Fyke Brook

996'

Camp Glen Gray

Lake Vreeland

pipeline facility

Fox Brook

Ramapo Valley Road

millstones

paleolithic shelter

Lake Tamarack

Camp Tamarack

water tower

202

Castle Point ruins

Ramapo Lake

Todd Lake

287

Crystal Lake

287

Ramapo River

202

287

208

**B** Blue Blaze
**O** Orange Blaze
**R** Red Blaze (Cannonball Trail)
**RS** Red with Silver Blaze
**T** Tulip Tree Blaze
**W** White Blaze
**Y** Yellow Blaze
**YS** Yellow with Silver Blaze

0   0.5   1   1.5 miles

0   0.5   1   1.5 kilometers

N

1,400 ft.
1,200 ft.
1,000 ft.
800 ft.
600 ft.
400 ft.
200 ft.

2 mi.   4 mi.   6 mi.   8 mi.   10 mi.   12 mi.

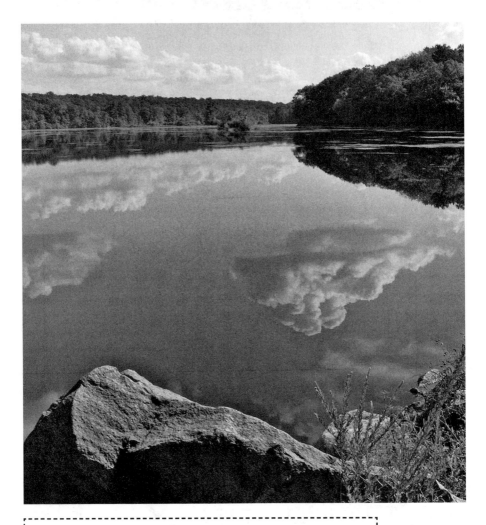

When placid, Ramapo Lake provides a perfect mirror image of these castle clouds.

atmosphere nearly around the clock. Rock crushers, too, worked all day reducing boulders to stones in the process of separating ore from tailings, while their ear-splitting racket resounded throughout the region.

By contrast, the most you are apt to hear these days, once the roar of traffic is behind you, are the dulcet notes of Mother Nature, including the territorial chirpings of birds and the siren songs of cicadas and crickets eager to find a mate. In a forest so filled with history and reflecting the myriad beauty of the Jersey Highlands, something worth photographing is always just around the corner. On one path or another, you may stumble upon a Paleolithic rock shelter or an abandoned swimming pool filled with wildflowers, frogs and turtles sunning themselves by a lily pond, an ancient outhouse perched precariously on the edge of a granite shelf, deer grazing in a grassy meadow, or a black bear gorging on blueberries. The following hike, interspersed with ponds and lakes, a number of ruins, and far-reaching vistas, serves as a colorful introduction to the Ramapo Mountains.

From the large parking area, turn around and walk to the opposite side of the road. Look for three white blazes of the Todd Trail (TT) on the telephone pole by a speed-limit sign, and head into the woods there. You descend initially over moss-padded bedrock through a setting of maple, chestnut oak, black birch, dogwood, and flowering azalea. In a couple of minutes, the TT levels off by a seasonal stream, darts around a large protruding slab of granite, and forks to the right, resuming its elevation loss. On hitting the bottom of this gully, the track meanders back toward higher ground, meeting in 10 minutes a slanted T with a forest road. Stay with the TT as it shifts first to the right, then left at a Y in 60 feet, succeeded immediately by a second right. Cruise left off the grassy forest road in another 80 feet onto a yellow-blazed trail (YT). That brings you quite rapidly to Todd Lake, an attractive lily pond surrounded by sheep laurel, dogwood, and ferns, where you shadow the shoreline clockwise to a fragmentary ruin of an old cabin (where we have, on occasion, surprised a pair of water snakes, a lizard, and several five-lined skinks sunning themselves on the rocks).

Moseying along, the YT rises to a grassy patch graced by the presence of a powder-blue water tower, only to drop away moments later, losing ground as it approaches a seasonal stream and minor cascade. The diamond-shaped yellow markings are clearly visible along this stretch as they lead higher up the hillside, cresting by a sign for the historic "Millstones," where such stones were quarried and carved decades ago. There are three discarded efforts to the right of the path, near the emergence of the white-blazed Millstone Trail, and another circular stone—the finest of the quartet—lies to the right as you begin to descend. The YT, now also bearing white tags, meanders downhill, eventually darting across the paved Glen Gray Road.

On dropping off the pavement, the path swings left by the old Tulip Springs Tent Site, dating to 1917, and parallels the road briefly before bending toward Fox Brook. It's an uphill march again, once you skip over the two bridges that span the rocky creek (look for cardinal flowers by its muddy banks in early August), with the yellow and white routes diverging in about 3 minutes. Steer right with the YT and continue upward, passing by a sizable erratic just as the track arcs to the left. In 10 minutes of steady walking, the trail levels off on the ridge and threads through a colorful area of rocks and ruins, including a ramshackle outhouse—use it only if you must! Forge onward over the bridge (an Eagle Scout project) and past the foundry foundations by the stream, then swing right at the slanted T with the grass-covered logging road, which also bears silver-on-yellow blazes. In 20 yards the YT breaks to the left, near the corroded framework of a collapsed fire tower, once more striking upward. At the false summit there are additional cabin remnants, barely discernible at ground level, but the real prize—a clear view of the Manhattan skyline to the southeast—awaits at the top of the crest.

Don't fret if haze or fog curtails the vista, for even without that New York eyeful, this remains, at 996 feet above sea level, an enchanting lichen-crusted shelf, decorated with knee-high grass, scrub oaks, and a smattering of chestnut snags. When you've had enough of the rarefied atmosphere, continue along the YT, which is joined at the summit by the MacMillan Trail (MT, orange markings). The Old Guard Trail (OGT, green tulip tree leaf on white blaze) appears a minute later on the left and can be used as a cut-through to the Cannonball Trail (CT, white C on red) if you want to slice 5 miles off the hike.

After fording a rocky debris field and a colorful seasonal runoff, the YT/MT shifts left onto a carriage road. In about 60 seconds the MT breaks to the right—follow it. Now trending downhill, this rocky route encounters a log cabin, its north end sadly collapsed and the tar-paper roof rapidly following suit, and a pair of appealing streams, only to emerge on a paved road. Go right on that and, once you have walked over the wooden car bridge, continue straight uphill with the orange blazes, back into the forest, entering a colorful clutch of high granite ridges topped by scattered cedars. This isolated area of striking rock formations ends too soon when the MT, having dropped down to a small stream, cuts sharply to the right toward MacMillan Reservoir. Your direction is over the trickling tributary to the left, on the red-and-silver-blazed Rocky Trail (RT). Before shuffling off on that, however, you might venture 10 minutes (just over half a mile) farther on the MT, through three successive trail intersections, for shore-side access to the picturesque lake.

That bit of sightseeing over, proceed along the RT as it gains nearly 200 feet over the next two-thirds of a mile. On leveling off, hold to the left side of the boggy wetland, then cross the pipeline break, churning right when you reach the patch of pavement. Scoot left at the Y, back on Bear Swamp Road, with Bear Swamp Lake beyond the trees to the right.

In hugging this side of the lake for 0.4 mile, you might pop down to the right and explore the ruins of lakeside cabins (be on the lookout for rusty nails, reclusive rodents, and slumbering snakes). The paved drive of one of these leads to an intact slate patio right by the water; the house, however, looks as though it were blown apart by a bomb. Farther on, a substantial stone foundation bristles with columbine in late spring. Cross the bridge by the dam pour-off and turn left on the CT, passing in the process yet another ruin, its chimney pointing skyward like a petrified snag.

Stick with this path for 4 miles, back to Skyline Drive. It is well marked and wide for most of that distance, overlapping old logging roads. It bypasses a couple of traces to the right, then bends right at a fork, en route to a small pond where purple irises bloom in spring and bullfrogs bellow throughout the summer. We spooked a wild turkey here once, its wings banging noisily against the close-growing birch trees as it struggled to take flight. The trail glides by a log cabin, an outpost of Camp Yaw Paw, and then swerves right, near the concrete dam of that shallow pond. *Vigilance* is your watchword for the ensuing 20 minutes, as the CT is intersected by a handful of paths, including the far end of the OGT. Fork to the right about 300 feet beyond a towering A-frame (just after a four-way junction), and lunge right again in another 3 to 4 minutes. Shortly thereafter, the path arrives at an open-topped, rectangular concrete tank, apparently an old bathing pool that now swims with lavender geraniums in May and orange jewelweed in August.

It's uphill from here, through a grassy woodland—a favorite haunt of white-tailed deer—before the path meets a small seasonal cascade that skips noisily from one stone to another. Jump to the right once you get through that rocky zone, making for the ridge. The CT merges shortly with the Hoeferlin Trail (HT, yellow blazes) and continues straight, crawling over the granite bedrock of the ridge, where spicebush and penstemon thrive, before tailing off to the left. Due to recent trail rerouting, you may have to look hard to note the three rusty trucks, circa 1945, below the slope: one upside down, another with a tree indenting its roof, all increasingly camouflaged by the forest. About a minute beyond the radio tower—100 yards away atop the ridge—the track joins the utility road leading to that tower. Dogleg left here and swing right in a few paces, pursuing the blazes back into the woods. Stride through the four-way intersection, ignore the trace that appears moments later, and continue directly between the two fenced-in gas outlets of the pipeline cut, with traffic noisily humming along Skyline Drive to the right. Hop over the concrete barriers and return to the shade of the trees. In about 5 minutes, the HT bounds to the left, and you may follow it to the parking area if you are ready to quit. (In doing so, look for the Paleolithic shelter around to the right on scrambling off the rocky bluff.)

Are you hanging with us on the CT? Great, because in addition to the lovely Ramapo Lake, a thrilling bit of drama awaits at Castle Point, not far ahead. When the CT crosses Skyline Drive, transfer to a white-blazed trail by the SLOW sign, 150 feet down the road to the left. There is a decent view to the west from a rock shelf, and then the path descends into a laurel-choked wetland, fords a serpentine stream, and slices to the left of a phragmites marsh. Next the trail swings left on a gravel track, reunites in a second with the gas-line cut, and starts up the hill. Just as the break threatens to become really steep, the path springs to the left by an easily missed, overgrown post. Blazes can be hard to spot, but in less than 3 minutes the trace slips to the left off this well-beaten track and continues over bedrock and grassy ground. Turn left at the T, under a string of power lines, and branch to the right in a few paces, leaving the wide cut. Near the top of the hill, the trail jogs left by an arrow painted on a rock, finally achieving the summit in another minute.

The views of the hills to the east—and especially of the Wanaque Reservoir, west of you—are wonderful. No less eye-catching, however, is the crenellated gray-stone tower that dominates this granite dome, where cedars and sycamores provide nominal shade and columbine and penstemon grow from the fractured bedrock. This muscular monument measures 30 feet high and a good 15 feet wide, but it is not the castle to which the name Castle Point refers. No, in spite of its medieval appearance, this is merely a cistern that once held drinking water for a nearby

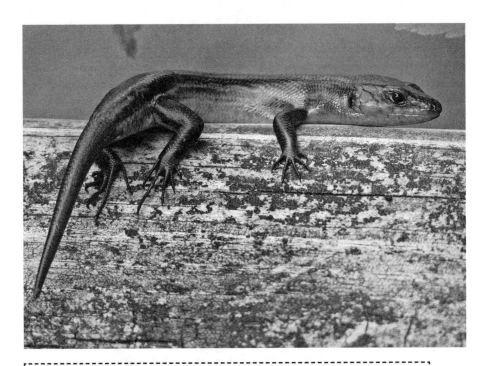

Five-lined skinks have the uncanny ability to disconnect their tail in order to escape a predator; the tail eventually grows back.

estate. The trail streaks south on the ridge, brushing by pitch pines, lilies of the valley, and, in a couple of minutes, an overgrown swimming pool, with a rickety set of stairs daring you to enter its weed-choked depths. Enough of these architectural hors d'oeuvres; the main course, the burned-out ruins of a colossal three-story fieldstone mansion, is just ahead. Now completely overgrown, this "castle" was built by William Porter (no relation to the master of short stories known as O. Henry; *this* Porter was a stockbroker) in circa 1910, but he died in a freak car accident just before his estate was finished. Porter's widow lived in the house, known alternately as Foxcroft, Oakland Castle, and Van Slyke Castle, until her death in 1940. Her heirs sold the property, and by the early 1950s it reportedly became tied up in a drawn-out divorce. Unoccupied, the mansion proved too tempting a treasure for trespassers, and by the end of the decade it was set on fire by vandals.

When you have finished exploring the ruins (and savoring the forsythia and daffodils, if you happen to be visiting in mid-April), proceed south, keeping to the east—or left—side of the ridge. The trail hops over the wall here (look for a blaze on the rocks) (GPS: **N41° 2.668' W74° 15.772'**). (Don't forget to enjoy the great view of Manhattan, and the lake below, before you start scrambling down the rocky slope.) Stay with the white blazes as they fork right, and in 1 minute head right on the forest road, which also bears the markings of the Cannonball Trail. This lane, North Shore Drive, arcs sharply to the east as it approaches Ramapo

Lake and continues clockwise around its shore. The white blazes end just before you reach the water, however, as the CT branches to the right. Remain with the forest road, now sporting blue tags, and proceed to the north end of the lake (which is, in fact, a glacial depression formed during the last ice age, between 12,000 and 15,000 years ago, a stone dam having helped to amass the remainder of the water). It is a very pretty setting, with yellow-flowering lilies on the surface, rocks around the shore, and a trickling cascade on the left.

Just as the dirt-surfaced North Shore Drive meets the lake, branch right, away from the blue blazes, circumnavigating the water counterclockwise. Bear right at the spur leading to shore access, then left as the Cannonball Trail merges from the opposite direction. Remain with the CT all the way to the south end of the lake, lurching left at the slanted T, where the CT finally breaks away. Vault left again at the subsequent fork, in 50 yards, and hang with the east side of Ramapo Lake all the way to the concrete dam, ignoring the red-blazed track that twice emerges on the right. Cross the dam, now escorted by the yellow markings of the Hoeferlin Trail (HT), and heave right onto Rye Cliff Road, leaving the pavement almost immediately when the HT (currently paired with blue ones) dives into woods to the right. After pivoting to the left, in a mere 2 minutes, and briefly paralleling Rye Cliff Road, the trail gradually delves deeper into the forest, climbing uphill on a wide, pebbly surface toward the north. Hang a right near the top of the slope, then left at a T, ignoring the trace that succeeds that. Go right at the ensuing fork, and as the path levels off, stick with the yellow markings all the way back to the parking lot, just a few stumbling steps farther on.

## NEARBY ACTIVITIES

Still have some stamina left? **Skylands Manor** and the **New Jersey Botanical Garden,** both within Ringwood State Park, make a wonderful combination of a Tudor-style mansion in a flowering environment. Gothic **Ringwood Manor,** also on the park grounds, contains 19th-century American paintings and furniture. For information and guided tours, call 973-962-7031 or visit **njparksandforests .org/parks/ringwood.html.**

In addition to Paleolithic hunters, mastodons once roamed Ramapo Mountain's verdant summit. **The Bergen Museum of Art and Science,** in Paramus, has two mastodon skeletons on display, as well as works by local and internationally known artists. For details, visit **thebergenmuseum.com.**

# 40 STERLING RIDGE TRAIL

## KEY AT-A-GLANCE INFORMATION

**LENGTH:** 14.8 miles

**ELEVATION GAIN:** 2,971 feet

**CONFIGURATION:** Balloon

**DIFFICULTY:** Very strenuous

**SCENERY:** Substantial ironworks relics, rugged mountain ridges with stellar highland views, a historic 1922 fire tower, a secluded pond, and a woodland maze of trails

**EXPOSURE:** Shady start succumbs to exposed slopes and ridges.

**TRAFFIC:** Rather solitary

**TRAIL SURFACE:** From packed dirt to densely rocky, with a few grassy patches

**HIKING TIME:** 8.5 hours

**DRIVING DISTANCE:** 32 miles

**SEASON:** Year-round, sunrise–sunset

**ACCESS:** Free; pets on leash not exceeding 6 feet, no bicycles, no motorized vehicles

**MAPS:** At visitor center at Sterling Lake (NY side); download from tinyurl.com/sterlingforestmap; USGS *Greenwood Lake*

**FACILITIES:** None, but visitor center has modern comforts.

**COMMENTS:** The park hosts a great deal of activities: snowshoeing, ice fishing, boating, and hunting. Call 845-351-5907 for information, or visit nysparks.com/parks/74/details.aspx.

## GPS COORDINATES

N41° 8.465'  W74° 18.956'

## IN BRIEF

"Alone far in the wilds and mountains I hunt," wrote Walt Whitman, in an example intrepid hikers might like to emulate here. Not to bag some of the rich range of wildlife that runs through these woods. No, the quarry to set your sights on consists of a thriving second-growth forest, boggy lowlands, fabulous vistas, and ridgetop rambles. Further explorations into the unsullied domain, which includes dramatic ruins of 18th- and 19th-century ironworks, are possible via a number of unblazed paths.

## DESCRIPTION

Just 35 miles from Central Park is one of the wildest, least-developed parcels of land in the entire metropolitan area. You want to see bobcats, black bears, coyotes, mountain lions, and rattlesnakes? They're all here, as well as red-shouldered hawks, red-bellied woodpeckers, red foxes, red-faced butterflies and, well, of course, white-tailed deer. And if you like to mix a little history with your hike, there are the sprawling ruins of a Civil War–era iron foundry to look forward to, with foundations dating back to the American Revolution.

This is Sterling Forest we're talking about, one of New York's newest state parks, a relatively undeveloped preserve of nearly

-------------------------------------------

## *Directions* ———————————→

**Follow I-95 over the George Washington Bridge and take Exit 72A onto NJ 4 West. Drive 8.3 miles, then stay straight and follow NJ 208 North for 10.2 miles before merging onto I-287. Take Exit 57 onto Skyline Drive and proceed 4.9 miles, bearing right onto the Greenwood Lake Turnpike. Continue 5.4 miles to the gravel parking lot on the left.**

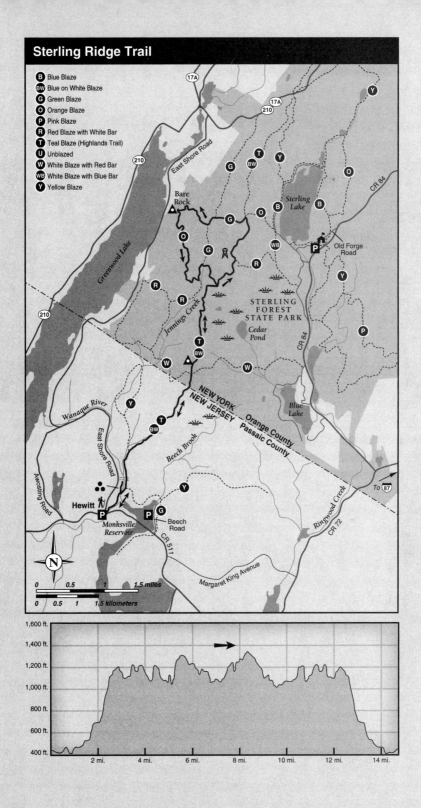

# Sterling Ridge Trail

**B** Blue Blaze
**BW** Blue on White Blaze
**G** Green Blaze
**O** Orange Blaze
**P** Pink Blaze
**R** Red Blaze with White Bar
**T** Teal Blaze (Highlands Trail)
**U** Unblazed
**W** White Blaze with Red Bar
**WB** White Blaze with Blue Bar
**Y** Yellow Blaze

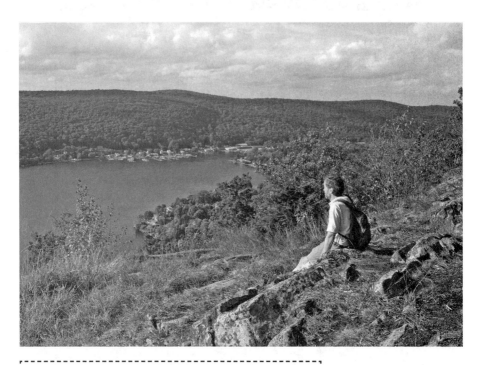

Not many hikers venture out to this solitary Greenwood Lake overlook, making it an ideal picnic spot.

20,000 acres. It wasn't always so. In 1702, the land was purchased from the Iroquois by the Earl of Stirling. Iron ore was soon discovered there, and as mining grew in importance, the trees of the forest—needed to fire the forges—dwindled proportionally. By 1885, when the property was bought by the Sterling Iron and Railway Company, hardly any trees remained. Left largely fallow, the land renewed itself, with the open fields succeeded by the dense forest you see today.

A system of trails is gradually being developed that allows the intrepid hiker to see much of the raw beauty within that forest, and a stop at the visitor center for a park map and route suggestions is highly advisable. Alternatively, you might consider the long, strenuous trek atop Sterling Ridge. To cover the entire 9-mile length of its spine, plan to leave a car at one trailhead (on the south side of Route 17A, for example) and shuttle in a second vehicle to its other end. Or, if you lack a shuttle car, try hiking in just beyond the fire tower (to roughly the two-thirds point), then out again over the same ground. The more interesting territory, arguably, lies south of the tower, and it is also the more rugged. The following write-up takes the second approach and includes a return loop through a marvelously rocky granite upland. Because of the physical demands of the terrain, think twice before bringing young children on this hike.

From the gravel parking area, walk east and cross CR 511 (Greenwood Lake Turnpike), going toward the street sign marking the right prong of East Shore

Road. Look for the steel guard rail and, near it, three blue-on-white blazes (and the teal diamonds of the Highlands Trail); those indicate the start of the Sterling Ridge Trail (SRT). Having located the trailhead, swing to the left of the guardrail and push off, heading directly under a mantle of maples. Within moments, the SRT scoots by a few concrete foundations and slag heaps (as well as vinca, violets, mayapple, and trout lilies), followed in 5 minutes by the substantial remnants of an ironworks. At the intersection just after that, keep to the left—make a mental note of this junction for your return—and you will quickly come to another ruin, known as "the company store," composed of large gray stone blocks, shored up with beams on one end. The path shifts right there and passes a couple of benches set in a nook overlooking a peaceful pond. Just upstream is a grassy meadow, with the mother lode of ironworks ruins off to the side. These massive stone buildings once housed foundry furnaces and the waterwheels to power them. Take five to explore the area, and be sure to check out the unblazed trace, to the left of and behind the second waterwheel, that leads upriver to more ruins and a powerful cascade with a 7-foot drop.

Back at the meadow, the path cuts right over a wooden footbridge—or at least it *used to* pass over a bridge. Tropical Storm Irene washed it away in 2011, and a year later it was still missing. It should have been replaced by the time this book goes to press, courtesy of an Eagle Scout project, but if it still isn't up, you will either have to wade across the stream or (if the water is low) rock-hop. Yellow blazes join those of the SRT and the Highlands Trail (HT) just across the stream, and then the trail bends left, beginning a steady uphill trend into the forest. Walking along this old road requires little effort initially, as maples are gradually displaced by hemlocks and the music of the river serenades you. Ignore the initial spur to the right, which leads downriver, but go left at the next fork, where the yellow blazes diverge with the right option. In 10 minutes a second yellow trail begins, with the spur to the left, while the SRT shifts right. And so begins the workout, as the track climbs steadily to a high ridge, veers left over a chunky streambed (usually dry by mid to late summer), hugs that swampy stream awhile, then continues the ascent up a rocky slope of scree. On approaching the stone plateau, where a couple of cedars cling to the sun-baked ground, scan the surrounding brush for wild turkeys, which frequent this area. Linger a moment, too, to enjoy the vista to the south, where the pond you brushed by earlier is so distant it might as well be a drop of dew, and if you're here in springtime, don't forget to look for Dutchman's breeches by the base of the scrub trees.

The climbing resumes via switchbacks around a craggy escarpment and a handful of shagbark hickory trees. A few dozen yards beyond is a bulging granite dome, 650 feet above the trailhead, with clear views over the hills to the west. This is the first of a series of interconnected ridgetops, and quite possibly the prettiest. Think about snacking on a sandwich here among the long golden grass, in the shade of dwarf oaks and sumac—you're going to need the energy! Moving onward along the grassy path, through maple, oak, and birch, in 10 minutes you'll see a discreet white tag on an oak indicating the state line "separating" New Jersey from New York.

Roll straight through each of the ensuing unblazed junctions, as well as the Lake to Lake Trail (LL, blazed with a red bar on white), and enjoy the next half-mile or so of fairly level, easy strolling. Then it's back into the saddle with a steep, sun-exposed climb up another 150 feet to one of the highest points of the ridge, and prime habitat for five-lined skinks. The views west from this pine-encircled rocky tor are the stuff that dream hikes are made of: that's the expansive Greenwood Lake just visible through the tree cover to the southwest, with the extended Bearfort Mountain range looming beyond. There is another scrub-pine plateau after this, with a carpet of blueberry bushes in between, and then an odd, altarlike erratic tucked under a hemlock.

Dropping into a boggy gully, the stone-spiked, mossy SRT slices first through laurels and oaks, then hits a thicket of rhododendrons prior to scaling another loose rocky embankment. This shelf is, like the previous, 850 feet above the road, and it extends for 200 yards before the path descends to a slowly defoliating hemlock hollow. Steer to the right at the intersection there, and march right through the following junction, where it meets, and is joined by, the Fire Tower Trail (FT, white bar on red). Perhaps 100 yards ahead and to the right is a high, rising series of rock fingers or granite tendrils. For a route that has yet to pursue any shortcuts and that hasn't seen a peak it didn't summit, the next move could hardly be a surprise. That's right: up and over the steepest section of those rocks. Having put that behind you, the fire tower is just minutes away.

At 5 miles out, this historic lookout post is, for many people, the return point of the hike. The 65-foot structure was built in 1922 and is still in service, as is the adjacent warden's cabin. Rather than retracing your steps back to the road, however, consider remaining on the SRT for further explorations into a lovely landscape that was slated until relatively recently to be "developed" into 15,000 homes. The hilly fun continues to the north, as the SRT hops on and off—then on again—the rocky, moss-crusted ridge. In time, the strikingly attractive trail rewards you with a clear vista of Sterling Lake, to the east, from atop an oak-studded granite shelf. A little beyond that high point, in a dip between ridge knuckles, is an important intersection, one in which the green blazes of the Western Valley Trail (WVT) fork to the left, the SRT (and Highlands Trail) maintains its northbound course, and the Bare Rock Trail (BR, orange markings) branches both to the right and left. If you are not at all interested in hiking through an unsullied area of dramatic granite uplift, highlighted by an eagle's view of Greenwood Lake, this is your turnaround stage, and you should now retrace your steps back to the south on the SRT. Otherwise hang a left on the BR.

Still with us on the orange-blazed BR? Wonderful, because some sensational scenery lies ahead. At first, the moss-rimmed track remains mostly level, passing among laurel, birch, striped maple, and a mix of oaks. You'll need to skip over a couple of narrow seasonal streams, sandwiched around an imposing talus slope, to the left. Ignore the wide, green-blazed track that merges from the right (almost immediately after the second stream), bearing left instead. In about 4 minutes (or 0.15 mile), break right, off the wide, grassy track, still following the orange blazes.

As the trail begins to gain elevation, the surroundings become noticeably wilder, with a forest floor of ferns and moss crisscrossed by an increasing number of fallen trees. This fun stretch threads through an intriguing area of glacial uplift, fractured fins, and impressive mounds, culminating in a ridgeline view through the trees of Greenwood Lake. Disappointed? Stick with the trail, and in a moment or two you will arrive at a well-signed spur that leads to Bare Rock, a short side trip to a thrilling ledgetop vista of the lake's north end.

Once again on the BR, chugging south, the trail climbs a bit, holding to the ridgeline for a while, then takes a sharp jag to the left, or north-northeast, only to circle round the highest node yet and resume its southbound course.

After perhaps 10 minutes, the BR again breaks east, descends slightly, shifts back toward the south, and, as it settles on the inland side of the western ridge, becomes more circuitous. Roundabout though it is, this route is also one of the more scenic stretches of the hike, dropping in and out of gullies, with stream crossings, and showcasing abundant rock outcroppings and erratics, several of them quite pleasing to the eye. Eventually, the BR dead-ends at a T with the Fire Tower Trail (white bar on red), a wide forest road, with an active stream gurgling alongside it. Swing left, trudging north, and in 5 minutes roll right, still on the FT, as the green-blazed Western Valley Trail proceeds straight ahead.

On making this turn, the trail edges by—and occasionally is subsumed by— an active beaver pond. To avoid the overflow, rerouting leads through the trees to the right, where it can be difficult to pick up the blazes. Once past the swamped path, look to hop back over the stream runoff and aim for the southeast corner of the pond, where the main trail resumes, forging uphill and back into forest. That challenge out of the way, you have only a few more minutes of sauntering before the FT slams into the SRT. Hang a right there, once again on Sterling Ridge, and remain on this familiar route all the way back to the trailhead.

## NEARBY ACTIVITIES

Long Pond Ironworks, on the Greenwood Lake Turnpike, has several remnants of the ironmaking industry from the 18th century, as well as a museum. Call 973-962-7031 for details, or visit njparksandforests.org/parks/longpond.html.

Skylands Manor and the New Jersey Botanical Garden, both within Ringwood State Park, make a wonderful combination of a Tudor-style mansion in a flowering environment. Gothic Ringwood Manor, also on the park grounds, contains 19th-century American paintings and furniture. For information and guided tours, call 973-962-7031 or visit njparksandforests.org/parks/ringwood.html.

# 41    STOKES SELECT

## KEY AT-A-GLANCE INFORMATION

**LENGTH:** 9.5 miles

**ELEVATION GAIN:** 1,587 feet

**CONFIGURATION:** Loop

**DIFFICULTY:** Moderate to strenuous

**SCENERY:** Marshes and wildflowers in lowland hardwood forests; stunted tree growth on mountain ridges; panoramic view of rural Sussex County atop Sunrise Mountain

**EXPOSURE:** Very little exposure, even on mountain ridges; medium exposure in winter

**TRAFFIC:** Light to moderate

**TRAIL SURFACE:** Dirt, roots, and endless rocks

**HIKING TIME:** 5 hours

**DRIVING DISTANCE:** 65 miles

**SEASON:** Year-round, sunrise–sunset

**ACCESS:** Entrance fee is charged Memorial Day–Labor Day. Residents: $5 weekdays, $10 weekends; double that for nonresidents. Dogs on leash.

**MAPS:** At park office; download from tinyurl.com/stokesmap; USGS *Culvers Gap*

**FACILITIES:** Restrooms, water, and public phone at park office

**COMMENTS:** Hunting is allowed; great camping available. For more details, call 973-948-3840 or visit njparks andforests.org/parks/stokes.html.

## GPS COORDINATES

N41° 12.184'  W74° 46.384'

## IN BRIEF

For fear of overselling a park, we normally resist assigning it too many superlatives. But in Stokes, we're stumped: this solitary, mountainous jaunt is so darn beautiful we can't help but beat the drum for it. It's a strenuous outing that alternates between lowland bogs and high-country terrain, providing several hours' communion with an extended patch of unspoiled nature. In spring, Kittatinny Mountain Ridge brims with wildflowers, while the autumn display of colors seen from this, New Jersey's highest natural point, is pure hiker heaven.

## DESCRIPTION

There are few animal sightings quite so exhilarating as an encounter with a bear. And in Stokes State Forest, visitors are constantly reminded that stumbling upon a black bear in the backcountry is a very real possibility. Although the odds are slim—these shy creatures are likely to scamper into the cover of the forest at the first sound of your approach—just the chance of seeing an *Ursus americanus* in the wild adds an extra frisson of danger to the hike. Not that this gem of a trek needs any gilding— not with the heart-stopping panorama atop Sunrise Mountain, and certainly not with much

---------------------------------------------

## *Directions* ———————————————→

Follow I-95 across the George Washington Bridge and take Exit 69 to merge onto I-80 West. Take Exit 34B, heading north on NJ 15. Continue 17.9 miles to the junction with US 206 North and follow it for 6.7 miles, then turn right onto the park road (Coursen Road). The park office is on the left. For the trailhead, proceed straight 1.8 miles, toward Stony Lake. At the T-intersection, turn right on Kittle Road and drive 0.25 mile to the trailhead parking.

# Stokes Select

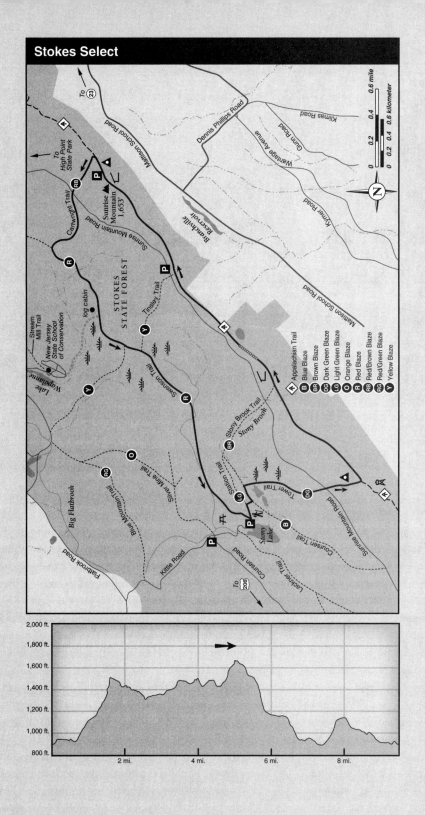

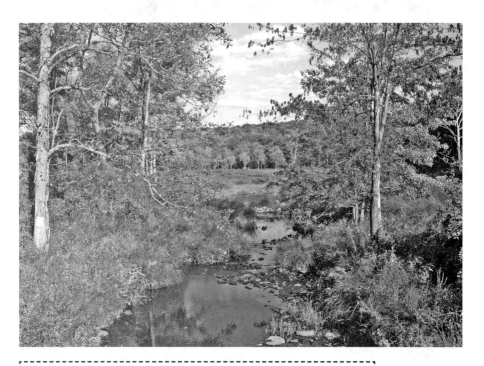

*Shhh!* Approach this watery spot quietly and you may just see blue herons, beavers, black bears, foxes, or fishers.

of your mileage accruing along the scenic Kittatinny Mountain Ridge, which erupts with wildflowers in the spring.

As you tramp over the trails, it may seem hard to believe that most of this beautiful park's 15,482 acres were completely denuded of trees as recently as a century ago. The damage began with the arrival of Dutch and English settlers who, on displacing the Lenape Indians in the early 1700s, carved large swaths of farmland out of the forest. The remaining trees came down in later decades, used up as firewood and charcoal. It is only from 1907, when an initial parcel of 5,432 acres was purchased by New Jersey, that Stokes underwent a renaissance. All that is left now of the old homesteads are ruins and rubble, largely overgrown by vast stands of oak, birch, beech, maple, and hemlock.

Your hike commences at the kiosk to the right of the paved parking area by Stony Lake. Six different colored blazes share the forest road initially as it plugs steadily upward away from the trailhead. The red markings of the Swenson Trail, your return route, break to the left within 100 yards, and a few steps later, the green-blazed Station Trail forks left, too. Hew to the right as the path narrows, and head left at the T. There is the capped well of an old cabin off the track to the left, tucked among a stand of white pines, with your turn to the right on the Tower Trail (TT, dark-green blazes) occurring just before that. Vestigial walls tumble through the swamp here, but in spring, your eyes will more likely be attracted to the abundance of wildflowers, including irises, mayapple, star-shaped anemones, violets, jack-in-the-pulpits, periwinkles, Canada mayflowers, and skunk cabbage.

For a couple of minutes, the rocky track remains rather level, sloshing through one wet spot and then another, past white birch, shagbark hickory, and some ash, as well as oak and maple, before grinding sharply upward. In slightly less than 10 minutes and a gain of 200 feet in elevation, the path levels off and cuts through a couple of seasonal streams. When it meets Sunrise Mountain Road, the TT shifts diagonally across the pavement to the right, with the steepest part of the climb still ahead. Don't let the exertion or the pebbly granola underfoot distract you from checking out the glacial deposits left and right of the trace, as well as the impressive bluff formation you are ascending. Near the crest, as you enter a concentration of mountain laurel, some fun hand-over-hand rock-scrambling is necessary to reach the top of the granite ledge.

The TT ends at a slanted T with the Appalachian Trail (AT), as the hike continues to the left. Take five, though, to catch your breath. It is possible to climb the fire tower dead ahead of you, though the hatch at the top is usually locked. Anyway, no extra height is necessary to enjoy the splendid views of the hills to the north and west, with Stony Lake far below looking no larger than a puddle. And in spring, this bald plateau is colorfully peppered with pink penstemon. Having finished your breather, walk northeast on the AT, staying with the white-blazed route for approximately 3 miles. Although the AT clings to the meandering Kittatinny Mountain Ridge at an average elevation of 1,400 feet, most of the year vistas are rather limited, due to the extensive scrub vegetation. Still, the forested scenery is quite appealing, with sheep laurel, serviceberry, and flowering azalea adding a welcome contrast to the mix of hardwoods, and occasional bog pots providing fertile ground for wildflowers and amphibians.

Your first glimpse of Sunrise Mountain comes shortly beyond the yellow-blazed fork of the Tinsley Trail to the left. At an altitude of 1,653 feet, it appears to tower above the surrounding ridge, but after a minor descent, the climb to its peak is accomplished in little more than 2 minutes. The massive stone picnic shelter that crowns this knob like an oversize tiara was built by the Civilian Conservation Corps in the latter half of the 1930s, while a U.S. Geological Survey crew later added the low obelisk. The stupendous panorama, meanwhile, has been provided by Mother Nature, with views extending in every direction but north, where the horizon is partially obscured by trees. While you are scanning the surrounding countryside for recognizable landmarks, you may hear hawks screeching and see other raptors or vultures soaring by at eye level.

The AT zips over a fin of rock on the east side of this ridge, descending momentarily toward an adjacent parking lot just off Sunrise Mountain Road. The spur to the right, as you near the lot, leads to a sun-struck rocky shelf, where two benches face the east, overlooking the lush farmlands of Jersey. The AT then drops down over a stone staircase and skirts to the right of the parking area. Aim your eyes left shortly after that, scanning the shrubs for the brown-over-red blaze of the Cartwright

Trail (CT) (GPS: N41° 13.280' W74° 42.896'). The start of this trace tends to be badly overgrown, making it all too easy to miss your turn. Much of the next mile is through wild, untrammeled terrain, contributing a healthy dose of natural beauty to what, for us, is one of the most delightful parts of the hike.

On gliding directly over a rising mound of bedrock (not to its right, as it first appears), the CT zigzags downward into a grove of pitch pines, descending abruptly from there into an avalanche of rubble and glacial erratics. Cross Sunrise Mountain Road and continue into the dense forest, where an occasional fallen tree or broken limb may require minor bushwhacking to proceed. In 10 minutes, the CT tapers lower over a chunky moraine field that doubles as a seasonal streambed. With blazes hard to see here, your best approach is to move due west, holding to the left of the streambed. The Cartwright trace ends at a T with the Swenson Trail (ST, red blazes), by a gravelike mound of stones, a tumulus that may explain, finally, what became of Adam.

Scoot to the left and remain with the ST all the way back to the trailhead, a distance of about 3 miles. The path swings through a boggy patch en route and hopscotches over a couple of seasonal streams, pulling up in a dozen minutes to a cabin. Stay straight, cruising to the left of the bog ponds, as the track begins to ascend into a rocky environment. Within 5 minutes of leaving the cabin, the ST hits the Tinsley Trail, whereupon Swenson jumps left, part of a delayed dogleg that is completed in about 3 minutes when it breaks to the right, leaving the wide track. Some rock-hopping over streams ensues, in part of a swampy precinct that attracts an abundance of birds (and bugs). The wandering trail finally enters into a concentration of laurels and white pines before merging with the main route. The trailhead is straight onward, a 3-minute stagger away.

The fun may not end with the unlacing of your boots. Seconds after driving away, on the completion of one of our hikes here, we had to hit the brakes as a 450-pound black bear abruptly lumbered out of the woods and shuffled across the park road. It was a humid summer afternoon, and he seemed in no hurry, but the forest had swallowed him up before we could extricate a camera from our pack.

*Note:* This park offers great camping—and fishing—near a trout-stocked stream and lake. In winter, bring your cross-country skis, snowshoes, or ice skates. A great, short alternative hike is a 2-mile foray into the **Tillman Ravine Natural Area,** a dense grove of hemlocks and rhododendrons featuring several species of endangered plants and animals. For further information, call 973-948-3820 or visit **njparksandforests.org/parks/stokes.html.**

## NEARBY ACTIVITIES

Take a cooling break at the **Newton Fire Museum.** The historic building dates from 1891, and its collection houses horse carriages, steamer engines, alarm systems, uniforms, and period photographs. For further details, call 973-383-0396 or visit **newtonfiremuseum.org.**

# TURKEY-EGYPT CONNECTION

## IN BRIEF

It doesn't take a trip on the Orient Express to experience exotic scenery, as this exhilarating hike proves. The myriad trails of this beautiful county park profile a wilder, untamed side of nature while leading to historic cabin ruins, a waterfall, countless swampy streams, mysterious erratics, far-reaching views, a grassy cedar grove, rich birding opportunities, and even the chance of seeing black bears.

## DESCRIPTION

Our hiking pals out West tend to rattle on with a peacock's pride about their treks through glacier-wracked terrain. Sure, there are still some glaciers on the Left Coast that haven't yet succumbed to global warming. But when it comes to seeing up close the impact a glacier can have on its environment, we in the New York region have no reason to hang our heads—not with so much of our landscape scooped and carved into gorges, gullies, gulches, kettles, and ravines by the last ice age. Not when so many mountain lakes and eccentric erratics have been left behind as reminders of those melting blocks of snow.

One block in particular, the Wisconsin Glacier, was responsible for much of the

---

### *Directions* ⟶

**Follow I-95 across the George Washington Bridge and take Exit 69 to merge onto I-80 West. Drive to Exit 43B and merge onto I-287 North. Continue to Exit 44 (Boonton) and turn right at the end of the ramp on Lathrop Avenue, and right again onto Main Street. In 0.3 mile, swing right on Boonton Avenue and proceed north for 3.3 miles to the parking lot and visitor center, on the left.**

---

### ⓘ KEY AT-A-GLANCE INFORMATION

**LENGTH:** 9.7 miles (can be broken into a smaller 5-mile loop and a 4.5-mile figure-eight)

**ELEVATION GAIN:** 1,517 feet

**CONFIGURATION:** Loop connected to a figure-eight

**DIFFICULTY:** Moderately strenuous

**SCENERY:** Humid wetlands, hardwood forests, grassy fields, huge rock formations, old farm sites, expansive views

**EXPOSURE:** Mostly dense canopy

**TRAFFIC:** Pyramid Mountain attracts far more visitors than Turkey Mountain.

**TRAIL SURFACE:** Rock-packed dirt with some grassy areas

**HIKING TIME:** 5 hours

**DRIVING DISTANCE:** 36 miles

**SEASON:** Year-round, sunrise–sunset

**ACCESS:** Free; foot traffic only, pets on leash not exceeding 6 feet

**MAPS:** At visitor center; morrisparks .net/aspparks/pyrmtntr.asp; USGS *Boonton*

**FACILITIES:** Portable toilets, public phone, and water at visitor center

**COMMENTS:** Guided trail walks are a great way to experience the area's geology and ecology. Call 973-334-3130 for further details, or visit morrisparks.net /aspparks/pyrmtnmain.asp.

## GPS COORDINATES

N40° 56.801'  W74° 23.320'

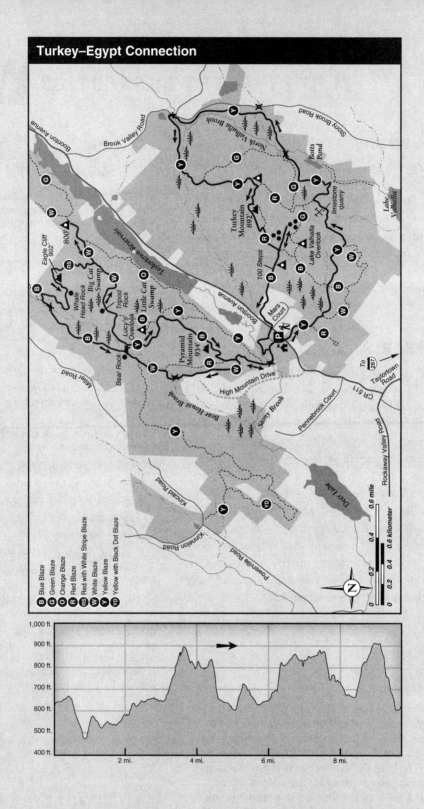

# Turkey–Egypt Connection

beauty on display at Pyramid Mountain Natural Historical Area, a Morris County park. When it disappeared about 18,000 years ago, the glacier deposited a number of extraordinary boulders, including Bear Rock, estimated to be the largest erratic in the Garden State, and Tripod Rock, a unique combination of one enormous stone supported by three diminutive ones. The numerous swamps and streams, as well as a dramatic waterfall, also reflect that climatic heritage. Those, in turn, help nourish the amazing array of wildflowers, in addition to the bears, bobcats, black-capped chickadees, and pileated woodpeckers (to name just a few) that dwell in this densely forested park.

When developers threatened to bulldoze Pyramid and Turkey Mountains in the 1990s, conservationists successfully teamed with Morris County officials to create this preserve. More than 1,000 acres of land are now protected—land so unspoiled, so beautiful, we know exactly where to take our Western hiking friends on their next visit. This prolonged trek incorporates both mountains, situated on opposite sides of Boonton Avenue. It may be broken into two shorter loops, though, if you lack the time for the full circuit. We like to start with Turkey Mountain, saving the more dramatic Pyramid Mountain for last. From the park exit, stroll to the other side of Boonton Avenue and step around the pipe gate (GPS: N40° 56.752' W74° 23.314'). Stay with this forest road, blazed yellow, as it passes a spur on the right and a bog on the left, then crosses a four-way intersection. Beech trees are the dominant hardwood in this shady hollow, with ample support from oaks, maples, black birches, and tulip poplars.

Remain with the yellow markings as they swing left at the T, at the bottom of the slope. Walk by the cabin ruins, and in a couple of minutes rock-hop over the confluence of swamp streams, a picturesque spot made all the prettier by the presence of skunk cabbage and ferns. The track begins to climb after that, leveling off in 5 minutes by flowering dogwoods, where it bends abruptly to the right. In a few steps the path brings you by the overgrown remnants of a limestone quarry, with trees growing out of the pits on either side of the path. Continuing onward, the yellow-blazed route arcs toward the northeast, skips by a spur on the left (red tags) and then breaks from the wide track, making a hairpin pivot to the left. Head that way, bounding over some small seasonal streams while approaching a broad swamp. The birding is great, incidentally, by Botts Pond, down the spur to the right, with warblers, scarlet tanagers, and indigo buntings among the warm-weather visitors.

There are numerous erratics in this vicinity, many impressively large, as you ascend to a power-line break. Look for a yellow blaze on the right leg of the stanchion, and bear to the right as the path returns to the woods a second later. This is a wonderfully wild nook of the bog, with oversize rocks rising off the fern-dappled ground and silver-barked beech saplings gleaming in the sunlight. A few minutes of rolling with the undulating terrain brings you to a four-way intersection. The hike proceeds to the right, but straight ahead there is a sensational

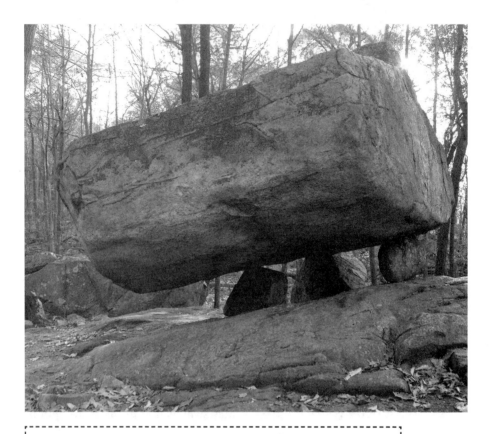

Massive Tripod Rock is but one of many dramatic geologic formations along this circuit.

waterfall, where you can see an extended cascade drop 12 feet to a dark pool, then gurgle noisily through a rocky streambed.

If you can pull yourself away from this splashy crasher, cross the bridge and cut up the middle of the three trails that appear immediately after it. This crawls above the falls, paralleling North Valhalla Brook while meandering up and down, through swamp and forest, for the next mile. There is so little foot traffic in this part of the park that you are just as likely to see the paw prints of bears, bobcats, or beavers in the muddy stream banks as anything left behind by the sole of a biped. You may also observe odd red stones larded with specks of white quartzite. These conglomerates, known colloquially as puddingstone (supposedly because it resembles English meat pudding), are common to Bearfort Mountain, in Wawayanda State Park.

In about 20 minutes, the path comes to a T and shifts right, then squiggles left, avoiding Stony Brook Road, visible through the trees. Several minutes hence, the trail merges with the road, glides left, crosses the bridge, and hops to the left back into the forest, still beside the lovely North Valhalla Brook. The resident naturalist reports that bears inhabit the woods higher up the slope, including some mamas with cubs, so remain vigilant and you may observe much more than the dark cup fungi that often dot the soil. The yellow blazes dart to the left at a fork that follows, gradually gaining elevation among mountain laurels and a fair peppering of glacial debris. Edge right at the ensuing fork, where a green-blazed route branches left. The path crests by a grassy knoll amid cedars and oaks, and ends at a T with a red-blazed track. Turn right on red, as they say at traffic school, and hop right again in a couple of yards at the ensuing wishbone intersection, where you may see white-tailed deer frolicking among the cedars. The altitude here, if you scale the gray rock that towers nearby, is 892 feet.

The trail forks in 3 minutes, with the diverging legs rejoining in approximately 800 feet on the other side of this grass-decked dome. The presence of flowering fruit trees by a stone wall reinforces the notion that this little patch of Eden was once cultivated turf. The path then descends to a marshy bog as cedars yield to chestnut oaks and other hardwoods before abruptly surging uphill again and ending in the open expanse of the power-line cut. You can pick up the Blue Trail in roughly 25 paces to the right. To the left, incidentally, just off a path that was closed as of our last visit for grass regeneration, lie two sizable cabin ruins. The first, through a scrub of sumac, sheep laurel, blueberry bushes, and dwarf oaks, lies the left of the trace, overgrown with wisteria. The second is to the right of a power-line stanchion, where the unblazed path ends. Tucked among spicebush and covered—in spring—with colorful columbine, this stone foundation was once the summer cabin of an artist who toiled for the American Museum of Natural History early in the last century. He reportedly abandoned the place when the power lines were installed. It's easy to understand the attraction of this setting, what with the vista to the east from atop the hill. On a clear day, you may not be able to see forever, but the Manhattan skyline is certainly a possibility.

Reverse course and scoot back down the cut, picking up the blue blazes as you cling to the exposed ground. There is yet another fine vantage point here, this time facing the hills to the west, beyond Pyramid Mountain. Immediately after that are the 100 Steps, a series of stones assembled like a staircase to simplify maintenance access to the utility lines. On different occasions, we've counted 138 and 147 steps—but never 100 (or 39, for that matter). No matter what the tally, though, this is a surprisingly fun descent, in part because the path threads through a thick overgrowth of maple, chestnut oak, spicebush, cedar, and flowering azalea, effectively concealing the power lines overhead.

You trough at a boggy wetland, surrounded by moss, ferns, and a few white birch trees, and in 5 minutes recross Boonton Avenue. The Blue Trail proceeds ahead, but if you are ready to call it quits, head left to the parking lot. In 20 yards, Blue doglegs left, then right and soon crosses a bridge. On meeting a yellow-blazed path, pivot left, still on Blue; then, as the climb becomes steeper, keep right of the power-line stanchion, staying with the blue markings until the junction with the White Trail (WT, white blazes), which you follow to the left. A dip ensues, with two wooden spans over a seasonal stream; then it's steadily uphill along the break to another stanchion, at which point the WT veers right, into the cover of the forest. The stone foundation by the crook of the brook is all that remains of the Morgan farmstead, once used as a hideout by the Tar Rope Gang, a group notorious for "liberating" merchandise from local stores.

In a short time the path arrives at the humongous Bear Rock, so named, some say, because the Lenape Indians associated the etched lines on the rock with the claw marks of a bear. (Others insist that the 25-foot-high, 45-foot-long erratic earned its sobriquet from its resemblance, seen at certain angles, to a sleeping bear.) When you are finished admiring this impressive monolith, head right over the bridge and boardwalk, then scamper left at the fork (where the yellow blazes angle to the right). That is Bear Swamp over your left shoulder, where the skunk cabbage is a backdrop to violets, yellow asters, gentians, and cardinal flowers. A steep ascent through a moraine field, requiring your best eggbeater gait, concludes in 4 minutes—and an elevation gain of 180 feet—at an oak-and-laurel-covered ridge. Go left with the WT at the next fork, where the blue markings diverge in the opposite direction.

There are a number of glacial erratics along this knobby ridge, but nothing quite so unique as Tripod Rock, 400 feet from the last junction. Some believe that Paleolithic peoples used it in conjunction with neighboring rocks as a kind of cosmic sundial to predict the summer solstice and best harvest time. To judge by the impromptu fire rings in the vicinity, primitive rites are still being observed here. The WT continues north on this shelf, rubbing up against Big Cat Swamp, where bobcats reportedly roam, and arrives in 8 or so minutes at your left onto the Red-with-White-Stripes Trail (RWS). Before you leave the ridge, though, we suggest you persist with the WT for another 5 minutes to its junction with the Orange Trail, where a granite-based vista point (800 feet elevation) overlooks the Taylortown Reservoir.

Back with the RWS, the stretch moving toward a low, rocky bluff known as Eagle Cliff is a colorful, visually appealing area of puddingstone and erratics, with many of the latter so oddly shaped they are easily assigned zoomorphic identities. After encountering an oversize elliptical erratic, known as Whale Head Rock, slip between a fissure in the bedrock and begin to descend. Slice to the left on the trace as you drop off that ledge, and in 3 minutes of navigating through a slanted rubble field, you should hit the bottom. The RWS then veers sharply right, avoiding a couple of boggy streams, and ends at a T. Swing left there, now with blue blazes, and in 10 minutes you will be back at Bear Rock, facing its north side. (Keep an eye out for deer on the rocky ridge to the right as you stroll this stretch.) Trot left there, once more crossing over the bridge and boardwalk. This time, though, keep to the right on the Yellow Trail and traipse on up the hill.

The jagged ledges flanking the rocky track are known collectively as Cat Rocks, for the bobcats that reputedly reside here. (The wild-turkey tail feathers we once found on this spot may have been evidence of a feline feast.) Heave to the right at the top of the ridge, as blue blazes coalesce with the yellow, and take a right

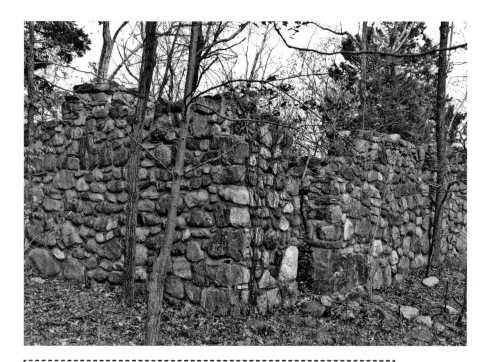

It's not hard to imagine that an artist once had a summer cabin on this solitary hilltop.

again in 150 feet, as the two colors diverge. With beech, oak, maple, and birch trees occupying much of the arable space, the autumn foliage season is a great time to do this stretch. A number of spurs to the left end at great viewpoints facing east to Turkey Mountain and the surrounding hills, with the blue-blazed path arriving at one momentarily. The peak of this plateau follows, though views in summer from its crown, at 934 feet, are limited by scrub oaks. And then it's down the side of the mountain over bedrock, loose rock, and dirt. The path swerves left at the power-line cut; hang with it all the way back to the bridge, rolling right on the broad track, which returns you to the nature center and parking area.

## NEARBY ACTIVITIES

Just up the road, near Pompton Plains, is **Mountainside Park,** renowned for its butterflies. Late May is the peak season for sightings of falcate orangetip, southern cloudywing, and a great variety of skippers, to name just a few. Year-round highlights include the ruins of an old Boy Scout log cabin, dating to the 1930s, and a stellar view of the Manhattan skyline from the crest. Aside from an occasional dog-walker, the 3-mile loop sees very little foot traffic. For further details, visit **naba.org/chapters/nabanj/sites/mtspark.html.**

# 43 WAWAYANDA 1: WAY WAY YONDER

## GPS COORDINATES

N41° 11.294'  W74° 25.518'

## IN BRIEF

If you feel pangs of pain on finishing this hike, those may owe more to the regret of leaving such a pristine environment than any blisters accumulated during the outing. From the heights of its granite-graced ridgetops to the depths of a sprawling rhododendron swamp, there is nothing run-of-the-mill about Wawayanda State Park. Spend a day on the vast network of trails of this wa-wa-wonderful property, and you're bound to see wildflowers and wildlife, but relatively few people.

## DESCRIPTION

There are about 6 miles of the Appalachian Trail coursing through Wawayanda State Park. We once asked a ranger what to expect of that stretch. "Views, I guess, but you might as well be hiking in Kansas," he huffed. His preferred stomping grounds were two of the natural areas, Wawayanda Swamp and Bearfort Mountain, tucked within the 16,679 acres comprising this wild, remote preserve. We offer the following trek as a hearty endorsement of that

------------------------------------------

## *Directions*

Follow I-95 over the George Washington Bridge and take Exit 72A onto NJ 4 West. Drive 8.3 miles, then stay straight and follow NJ 208 North for 10.2 miles before merging onto I-287. Take Exit 57 onto Skyline Drive and proceed 4.9 miles, bearing right onto the Greenwood Lake Turnpike. Continue for 8.1 miles and stay straight onto CR 513/Union Valley Road. After 0.3 mile, bear right on the Warwick Turnpike. The park entrance is 4.7 miles ahead, on the left. Follow Wawayanda Road for 2.2 miles to the left turnoff for the lake beach, and drive to the boat launch/rentals parking area, to the far left.

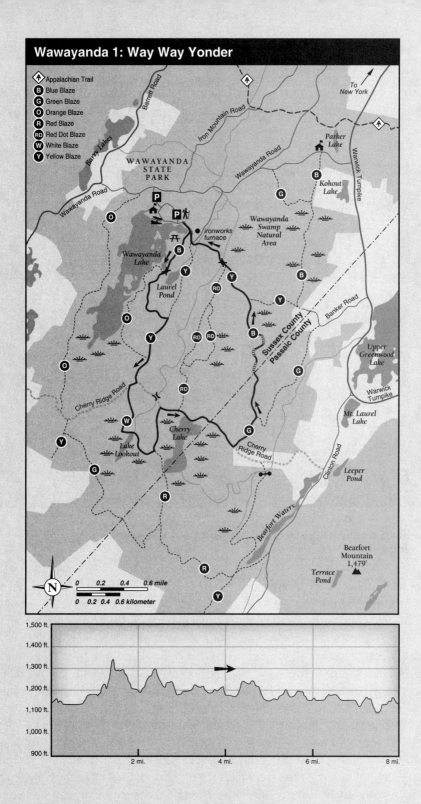

# Wawayanda 1: Way Way Yonder

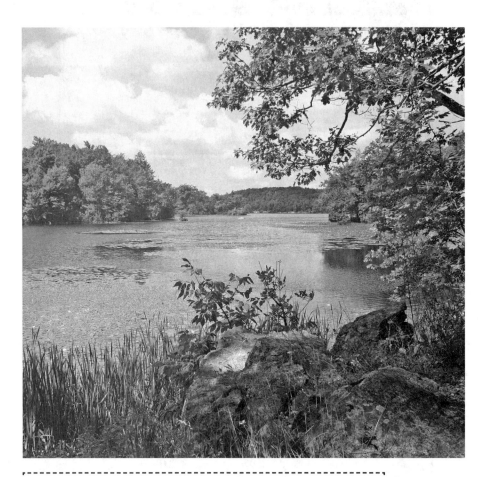

Wawayanda Lake draws all types of people, from boaters, fishermen, sun lovers, and picnickers to artists. And swimmers, of course!

recommendation. This lengthy jaunt is peppered from start to finish with an awe-inspiring beauty that reaches its pinnacle numerous times atop granite-graced ridges, and in the magical setting of a vast rhododendron swamp. It is the hike for which you've been waiting—one so enchanting it's likely to draw you back again and again.

Just 300 feet from the north shore of Wawayanda Lake are the disintegrating remnants of Double Pond, a 19th-century iron-smelting village. The most striking survivor from that distant era is the charcoal blast furnace, a mortarless stone-block behemoth that measures 30 feet across at its base and a staggering 37 feet high. The furnace was in use from 1846 to 1857, producing pig iron of such high quality that it was formed into train wheels, as well as Union cavalry swords during the Civil War. More recently, during the first half of the 1900s, the New Jersey Zinc Company logged this region, using the timber for props to strut up its far-flung mines. The vast network of forest roads here dates from that time.

For some people, the name of this park easily takes the form of "way-way-yonder," in part because of its remote position in the Highlands of New Jersey, and partly due to the ambitious hikes engaged in here. In truth, though, *Wawayanda* is a Lenape Indian word that means "winding, winding water." No question about it: an exhilarating all-day trek through this wilderness wonderland will wind you from one watery spot to another. If you lack the sole for that sort of distance, try splitting the walk into shorter segments, doing the following hike one day, for instance, and coming back another time to concentrate on the Bearfort Mountain Natural Area, described in our next hike.

This colorful hike begins at the parking area by Wawayanda Lake's boat-rental facility. Facing the water, stroll to the far left corner of the lot and proceed along the gravel lane through the picnic area, staying near the cattail-rimmed lake. Keep to the right, by the railing, where the Wingdam Trail (WT) starts, and follow its blue blazes over the grass-covered dam. Once across that dam, the WT surges straight ahead, while the option to the left is your return route (skip the unblazed trace to the right). For the next mile, the WT rises and falls, mimicking the undulations of this hilly terrain. It drifts between two ridges, well shaded by hemlock, cedar, beech, black birch, and oak trees, and (just after an unblazed trail appears on the right) brings you to a lily marsh, fringed with rhododendrons and fed by spill-off from the lake. There is a brief opening in the canopy as you stride over a bridge, and then it's uphill among rhododendrons, with granite boulders on either side of the path and dirt and stones crunching underfoot. In 5 minutes, after passing the start of the orange-blazed Sitting Bear spur, the trail levels off on a grassy plateau at an altitude of 1,200 feet.

The WT arcs east from there, passing over rocks, partly descending the hill, and ends in about a minute at a junction with the Laurel Pond Trail (LPT, yellow blazes). Hang a right, as the path hugs an impressively rocky ridge with a great view across a gaping ravine. As is common in these highland woods, the scenery changes from moment to moment, with the beech trees and boulders being replaced by a resurgence of rhododendrons and hemlocks—part of the sprawling Wawayanda Swamp. The LPT ends at a forest road, where your route hooks right, toward a pair of red gate posts on an unpaved piece of the Cherry Ridge Road. Slip by those pillars, and in less than 60 seconds bound left, onto the Lookout Trail (LT, white blazes). This lovely, narrow track, sided by ferns and shaded by a mix of hardwoods, passes a negligible trace under a clutch of hemlocks, where it surges downhill to the left, drawing you to the north end of Lake Lookout. Do as its name suggests and look out for blue herons and other waterfowl, for beavers, for milkweed flowering around its rim, and for a comfortable spot in which to indulge in a snack or a sip of water. Having taken care of such niceties, proceed across the grassy dam (try to ignore the ugly mess that local partiers have left behind) and walk straight back into the shady embrace of the forest, through a patch of pines and hemlocks, reaching a junction with the Old Coal Trail (OCT, red blazes) in approximately 6 minutes. Turn left and plan on

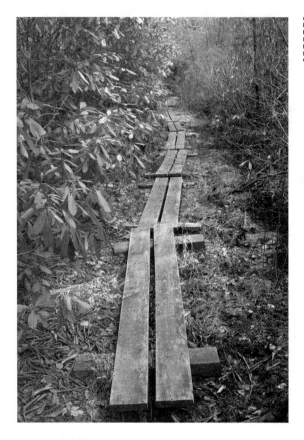

Duckboards help ease the way through the often-flooded swamps of Wawayanda.

remaining with this wide path for the next 5 to 10 minutes, until it meets Cherry Ridge Road, an unpaved forest track.

Turn left on Cherry Ridge Road and continue along it for about 1 mile. (If you're looking to end the hike early, you can take the Red Dot path, surfacing on the left in a handful of minutes.) Although less scenic than most other areas of the park, this route does rub up against an appealing swamp (to the right), just before you arrive at another pair of red gate posts. Keep trudging along the road until you reach yet another set of posts, taller yellow ones, and just up the road, at a convoluted turnaround, swing left onto the green-blazed Banker Trail (BT).

Heading directly into the woods, the grass-verged BT is a welcome return to nature as it brushes by an abundance of boulders, laurels, and occasional clumps of squaw root. The dense patch of rhododendrons that follows, as well as a reed marsh and overall boggy conditions, are reminders that you are back in the Wawayanda Swamp Natural Area. It may not have the high drama of the Bearfort region, but there is a certain serenity to this secluded swale, and a subtle beauty, too. As the conifers recede amid a lustrously luminous bower of beech saplings, a fork materializes to the left—take it. This is the Cedar Swamp Trail (blue blazes), which travels at times through rhododendron alamedas (with a fabulous display of pale-pink flowers in mid-July), alternately gaining and losing ground, occasionally relying on moss-covered stones and pontoon roots to get by the swampy overflow.

All of which is just a warm-up to the real treat of trucking through the natural area. Shortly after the trail jogs left by a rusty old car being swallowed by vegetation, it enters the cedar swamp in earnest. Here commences a quarter-mile of continuous planks (they're too narrow to be described as a boardwalk!), a string of lumber that would make it possible, under ideal conditions, to wander this wild, uncorrupted bayou without getting one's feet too wet. This swamp being a reflection of real nature, not a theme park, conditions are seldom ideal, and the last several times we've ventured into it, lengthy sections of the boards have resembled badly distributed dominoes, forcing us to stretch, leap, and otherwise improvise in order to get through with only mildly moistened boots. From early spring through midsummer, the air is filled with the alien calls of peeper frogs and sundry birds hunting for insects. When the path rises from this sweet locale (be alert for deer, and wild turkeys on the embankment to the right), it merges with the Double Pond Trail (yellow blazes), bending to the left. Some broad swamp pools often engulf the trail ahead, requiring additional contortionism on the part of hikers. Skip the Red Dot Trail, which appears on the left in a couple of minutes, and cruise past an extension of the swamp and over a boardwalk–cum–wooden bridge. While doing so, be sure to look for the beaver lodge 300 feet to the right, concealed among the scrub.

Finally back on higher turf, the path slips around a green gate, bringing you to the paved road of the group campsite. Stay with that as it drifts left briefly, then right, crossing a bridge and then going straight by the vaulted toilets to a five-way intersection. Dominating this scene is the massive stone blast furnace of the Wawayanda ironworks that once filled the sky with black smoke. To return to the parking lot, seize the second trail from the left, an uphill route. In 2 minutes, it drops you by the dam at the edge of Wawayanda Lake, where you trot to the right, back on the WT.

## NEARBY ACTIVITIES

For something warmly rewarding after your rhododendron-jungle experience, there is an alluring winery, just across the New York border, that might entice you. The **Warwick Valley Winery & Distillery** not only produces, ah, wine, it also crafts fruit nectars, ciders, and gin in elegantly labeled bottles. As if that's not enough, there's also house-made bread, baked from scratch! Indulge yourself with a first impression at **wvwinery.com.**

# 44  WAWAYANDA 2: TERRACE POND

### KEY AT-A-GLANCE INFORMATION

**LENGTH: 4.8 miles**

**ELEVATION GAIN: 638 feet**

**CONFIGURATION: Loop**

**DIFFICULTY: Moderate**

**SCENERY: Rocky puddingstone ridges, beaver swamps, a lush lake, laurel and rhododendron thickets**

**EXPOSURE: Mainly shady, with exposure on ridges**

**TRAFFIC: Well trafficked in summer, mostly by lake visitors**

**TRAIL SURFACE: Rocky ledges, packed dirt, grassy stretches**

**HIKING TIME: 2.5 hours**

**DRIVING DISTANCE: 39 miles**

**SEASON: Year-round, 8 a.m.–8 p.m.**

**ACCESS: Free; no bikes, no motorized vehicles, dogs on leash**

**MAPS: At park office; download from park website below; USGS *Wawayanda***

**FACILITIES: At park office, but none at trailhead**

**COMMENTS: Hunting is allowed. Beaver activity calls for waterproof boots. For further details, call 973-853-4462 or visit njparksandforests .org/parks/wawayanda.html.**

## GPS COORDINATES

N41° 8.578' W74° 24.452'

## IN BRIEF

The high point of this short outing, both literally and figuratively, is an extended rocky ridge overlooking beautiful, pristine Terrace Pond. Sure, there's also an antediluvian swamp and miles of scenic, secluded backcountry trails. But what you're likely to savor most will be the exhilaration of scrambling through the puddingstone formations that compose that rocky ridge.

## DESCRIPTION

No visit to Wawayanda State Park can really be considered complete without hiking through two of its natural areas, the cedar swamp and Bearfort Mountain. The cedar-swamp area, described in detail in the preceding hike, features a prolonged passage via duckboards through the bayoulike conditions of a rhododendron jungle. In short, there's nothing like it anywhere else. The same superlative may fairly be applied to the Bearfort Mountain side of the park. Trails forge over and around an extended—and quite extensive—ridge of puddingstone fins and uplift, leaving most hikers agog at the otherworldly beauty of this unique

-------------------------------------------

## *Directions* ——————————————➤

Follow I-95 over the George Washington Bridge and take Exit 72A onto NJ 4 West. Drive 8.3 miles, then stay straight and follow NJ 208 North for 10.2 miles before merging onto I-287. Take Exit 57 onto Skyline Drive and proceed 4.9 miles, bearing right onto the Greenwood Lake Turnpike. Continue for 8.1 miles and stay straight onto CR 513/Union Valley Road. After 0.3 mile, bear right on the Warwick Turnpike. Proceed 2.3 miles and turn left on Clinton Road. The trailhead parking is 1.7 miles ahead on the right, across from the trailhead.

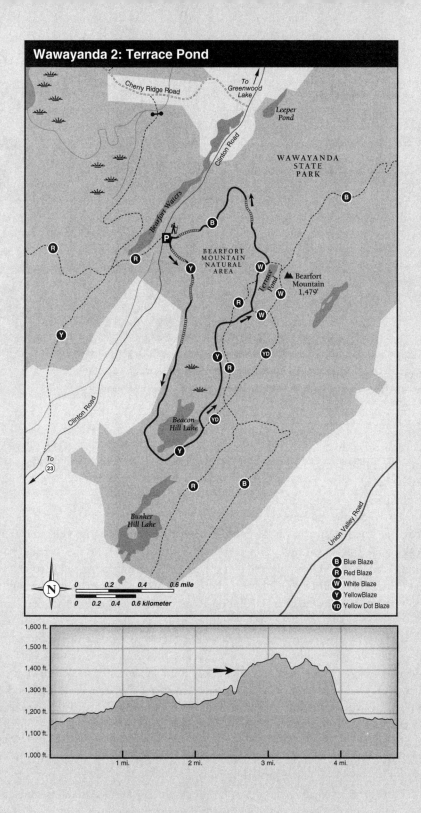

# Wawayanda 2: Terrace Pond

Cherry Ridge Road

To Greenwood Lake

Leeper Pond

Clinton Road

WAWAYANDA STATE PARK

Bearfort Waters

P

BEARFORT MOUNTAIN NATURAL AREA

Terrace Pond

▲ Bearfort Mountain 1,479'

Beacon Hill Lake

Clinton Road

To 23

Bunker Hill Lake

Union Valley Road

**B** Blue Blaze
**R** Red Blaze
**W** White Blaze
**Y** YellowBlaze
**YD** Yellow Dot Blaze

N

| 0 | 0.2 | 0.4 | 0.6 mile |
| 0 | 0.2 | 0.4 | 0.6 kilometer |

1,600 ft.
1,500 ft.
1,400 ft.
1,300 ft.
1,200 ft.
1,100 ft.
1,000 ft.

1 mi.    2 mi.    3 mi.    4 mi.

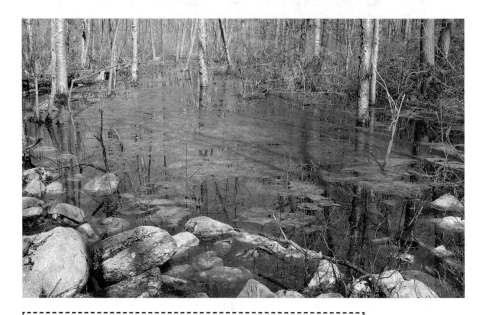

Spring peepers cheerfully announce their presence in this shallow vernal pond.

environment. Much of that puddingstone involves the sort of hand-over-foot scrambling that brings out the child-playing-explorer in all of us. The hike itself may be rather short, but the thrill of doing it is likely to linger long after you've left the park.

To reach the puddingstone paradise of Bearfort Mountain, walk directly across the road from the dirt-surfaced parking area and pick up the trail in the break of the thicket. Almost immediately, the path forks. Take the Terrace Pond South Trail (TPS, yellow blazes) to the right, a narrow, moss-sided route that meanders up the slanted hill. The trees here are similar to what you will find in the larger part of Wawayanda across Clinton Road, but the terrain is far wilder, partly due to its corrugated, rock-and-ridge texture, and in part because fewer of the trails overlap forest roads. Also, several of its swampy sections rise like floodwaters from late winter through midspring, requiring a fun rock-hop two-step to ford them. One such boggy stretch occurs within a few minutes, where duckboards, log corduroys, and a long series of rocks ease the way. As the serpentine TPS slithers uphill, it showcases a number of appealing boulders, many split by vertical fissures, as well as a head-high thicket of rhododendrons. Ignore the trace to the right atop the rocky plateau, and lean left in another minute as a forest road merges from the right. Stay with the yellow blazes, bypassing the next pair of overgrown traces, both on the left, and then steer left at the wide intersection.

Next up is an algae-covered pond, though not the Terrace Pond to which this trail's name refers. Nor is the black body of water that follows, which you reach after holding to the left at a Y. From that second dark pool, where glacial erratics, mountain laurels, and white pines flavor the setting, the bayou expands, with huge, stride-stopping puddles often straddling the path. The TPS has been rerouted to the right, scuttling over the rocks to get by these obstructions, saving your boots from a dunking—for now. The whittled twigs by the water's edge, incidentally, are the work of beavers, and a lodge lies cloaked by foliage to the left as you bolt over a pair of large drainage pipes. When the Yellow Dot Trail (yellow spots on white rectangles) surfaces on the right, vault left, still with the TPS.

Gradually, the track draws away from the watery bog, rising circuitously to the top of the hill, part of an extended ridge of accordion compressions and rocky fins that compose Bearfort Mountain. This is one of the most exhilarating stretches of trail *anywhere,* and not solely because the bedrock, a quartzite-spiked red stone, is of an unusual conglomerate known as puddingstone (think of liver larded with quail eggs). Nor is the main attraction the yellow and pink penstemon that covers the mount in spring, nor even the surprising appearance of pink lady's slipper orchids at the base of the rocks. No, those are all gravy on the feast of near-continuous scrambling from rocky point to rocky point, with far-reaching views and access to the pristine Terrace Pond tossed in as a sweet dessert. Any wildlife you may stumble upon, like bears, otters—or the barred owl we once startled—simply add to the thrills of a breathtaking area that puts the *F* in "physical."

Switch left at the junction with the Terrace Pond Red Trail (red markings), navigating further through this outdoor palace of puddingstone. Take your time, snack on a sandwich, and enjoy the crow's-nest vistas and the uniqueness of this otherworldly landscape. Canter left at the slanted T, at the bottom of a steep fin of rocks, exchanging red blazes for white ones, and persevere with the white-blazed trail to the edge of Terrace Pond, elevation 1,380 feet, where hooded mergansers frolic and fish. If you've braved this sun-struck area in summer, go ahead and refresh yourself with the cool water of this Castalian fountain—just remember that swimming is not allowed.

On finishing with that backwoods baptism, lope left at the north end of the pond onto the blue-blazed track. More craggy crossings ensue, capped in many cases with spicebush, sheep laurel, scrub oak, and pitch pine. Eventually, the path leaves this memorable mountain, diving left on a pipeline cut. Descend via the overlapping traces to a fairly level spot near a cluster of hemlocks and black birches, where the blue blazes veer left into the cover of trees (GPS: **N41° 8.800' W74° 23.966'**).

In a handful of minutes, and a leisurely bog slog, the trail emerges where you started, at Clinton Road.

## NEARBY ACTIVITIES

What was once known as the Sterling Hill Zinc Mine now has been molded into a rather intriguing museum. Underground mining tours, fluorescent exhibits, fossils, ores and minerals, an astronomical observatory, and much more make for an entertaining and educational visit. Go dig at **sterlinghillminingmuseum.org**.

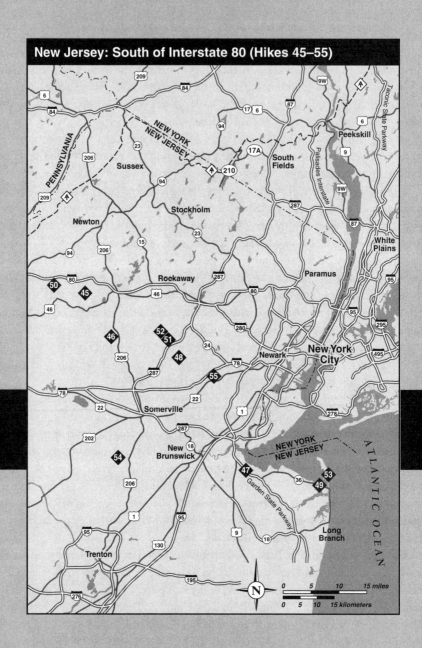

## New Jersey: South of Interstate 80 (Hikes 45–55)

# NEW JERSEY:
## SOUTH OF INTERSTATE 80

# 45 ALLAMUCHY NATURAL AREA AMBLE

 **KEY AT-A-GLANCE INFORMATION**

**LENGTH:** 8.2 miles

**ELEVATION GAIN:** 1,171 feet

**CONFIGURATION:** Loop

**DIFFICULTY:** Moderate

**SCENERY:** A succession of mixed hardwood forests, grassy fields, marshlands, and a lovely fishing pond in the center

**EXPOSURE:** Half-exposed, half-shady

**TRAFFIC:** Light on weekdays; popular summer spot, weekend mountain biking

**TRAIL SURFACE:** Dirt with alternating grass, rocks, and roots

**HIKING TIME:** 4 hours

**DRIVING DISTANCE:** 57 miles

**SEASON:** Year-round, sunrise–sunset

**ACCESS:** Free; no motorized vehicles, dogs on leash

**MAPS:** At trailhead kiosk

**FACILITIES:** Portable toilet

**COMMENTS:** Hunting is allowed. In spring, a wild variety of feathered creatures can be spotted—a true birder's special. For more information, call 908-852-3790 or visit njparksandforests.org/parks /allamuch.html.

## GPS COORDINATES

N40° 53.263'  W74° 48.847'

## IN BRIEF

Whether the quarry is birds, the backwoods, or beautiful bodies of water, Allamuchy has what it takes to make your outing a success. In fact, the combination of a wild, untended woodland with countless streams, several swamps, and a couple of lakes adds up to an environment that birds find irresistible. A good many hikers do, too, what with the miles of trails that snake through an underpopulated backcountry.

## DESCRIPTION

Most people who are aware of Allamuchy Mountain State Park know of it only parenthetically as the setting for Waterloo Village. Within the loose structure of an early 1800s community, visitors there pass through time, from a re-created Lenape Indian settlement to a thriving port by the once-bustling Morris Canal. There are sawmills, gristmills, a blacksmith shop, and a general store, along with a variety of historic homes. Everything, it seems, except the mountain to which the name of this park refers. For that—and a highly enchanting hike—you need to venture into the Allamuchy Natural Area, a 2,440-acre chunk of hilly hardwood forestland tucked into the western part of the park.

Allamuchy draws its name from Chief Allamuchahokkingen ("place within the hills")

------------------------------------------------

*Directions* ⟶

**Follow I-95 across the George Washington Bridge and take Exit 69 to merge onto I-80 West. Take Exit 19 and drive south on CR 517 for 2.1 miles to Deer Park Road. Turn left on Deer Park Road and proceed straight for 0.7 mile to the parking area.**

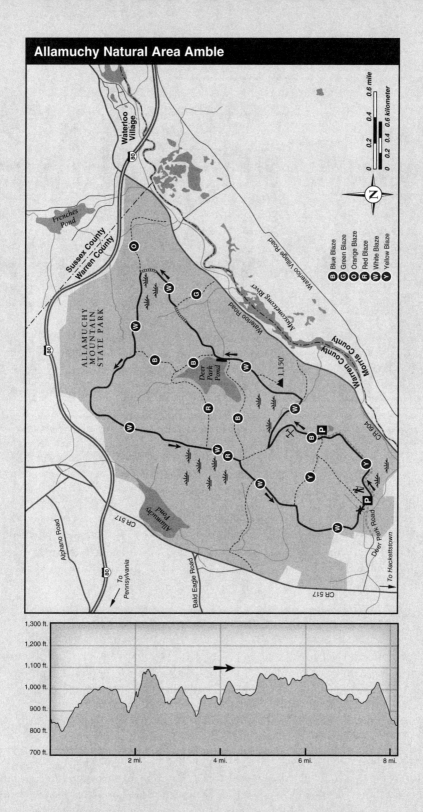

# Allamuchy Natural Area Amble

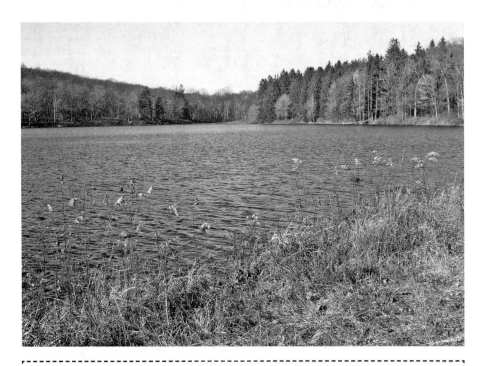

Perch, pickerel, and largemouth bass lure anglers to this pond, whereas a variety of spring migrating birds attract the binocular-sporting crowds.

of the Lenape tribe. After the natives were displaced by European settlers, most of this locale was absorbed by the estates of the Rutherford and Stuyvesant families, descendants of New Amsterdam's final governor, Peter Stuyvesant. More recently, the Musconetcong River, south of the park, has become renowned as one of the best trout fishing spots in New Jersey. The Allamuchy Natural Area—as already noted—enjoys no such fame, which works to the advantage of anyone with an interest in great birding opportunities, unsullied beauty, and a secluded system of trails.

The first part of this hike follows yellow blazes along the dirt road by the kiosk. It is usually possible to drive a mile farther to a different parking lot, one that is closer to Deer Park Pond, but we suggest you walk this stretch. It is attractively overgrown by cedar, maple, flowering dogwood, oak, apple, and tulip trees, with a lowland swamp below the road's right shoulder. This combination makes for an amateur ornithologist's wonderland, one in which we've seen a rose-breasted grosbeak, a redstart, an oriole, and a flock of goldfinches, among many species. You should also see, if you're here in spring, lavender-colored wild geraniums, yellow asters, violets, and white anemones, to name just a few of the wildflowers that highlight the ground cover. The spur to the right, after 15 minutes of walking, dead-ends in a few paces at a picturesque pond, with sheep laurel and chokeberry encroaching and purple irises thriving in the mud. We've also observed half a dozen painted turtles slumbering on the rock to the left, their wet carapaces glistening in the morning sun.

Back on the main track, the dirt road skims by a ranger's residence and then swerves to the right, just as the yellow blazes veer left onto a side trail. Remain with the road as it proceeds past a parking area and slips around a pipe gate. In a couple hundred yards there is a spur to the left, with the shallow tunnel of an old mine a few feet away; swallows like to nest in its carved-out ceiling. Your turnoff, the Deer Path Trail, is just beyond the quarry, on the right side of the forest road. (If you reach parking area 2, you've gone too far.) Though it starts out as an overgrown trace, this white-blazed route soon widens to comfortable single-file dimensions, snaking through a swamp made all the more colorful by a scattering of glacial erratics among the flowering azaleas, mayapple, skunk cabbage, and ferns. You may even see tiger and spicebush swallowtail butterflies brightly fluttering through this zone. As the trail begins to descend, high water or muddy conditions often require that you hop from one moss-coated rock to the next to keep your boots dry. Swing left at the fork (GPS: N40° 53.704' W74° 47.888'), now heading uphill.

The blazes along this somewhat rocky stretch were once red, and you may still see a few that are weathered to salmon or orange. The prevailing markings, however, are now white, a color you will stick with for the remainder of the hike. The serpentine ascent rapidly threads through a rather open forest, with an appealing amount of glacial debris littering the slope up to the right, until the path levels off and then descends, with Deer Park Pond straight ahead, partially screened by maples and oaks. Bear left at the fork, still treading downward, and hang a right when you reach the forest road. Stay with the road as it crosses the dam, and if you brought a lunch along, you might avail yourself of the hemlock-shaded spot by the pond, where a low rock makes a comfortable seat.

Heave to the right at the fork, just as the wide dirt road enters tree cover. White blazes replace older blue ones over this next leg of the hike, but as noted previously, you may find some defunct color swatches still sticking to trees, leading to possible confusion. This path gains ground initially, then loses it, while meandering from rock-pocked forest to fern-flecked swamp, from glacial erratics to a muck-crusted boardwalk. Just after the latter, the track swerves left; 15 feet beyond, a spur (green markings) to the right heads to Waterloo Road. Stay with the main trail as it commences to climb, passing by great, granite-struck leavings of the last glacier to scrape through New Jersey. More erratics follow as the path dips into another bog patch, fording the muck via a second narrow boardwalk. In a little more than a mile, this enjoyable track ends at a fork, with white blazes going to the right, or west.

At first the wide, rocky path resembles an old forest road until, having gently ascended for a few minutes, it narrows significantly to single-file. A few metal posts to your right remain from a long-gone boundary fence, as the path arcs toward the south, with a couple of traces leading that way a few steps later. Stay with the main trail as it again rises slightly, cresting in 60 seconds among rocky mounds—terrain that is strikingly similar to the undulating earlier stretch. A notable difference, however, is that this region is a bit more open, with an increasing number of dogwood, white birch, and cedar trees entering the arboreal mix. In due time, you arrive at a junction with a red-blazed track merging from the left. Continue straight, with concurrent markings of red and white, as the pebbly path drops through another bog, where purple irises flower in spring. At the ensuing fork, the white route breaks to the right (the left-hand option was unblazed when last we hiked here), and you should, too.

From this swampy setting, the path gradually moves toward an attractive mound of fractured granite, with a seasonal bog stream serenely rippling by its base. The trail climbs from there, expeditiously entering a boulder-blasted landscape before tapering downward again to yet one more boggy patch. Bear to the right at the fork with a yellow-blazed track, still hanging with white blazes. This is the home stretch of the hike, where the fence to your right is so rusty it is hardly noticeable in an area choked with sarsaparilla and pricker bushes, and large-trunked black birches are the dominant tree. After drifting under a pair of power lines, the path bottoms out by a sweet little pond. Step around the reeds and ferns for a closer look at the shallow water, and you just might spy a few spirited trout and possibly some frogs. A couple of yards farther on is a mowed lawn. Scoot left there to return to your car.

## NEARBY ACTIVITIES

A bustling port in the 19th century, the handsomely restored **Waterloo Village** is now a living-history museum. It contains a working mill complex, several historic buildings, a re-created Lenape Indian village, and a preserved farm site, with costumed interpreters demonstrating traditional trades. It is also a great venue for summer music concerts. For details, visit **winakungatwaterloo.com.**

# BLACK RIVER TRAIL  46

## IN BRIEF

Take a pinch of iron-mining history, combine that with a highly scenic river, add a few successional fields, a conifer-covered hillside, and the possibility of seeing wildlife, and what do you have? The makings of a tremendous hike along the Black River Trail. This one manages the neat feat of carrying you deep into a wilderness and back in time, all within the confines of a well-populated suburban community. A cabin ruin and hidden cascade add to the fun in a trek you are likely to savor long after its finish.

## DESCRIPTION

The folks at New Jersey's Morris County Park Commission are a modest lot. We conclude so, anyway, not from having met them—we haven't!—but because they manage one of the most beautiful trails most people have never heard of. That's the Black River Trail system we're referring to, as fine a parcel of real estate as you are likely to find in this part of the state. A good piece of this hike hugs the photogenic banks of the Black River, some of

---

## *Directions* ⟶

Follow I-95 across the George Washington Bridge to Exit 69 to merge onto I-80 West. Take Exit 27A and drive south on US 206 for 8.1 miles. Turn right (west) on CR 513/NJ 24 and continue for 1.2 miles to the large parking lot on the left, by the Cooper Gristmill. If you have a shuttle car, park it first at the Willowwood Arboretum. From the intersection of US 206 and NJ 24, proceed south on US 206 and drive 3.8 miles to Daly Road. Make a right on it and, after 0.7 mile, turn right on Union Grove Road, which becomes Longview Road. The arboretum entrance is 0.2 mile away, on the left.

### KEY AT-A-GLANCE INFORMATION

**LENGTH:** 6.6 miles for the balloon (7.8 miles for the one-way stretch from Cooper Gristmill to the Willowwood Arboretum)

**ELEVATION GAIN:** 1,079 feet

**CONFIGURATION:** Balloon

**DIFFICULTY:** Easy to moderate

**SCENERY:** Cascading river, grassy meadows, dark conifer forests, thick deciduous woods, and a gristmill

**EXPOSURE:** Mostly shady with a few open-road and meadow stretches

**TRAFFIC:** The farther you hike, the lonelier it gets.

**TRAIL SURFACE:** A lot of dirt, but also grass, pavement, rocks

**HIKING TIME:** 3.5 hours

**DRIVING DISTANCE:** 56 miles

**SEASON:** Year-round, sunrise–sunset

**ACCESS:** Free; pets on leash not exceeding 6 feet, no biking, no horseback riding

**MAPS:** At kiosk and visitor center; download from morrisparks.net/asp parks/coopermilltr.asp

**FACILITIES:** Vault toilets

**COMMENTS:** The Black River is a popular trout-fishing spot: anglers—not bears—are commonly seen darting in and out of the bushes. And in spring, you may be so lucky as to find a pink lady's slipper orchid. For further information, visit tinyurl.com/blackriverpark.

## GPS COORDINATES

N40° 46.703'  W74° 43.207'

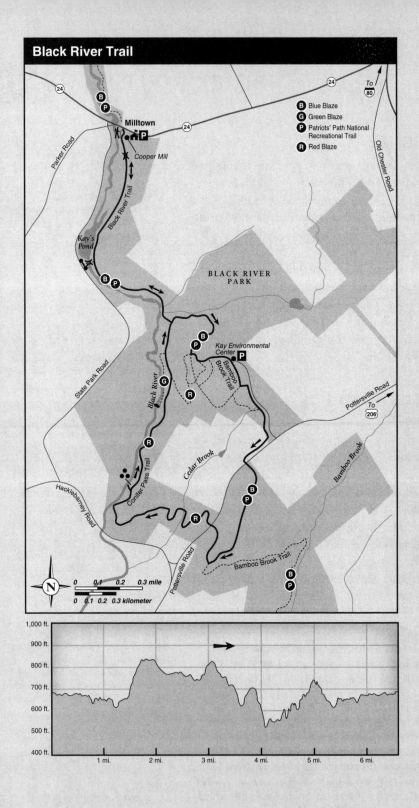

# Black River Trail

**Milltown**

*Cooper Mill*

*Parker Road*

24

24

**B** Blue Blaze
**G** Green Blaze
**P** Patriots' Path National
Recreational Trail
**R** Red Blaze

24

*To* 80

*Old Chester Road*

*Black River Trail*

*Kay's Pond*

**B** **P**

BLACK RIVER PARK

**B**
**P** **Kay Environmental Center** **P**

*Bamboo Brook Trail*

*State Park Road*

**G**
**R**

*Black River*

**R**

*Cedar Brook*

*Conifer Pass Trail*

*Pottersville Road*
*To* 206

*Bamboo Brook*

**R**

**R**

**B**
**P**

*Hacklebarney Road*

*Pottersville Road*

*Bamboo Brook Trail*

**B**
**P**

**N**

0   0.1   0.2   0.3 mile
0   0.1  0.2  0.3 kilometer

1,000 ft.
900 ft.
800 ft.
700 ft.
600 ft.
500 ft.
400 ft.

1 mi.   2 mi.   3 mi.   4 mi.   5 mi.   6 mi.

it passes through meadowlands rich in birdlife, and a fair portion winds over a conifer-covered hillside. From dynamic cascades to a placid pond, from cabin ruins to a historic mine, there is hardly a dull moment on this relatively easy trek.

The entire length of this trail, from Chubb Park to Willowwood Arboretum, is 8.2 miles one-way. Thus, if you have an extra car, you might use it as a shuttle, leaving a vehicle at one end of the route and starting the hike at the other. Otherwise, we suggest a shorter loop of 6.6 miles, beginning at Cooper Gristmill. This solid limestone block construction, incidentally, is a remnant of the community of Milltown, which thrived during the 19th century. Don't bother to look for it on your Rand McNally: Milltown is gone, along with the blacksmith shop, distillery, sawmill, and general store that once shared the shoulder of the road with Cooper Gristmill. Iron mining was the local industry then, with the Chester Furnace, a mile to the north, producing 300 tons a week at its peak, and locomotives loaded with the stuff rattling through town every day. Miners netted three bucks a week in wages and lived in a shantytown at the fringes of the community. The first mile of this hike showcases relics of that halcyon era.

Pick up the blue blazes of the Black River Trail (BRT) at the mill. Chubb Park is to the north, through the tunnel that runs under NJ 24/124. Your destination lies in the other direction, but take a moment to walk up the tunnel for a glimpse of the river on the other side of the road, where it is dammed above the mill. Having finished that detour, descend the wooden stairs behind Cooper Gristmill and cross the rivulet, nearing the river's east bank before the path veers away, via a series of short bridges, in the direction of a scenic swamp. The stream here slithers by skunk cabbage and irises toward the Black River, with an array of granite boulders littering the dark soil and a couple of benches, well shaded by maple, beech, black birch, and a mix of oaks, ideally situated to soak up the serenity of the setting.

The BRT is clearly marked and very easy to follow as it swings left and parallels the river, tripping over a series of short bridges in the process. For the next half-mile, the well-graded track overlaps the old Hacklebarney branch of the Central New Jersey Rail Road, which was constructed in 1873 to transport ore from the mines. Beyond a bit of gravel here and there, nothing is left of the tracks, but if you look closely to the right on passing the bog, you may see some terrapins and frogs among the ferns, violets, ramps, trout lilies, and jack-in-the-pulpits. Then there is Kay Pond, where the river is bottled up. Generations ago, this was the community swimming hole, but unless it's really hot, you would now be better off leaving it to the snapping turtles that lurk around the perimeter. The fenced-in building below the dam—originally a mill—was later converted into an electric plant.

Moving onward, the trail nears a chain-link fence where the overgrown, rubble-filled slope is all that remains of the Hacklebarney Mine. During its peak, from 1879 through 1892, the mine yielded around 20,000 tons of ore annually. It now produces birch trees, maples, and chokeberry—and Dutchman's breeches in spring. On departing that area, the hike heads into a wilder environment, with the rocky embankment to the left soaring 30 feet (keep your eyes peeled for wild

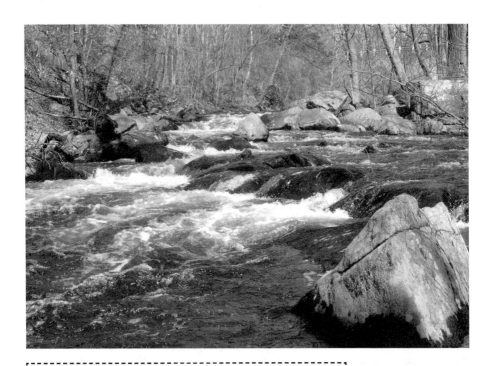

The roaring Black River feeds the illusion of being deep in the wilderness.

turkeys), and the river opposite crackling merrily along. Several additional short bridges and boardwalks appear here, as the path hovers around an attractive bog. Finally, after passing concrete pilings that once supported a bridge, the track tapers uphill toward the east, leaving the water behind. The climb tops out at a fork in about 100 yards, with the blue blazes leading left, toward the Elizabeth Kay Environmental Center (EKEC).

In addition to the wild turkeys, red foxes, and coyotes that crisscross this hillside, remnants of walls prove that this hardwood forest was formerly open farmland. You may smell the sweet perfume of honeysuckle near the end of your ascent, part of a vast array of successional plants, like cedar, sarsaparilla, dogwood, and ash, that have resurfaced in what was formerly known as Hidden River Farm. Hidden River was purchased by Alfred and Elizabeth Kay in 1924, who maintained it as their summer retreat. Much of what they raised, including cows, chickens, pigs, herbs, miscellaneous grains, and vegetables, was shipped to their Florida residence. Eventually, the property was donated to Morris County, which converted the farmhouse into the EKEC.

Cross the grassy patch at the top of the hill and turn left at the intersection, moving toward the EKEC. Stay with the gravel drive for 0.2 mile to the parking area, and once there walk from the public telephone, marked with a blue blaze, to the far side of the house. Transfer to the Bamboo Brook Trail, straight over the aisle of mowed grass and under a large maple by an orchard of flowering dog-woods. The path hits a T at a dilapidated rail fence, where it jogs to the left, still blazed with blue. Go through the green wooden gate (it is usually open), emerging by a field speckled yellow with flowering lupine and goldenrod, and jog to the right, merging with the farm's entrance road. Bluebirds often cavort in the grassy meadow to your left, while butterflies favor the scrub growth over the fence. Remain on the driveway until it meets Pottersville Road and veer right there. Within 3 minutes, blue blazes marking the entrance back into the forest appear on the left side of the road (GPS: **N40° 45.458' W74° 42.596'**).

Even in an expanding neighborhood where modest homes are being replaced with McMansions, there is a secluded feel to this lightly trafficked section of the woods. After a bit of meandering, the path arrives at a grassy breach in the trees, where deer frequently graze. A fork in the trail occurs a minute later, as the blue-blazed route continues to the right. Hang with this track as it traverses an old forest lane, moving upward over increasingly rocky turf. In 5 minutes, that climb is done and—what else?—a descent commences. Partway down the hill, the Conifer Pass Trail (red blazes) forks to the right—take it, moving now west-northwest. There are a few knee-high stone cairns spaced out along the way to help guide you through the rocky terrain, and within 4 minutes, the path recrosses Pottersville Road.

On the other side of the blacktop, the hardwood forest evaporates as it is transformed, miraculously, into a wide, tilting plain of white pines. Ferns and false lilies grow by the feet of these silent giants, as well as Virginia creeper and barberry, while a piney scent, mingled with honey, often fills the air. The trail continues downward, swiveling from the west toward the south and then back to the west, ultimately hitting the trough at a pleasant little glade by Cedar Brook, which you hop over. It's uphill from there, steeply so for 60 seconds, with a leveling off among hardwoods and a fading complement of conifers. The descent that follows tapers toward the southwest before shifting northward. In a handful of minutes, as pines resurface with laurels, the path returns to the Black River.

In keeping to the right, alongside the dark, eddying water, you enter a fabulous part of the hike. Much of the thrill here derives from the finely chiseled rocky setting, one in which the river explodes by boulders and crashes over a series of erratics for a prolonged, voluptuous cascade. With the presence in early June of pink lady's slipper orchids popping out of the peat up the slope to your right, all that is needed to complete the fairy-tale image is an elf sitting on a giant toadstool. You, too, may feel inclined to sit, with a rock by the dark river an ideal perch for immersing one's thoughts in the sound and fury of the scene. Gradually, the trail weaves away from the Black River, hugging the hemlock-covered hill, and swings right on a wide forest road. First, though, take five and stroll a few hundred feet to the left, to the stone foundation of Elizabeth Kay's old cabin, its pinnacle of a chimney still intact. With tiny yellow violets carpeting the ground in spring and the river bending just below, it's hard to imagine a more idyllic spot in which to build a rustic retreat, tucked as it is among rhododendrons.

Back on track with the red blazes, walk uphill to the slight leveling and take the hairpin turn to the left. Keep left again in 250 feet, dropping off the dirt lane. Hemlocks are mingled with hardwoods here, and yellow penstemon speckles the forest floor. On reaching a ridge, the path tapers back toward the water, where the latter lustily crashes against protruding rocks, then resumes its upward trend. As the mountain laurels and pines recede, the track merges into a broad forest road, blazed green; continue straight on that (instead of following red sharply to the right, back up the ridge). You may notice that the land to the left of this hard, pebbly lane has been signposted as an "environmentally sensitive area." To hike the trails and bushwhack there, you'll need to obtain a permit at the EKEC or from the Morris County Park Police. You may also observe, as you amble along, an old bathtub by the side of the trail, a sight that isn't as odd as it may at first seem. Back when forests such as this were open planting and grazing ground, thrifty farmers recycled their spent bathtubs as watering or feed troughs for livestock. The tubs remain, long after the farms have folded and the cleared land has been reclaimed by nature. Now, if only someone could explain why we're forever finding fridges and bald tires in swamps. . . .

Stay with the green markings at the ensuing fork as they branch to the left, then switch to the unblazed trace on the right. This single-file forested path, overhung by beech saplings, oaks, and tulip trees, merges in a moment with a wide track. A left turn there puts you back on the Black River Trail, the first leg of the hike. Cooper Gristmill is 1 mile ahead.

## NEARBY ACTIVITIES

You might start the hike with a guided tour and demonstration of the restored **Cooper Gristmill,** which was a state-of-the-art operation when it was built in 1826. For details visit **morrisparks.net/aspparks/coopermillmain.asp.** And consider ending the day at the **Willowwood Arboretum,** surrounded by rolling farmland, crosscut by informal walking trails, and sporting 3,500 varieties of native and exotic plants. For detailed information, visit **morrisparks.net/aspparks/wwmain.asp.**

# CHEESEQUAKE NATURAL AREA TRAIL

## IN BRIEF

Do you enjoy traipsing through cedar swamps and backwoods bayous while bounding over boardwalks? Cheesequake is well endowed in each of those categories, with plenty of raw, natural beauty left over to appeal to other tastes. The birding is great by its lake and marshlands. Then there are several notable forests, populated by stands of monumental oaks, tulip trees, and white pines. And the wide, swiftly flowing Cheesequake Creek is so alluring you may be tempted to portage your own canoe.

## DESCRIPTION

For most people, Cheesequake State Park is little more than a green spot on the roadmap, with the Garden State Parkway cutting across it like a bull charging through a red-ribbon fence. On the way to or from the Big Apple, few motorists give the slightest thought to stopping. That's their loss, because this 1,274-acre park is extravagantly beautiful, partly because it straddles a transitional zone between two major ecosystems. Miles of trails (and a hefty number of boardwalks) meander among pine barrens, a cedar swamp, marshlands, and open fields. In

----

### *Directions* ⟶

**Follow I-95 across the George Washington Bridge and drive south to Exit 11 to merge onto the Garden State Parkway South. Proceed to Exit 120 and make a right on Matawan Road/Laurence Harbor Road, followed by another right, in 0.2 mile, on Cliffwood Road/ CR 689. Drive 0.3 mile and turn right on Gordon Road, which leads, in 0.6 mile, to the park entrance. The park office is on the right. For the trailhead parking, go straight to the next lot on the left.**

## (i) KEY AT-A-GLANCE INFORMATION

**LENGTH:** 5.5 miles

**ELEVATION GAIN:** 424 feet

**CONFIGURATION:** Loop with spur

**DIFFICULTY:** Easy

**SCENERY:** Pine barrens, swamps, boardwalks, water features, and hardwood forests

**EXPOSURE:** Mostly very shady

**TRAFFIC:** Hectic in summer

**TRAIL SURFACE:** Dirt, roots, sand

**HIKING TIME:** 3 hours

**DRIVING DISTANCE:** 44 miles

**SEASON:** Year-round, 8 a.m.–sunset

**ACCESS:** Entrance fee is charged Memorial Day weekend–Labor Day. Residents: $5 weekdays, $10 weekends; double that for nonresidents. Dogs on leash.

**MAPS:** At park office and interpretive center; tinyurl.com/cheesequake map; USGS *South Amboy*

**FACILITIES:** Restrooms, water, and phone at office

**COMMENTS:** Hunting is allowed. The fall colors are spectacular, and in winter sledding and skiing are popular. Trout are stocked at Hooks Creek Lake in spring. Would-be overnighters take note: campers at Cheesequake have reported incidents of violent nighttime assaults and tent vandalism. Call 732-566-2161 for information, or visit njparksandforests.org/parks/cheesequake.html.

## GPS COORDINATES

N40° 26.184'  W74° 15.920'

# Cheesequake Natural Area Trail

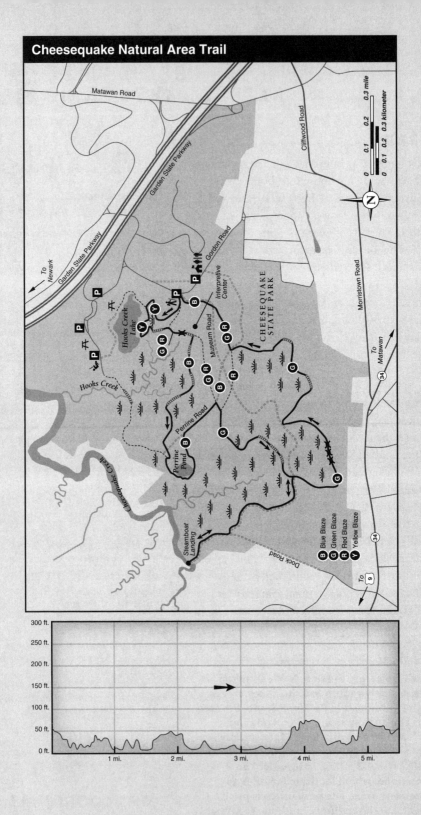

fact, there is so much eye candy in this diverse terrain that at the end of a day of hiking, many trekkers don't want to leave—so they set up a tent and camp.

Cheesequake's name, incidentally, is not a phonetic misspelling of some heavy sort of dairy-based dessert. Back in June 1940, when the preserve was first opened to the public, park officials plucked the word from the language of the Lenape Indians, who hunted and fished these grounds into the 1700s before being wiped out by white settlers. The Lenapes were but the last in a long line of Indian tribes who found the Cheesequake (properly—if seldom—pronounced CHESS-quick) area inviting, with the earliest traces of occupation dating back 5,000 years.

The trailhead and map kiosk are to the far left of the parking area. Of the many overlapping and intersecting circuits within the park, the following 5.5-mile trek provides a broad overview of Cheesequake's natural attractions and varied habitats. Head out on the wide path and turn right at the fork, in 150 feet, onto the Yellow Trail (YT), where blueberry bushes and sassafras compose the under-story and maples, mountain laurel, and various oaks provide shade. Bear left in a few minutes at the slanted T, as the moss-sided track hugs a ridgeline that tapers toward Hooks Creek Lake. Enjoy the vantage point high over the water, then descend the wooden staircase. The YT continues to the left, near the bottom of the steps, but first hover a moment by the edge of the lake, which is attractively framed by pitch pines, cattails, and other reeds.

If you can resist the urge to cast out a line—the trout fishing is great in the spring, while perch and bass are the trophies in summer—return to the path and keep moving. A few pitch pines pop up by the side of a salt marsh, where you may spot cormorants, snowy egrets, pine warblers, and other shorebirds partly con-cealed behind salt hay and cordgrass. After pulling away from here, the path arcs to the right and hits a boardwalk, bringing you to a freshwater floodplain (another fine place for birding). Half a minute later, take the fork to the right to the inter-pretive center. In walking under the wooden archway, crossing a bridge, and steering toward the modern, wood-sided pavilion, you have exchanged yellow blazes for red and green ones. Pick up the Blue Trail (BT) to the right of the build-ing, and stay with it along the spine of a sheep laurel–cloaked ridge. Those small platforms set within the cover of trees, by the way, are known as quail roosts, which are used, curiously, by bobwhites.

On descending back to the level of the marsh, the path meets a boardwalk, with a stream running under it. Atop the stairs that follow, transfer to the right at the T, sticking with the BT as it breaks off from the red and green blazes. From this highland stretch of turf, you gain a fine vista—in winter—of the expansive marsh below. Enjoy it—you'll be brushing against marsh grass again momentarily. First, though, it's down another set of stairs, over a short boardwalk (surrounded by the murky muck of an attractive swamp), and up some steps, succeeded by a similar descent and ascent. Stomp down yet another set of stairs, and the marsh will now be on either side of you, as the track morphs into a 5-foot-wide board-walk, 2.5 feet off the ground. The highway is visible (but barely audible) far off

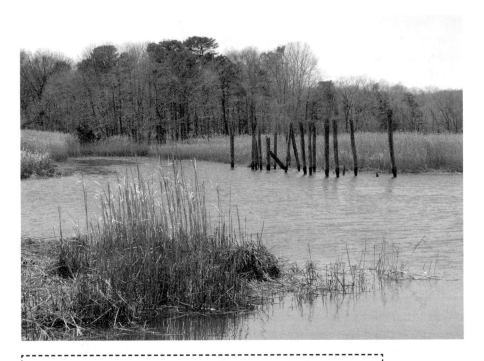

The pier of the old Steamboat Landing is long gone, but a strikingly beautiful setting, and an occasional osprey, remain.

in the distance, although you may find it more rewarding to scan the horizon—and underbrush—for birds. On one foray here, we spotted seven great egrets on one side of the long walkway and a red-winged blackbird on the other.

Atop the next staircase the BT jogs right, overlooking the marsh, then left, adhering to the contours of a ridge. Ignore the traces as the path dips again toward the marshland, sticking with the blue discs that are posted among a mini–pine barrens of bayberry, holly, maple, black birch, and—naturally—pitch pine. After puttering left, the path delivers you to an unpaved road, where you slip under the wooden arch and hang a right, followed by a quick left (GPS: **N40° 26.218' W74° 16.656'**), still with the BT and overlapping a wide, sandy forest road. Check out the bird blind on the left, where you can spy on black-crested cormorants, ducks, and gulls on Perrine Pond. Then, on continuing along the path, don't forget to scan the sky for ospreys swooping over the marsh to the right. Swallows also tend to mingle among the reeds, and in the loamy ground to the left, as the now-gravel surfaced track pulls away from the water, you may be able to discern the freshly burrowed holes of fox dens. At the T with a forest road, motor to the right and, in 2 minutes of rapid walking, veer right on the Green Trail (GT).

The path still clings to a ridge when it departs the gravel road, bobbing and weaving through an attractive setting of laurel, serviceberry, and pink flowering azalea. In hilly terrain such as this, of course, it is only a matter of time before high ground becomes low, and sure enough, the trail soon drops down to a swamp speckled green with ferns and skunk cabbage. A boardwalk here stretches for a whopping 100 yards, ending at a wooden staircase. Tread up that, then down the steps that follow, onto the next boardwalk, surrounded suddenly, marvelously, by cedar trees. The walkway, which can be treacherously slick, snakes through this cedar swamp, where the water has been dyed orange by tree tannins leaching into the underlying soil. The planks end briefly—keep to the right—only to resume for a short spell longer. Then it's briskly uphill, back among laurels and oaks.

On hitting the park road, you have three choices: proceed directly across on the GT, swing right for Steamboat Landing, or left for an early bailout. The detour to Steamboat Landing is highly scenic and requires only about a half-hour for the round-trip. As the conifers growing on the embankment to the left and right of the dirt road give way to hardwood trees, peer sharply left, about 70 yards in, for one of the park's largest white oaks. After coming abreast of a marsh, the lane forks: dogleg left around the barrier and lunge immediately right onto Dock Road. In 3 minutes, the unpaved lane dead-ends at a bend in Cheesequake Creek, by a confluence of streams, with the rotting pilings of an old steamboat landing 70 feet across the swiftly flowing water. There is a subtle, almost subliminal serenity to this delightful spot that makes it well worth visiting. The osprey-nesting platform, installed in April 2007, serves as an additional attraction.

Back at the four-way intersection, venture right on the prolongation of the GT. As you shuffle along, check out the spectacular stand of white pines, concentrated primarily to the left. Too soon you leave that behind and ascend a slight slope that is well scarred with roots, followed by a wooden staircase—yet another example of the prodigious efforts at trail maintenance made by park staff and volunteers. The GT dips again shortly and meanders over three bridges, then bends left by some wooden rails. In time the path, which occasionally resembles a grooved toboggan run, approaches Museum Road, only to swerve right just before meeting it.

The ensuing segment of the hike showcases a few kettle-hole depressions to the right of you and, in the swamp on the left, an impressive grove of tulip trees, many quite monumental in size. The GT soon arcs left toward the heart of that swamp and slips over 175 feet of boardwalk, jumping to the left at the end of the planks. With gigantic skunk cabbage leaves rising up from the mud and a thickly shrouded wetland to rival the swamps of Florida, you may not see many birds here; listen attentively while strolling over three additional boardwalks, though, and your ears might detect (along with the chirruping of frogs) the alien call of a red-bellied woodpecker or the hooting of a barred owl. After treading through a deeply rutted patch, look to the right for a giant beech tree, an icon among the many hardwoods in the area.

The group camping area is directly ahead when you pass under the wooden arch. Instead of entering it, go left on the paved road, and in a couple of minutes scamper right under the next archway. The Red Trail joins Green here, as the path

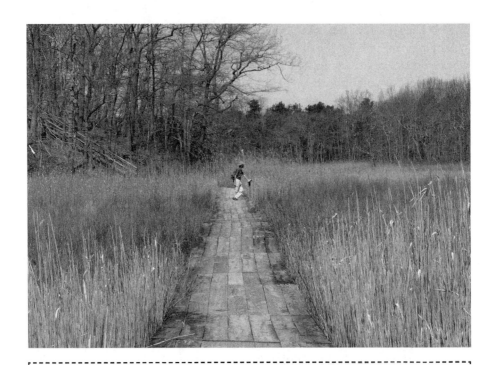

If you don't see egrets or herons fishing in this saltwater marsh, you'd better have your eyes examined.

circumnavigates the backside of the campground, scooting to the left as it approaches the second camping field. Mosey right on the paved Museum Road and, remaining with that, you will be back at the parking area in 2 or 3 minutes. Don't imagine, though, that you are finished with Cheesequake. Like many of the better hikes, this is one to experience in each of the four seasons.

## NEARBY ACTIVITIES

A short distance down the Garden State Parkway is **Holmdel Park,** a 350-acre domain whose fully developed trail system showcases a great deal of eye-catching scenery in 3 or so miles of pathways. Hardwoods and pines, hills and bogs, streams and wildflower meadows are all a part of what makes walking there so pleasant and diverting. A few sustained uphill stretches will get hearts a-thumping in all but the most hardy of hikers, and with a petting zoo on park land, this is a can't-miss for the youngest trailblazers in your crew. You'll also find an arboretum and the historic Longstreet Farm, where interpreters in period costume help bring the area's agricultural past to life. For more information, call 732-946-9562 or visit **tinyurl.com/holmdelpark.**

# GREAT SWAMP WILDERNESS TRAIL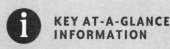

## IN BRIEF

*Walk in a wilderness of swamps and bogs,*
*Under the beech trees or over moss logs.*
*Admire the lily,*
*On ground that's not hilly,*
*While looking for otters, turtles, and frogs.*

## DESCRIPTION

History records that, in 1708, what is now the Great Swamp and much of the land around it was purchased from the Delaware Indians for four cutlasses, a like number of pistols, 15 cauldrons, 30 pounds sterling, and a keg of rum. As you set off into the swamp and commence with involuntarily donating your blood to the swarms of mosquitoes that thrive in this muggy marsh, you may feel the Indians got the best of the deal.

Come on, rub in some DEET and give the Great Swamp a chance: there is a subtle beauty to this place that grows on you as you stroll along its beech-and-oak-lined trails. Peer intently beyond the ferns, cattails, and many mushrooms, and you may spot a frolicking river otter, red fox, coyote, or mink. The endangered salamander and threatened blue bog turtle also make their homes here, and 222 species of birds wing through the refuge at different times of the year.

### *Directions*

Follow I-95 across the George Washington Bridge and take Exit 69 to merge onto I-80 West. Go to Exit 43A and merge onto I-287 South. Proceed to Exit 33 and turn right onto Harter Road. After 0.4 mile, go right on James Street. Continue 1.1 miles and bear right on Blue Mill Road, which becomes Lees Hill Road in 0.8 mile. Drive on for another 0.4 mile and veer left on Long Hill Road. The trailhead and parking are 1 mile ahead, on the left.

## KEY AT-A-GLANCE INFORMATION

**LENGTH:** 4.7 miles

**ELEVATION GAIN:** 26 feet

**CONFIGURATION:** 2 connected loops

**DIFFICULTY:** Very easy

**SCENERY:** Level trail skirts open marshland, quiet canals, hardwood forest, and shallow ponds.

**EXPOSURE:** Canopy cover mostly throughout

**TRAFFIC:** Fairly light

**TRAIL SURFACE:** Dirt and roots with a few grassy stretches

**HIKING TIME:** 2 hours

**DRIVING DISTANCE:** 45 miles

**SEASON:** Year-round, sunrise–sunset

**ACCESS:** Free; foot travel only, no pets on trails. Boardwalks at the Wildlife Observation Center are wheelchair-accessible.

**MAPS:** Download from tinyurl.com/greatswampnwr; USGS *Chatham*

**FACILITIES:** Vault toilets at Wildlife Observation Center

**COMMENTS:** The grounds are closed to nonhunters during a brief annual deer-hunt period. The refuge manages two education centers that introduce visitors to the area's geology and offer classes and guided tours. For information, call the refuge at 973-425-1222 or visit fws.gov/refuge/great_swamp.

## GPS COORDINATES

N40° 43.644' W74° 29.685'

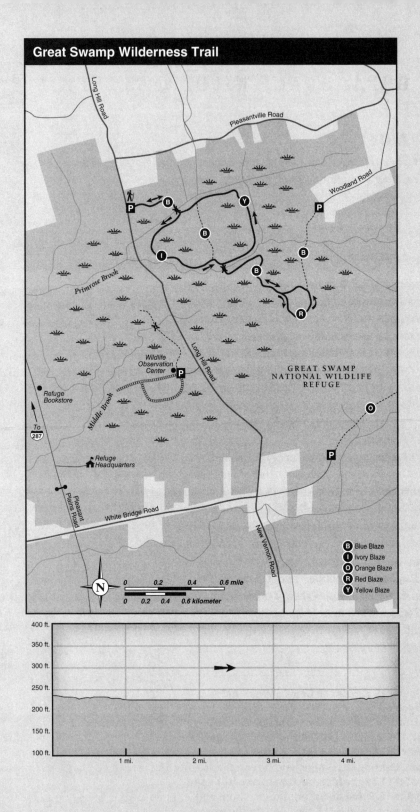

# Great Swamp Wilderness Trail

Long Hill Road

Pleasantville Road

Woodland Road

P

B

Y

B

P

I

B

Primrose Brook

B

R

Long Hill Road

Wildlife
Observation
Center

P

GREAT SWAMP
NATIONAL WILDLIFE
REFUGE

Refuge
Bookstore

Middle Brook

O

To
287

P

Refuge
Headquarters

Pleasant
Plains Road

White Bridge Road

New Vernon Road

N

| 0 | 0.2 | 0.4 | 0.6 mile |
| 0 | 0.2 | 0.4 | 0.6 kilometer |

B  Blue Blaze
I  Ivory Blaze
O  Orange Blaze
R  Red Blaze
Y  Yellow Blaze

400 ft.
350 ft.
300 ft.
250 ft.
200 ft.
150 ft.
100 ft.

1 mi.    2 mi.    3 mi.    4 mi.

A proposal in 1959 to build a jetport on this land spurred a grassroots effort to save the swamp, which brought about the purchase of 3,000 acres. That parcel was donated to the U.S. Department of the Interior, which has since increased the size of the refuge to just under 7,500 acres, with roughly half of that designated as wilderness. The level, easy trail we describe is one of four options that run through the wilderness area. Note that in early spring the ground can be quite muddy and flooded with water, Mother Nature's reminder that this is indeed swampland.

Take a good gander at the map posted at the trailhead by the car park. This double loop of 4.8 miles begins and returns on the Blue Trail (BT, blue blazes), switching off it three times along the way to investigate short side circuits. You'll be in a shady forest environment at the outset, among cedars, maples, and the more dominant beeches and oaks, the trunks of many coated with moss. Within 10 minutes, the rather rooty path crosses two canals, and after the second sluice, bear right on the Ivory Trail (IT, white blazes). The forest opens up a tad on this 0.8-mile leg, and it is tempting to sit off to the side on a good-size rock and wait for deer to come grazing through the knee-high grass. A small pond, farther along the IT, also offers the chance of seeing wildlife, and even the diminutive bog pots that pepper the sides of the path are active turtle and salamander habitats.

As the IT ends, the BT continues to the right and swerves over a wooden bridge, entering an area of white birches and, from spring through summer, a kaleidoscope of colorful wildflowers, including trout lily and spring beauty. If most of the blossoms are gone when you mosey through, console yourself with the multitude of mushrooms clinging to many of the downed logs. Beware of poison ivy, though, which grows abundantly in this sanctuary. The BT then sputters by an appealingly wild, overgrown thicket that is reminiscent in some ways of a Florida swamp, lacking only cypress trees and alligators to complete the subtropical illusion.

In a few strides, you're out of Florida and back into a grassy grove of beech trees, ferns billowing by the ground, and a canal of murky water stewing silently to the left. The right fork by a fairly hefty beech marks the start of the red loop (RT, red blazes), which rejoins the BT in half a mile. As you move along that spur, you'll see catbrier, cattails, and maybe even a bobcat (but only if your imagination is lively). Otters near a phragmites marsh are a more likely sighting, and if you pad the path with soft steps you might even catch a glimpse of an elusive wood duck. The RT expires at a massive oak, where you turn left, back with the blue blazes. (The other direction takes you to the Woodland Road parking area.)

Within 5 minutes, you will see the earlier turnoff onto the RT and, shortly after that, recross the wooden bridge. Instead of turning left, though, which would bring you back toward the IT, veer right onto the Yellow Trail (YT, yellow blazes). This 0.9-mile segment meanders by a boggy patch, then straightens out and for perhaps 120 yards passes through a bower of oaks, aligned as if they had been planted to shade a carriage lane. A dense thicket succeeds that, with a small,

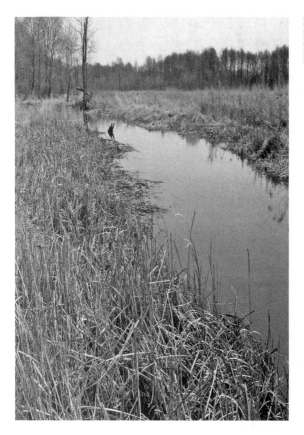

> You may not see the forest for the trees, but you can't ignore Loantaka Brook for the swamp.

grass-rimmed pond 60 feet to the right of the path. Silently follow the slight trace to the water's edge and you may spy mergansers or other birds bobbing about the inky surface.

As the YT bends to the left, it encounters a more extended stretch of swampland, with bog pots and mossy roots serving as land mines on the trail. If you opted to wear boots instead of sneakers, this is where that decision pays off, as the ground can be very moist (downright muddy in spring). Keep right at the ensuing fork, cross through the narrow canal and over the bog pots, and proceed past the ivory spur. The trailhead is 0.5 mile ahead.

## NEARBY ACTIVITIES

If you have some stamina left, check out the other worthwhile trails in the refuge.

The **Museum of Early Trades & Crafts,** in Madison, is housed in a building listed on the National Register of Historic Places. Its many exhibits focus on New Jersey's rural past and the tools used by 18th- and 19th-century farmers and craftsmen. Call 973-377-2982 for details, or visit **metc.org.**

The **Raptor Trust,** on White Bridge Road in Millington, is a fascinating rehabilitation facility for birds of prey and other wild avians, and well worth a visit. For information, call 908-647-8211.

# HARTSHORNE WOODS
# GRANDEST TOUR

**49**

## IN BRIEF

The rolling terrain of this densely forested county park provides a pretty fair workout over a modest amount of miles. Much of the land is covered by mountain laurel, which breaks into blankets of pink blossoms in early June. For far-reaching views of the Navesink River, consider visiting in late autumn through early spring, when the broad mix of hardwood trees is bare of leaves.

## DESCRIPTION

Take a stroll any day of the week along the 16 miles of trails in Hartshorne Woods, and you are likely to have company. Bikers, hikers, and even equestrians visit this 736-acre park with a regularity that a Metamucil consumer could only envy. As a well-kept secret, Hartshorne Woods ranks well below the secure, undisclosed locations in which some political big shots may soon be spending their retirement. But then, a romp in this Monmouth County property is a lot more fun than bouncing off the walls of a concrete bunker.

If, on the other hand, bunker-hunkering is what makes you tick, Hartshorne has its share of such shelters, too. Its Rocky Point section was once a key piece in the Atlantic Coast Defense System, and paved trails there circle Battery Lewis, where artillery guns protected

### KEY AT-A-GLANCE INFORMATION

**LENGTH:** 7 miles

**ELEVATION GAIN:** 1,100 feet

**CONFIGURATION:** Double loop

**DIFFICULTY:** Easy to moderate

**SCENERY:** Rolling Monmouth hills covered by mixed forest, offering scenic glimpses of Navesink River, and a side trip through military history

**EXPOSURE:** Almost completely sheltered

**TRAFFIC:** Heaviest on weekends, but plenty of visitors come to exercise midweek.

**TRAIL SURFACE:** Mostly rock-filled dirt

**HIKING TIME:** 3.5 hours

**DRIVING DISTANCE:** 55 miles

**SEASON:** Year-round, 7 a.m.–sunset

**ACCESS:** Free; pets on leash. The multiuse path is wheelchair-accessible.

**MAPS:** At trailhead kiosk; download from tinyurl.com/hartshornemap; USGS *Sandy Hook*

**FACILITIES:** Portable toilet at the trailhead, water fountain

**COMMENTS:** *Hartshorne* means "horn of the hart" or "stag," and if you're lucky, you'll encounter not just an antler but an entire deer. The park recently opened a new trail in the Claypit section, south of Hartshorne Road, with a connector to the existing trail system. For information, call 732-872-0336 or visit tinyurl.com /hartshornepark.

### Directions

Follow I-95 across the George Washington Bridge, proceed south and take Exit 11 to merge onto the Garden State Parkway South. Take Exit 117 and merge onto NJ 36 East. In 11.5 miles, turn slightly right and right again onto Navesink Avenue/CR 8B. Proceed for half a mile to the trailhead parking on the left.

## GPS COORDINATES

N40° 24.121'  W74° 0.757'

# Hartshorne Woods Grandest Tour

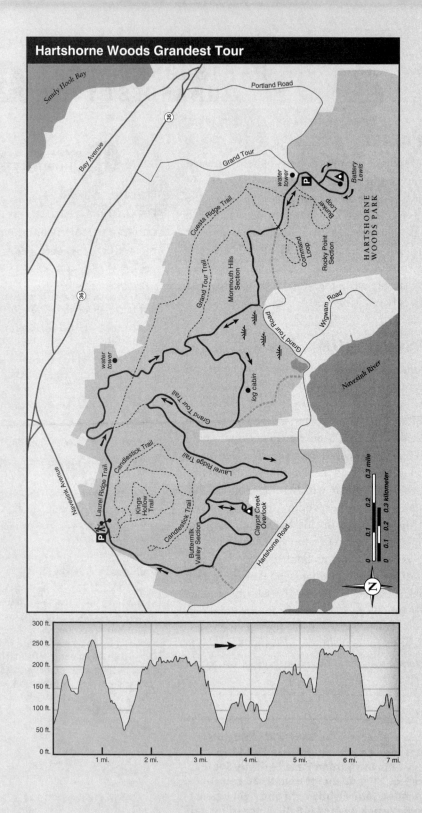

the Jersey Highlands and New York City during World War II. The other two sections of the preserve are more nature-oriented, with dirt and pebbly pathways flowing from swampy swales to oak-and-laurel-laced heights, with occasional views of the Navesink River tossed in for good measure. Hartshorne, incidentally, is named for Richard Hartshorne, who, after spying this land from on board a ship in 1670, went on to purchase it from the local natives. Some of his descendants still reside in the area.

This double loop encompasses the Monmouth Hills and Buttermilk Valley parts of the park, with a short stop by Battery Lewis. The most challenging aspect of the fairly easy, up-and-down tour is keeping to the correct trail, as blazes only appear at intersections—sometimes not even then—and the park map is unreliable. From the Buttermilk Valley trailhead on Navesink Avenue, go to the kiosk and take the Laurel Ridge Trail (LRT) to the immediate left. For 5 minutes, this wide gravel walkway slowly ascends through oaks and laurels before a minor cresting; lope left there onto the Grand Tour Trail (GTT, black diamond blazes). The moss-sided track persists down the slope for a bit, then shifts toward the east-southeast, gradually gaining ground.

Expect a grinding climb of 5 to 10 minutes, one that will carry you through a four-way intersection with a dirt road. On reaching the ridge, the path approaches a second road but zigs left just shy of it, lunging toward a looming water tower, only to cross the gravel surfaced lane and spurt downhill well short of that aquatic eyesore. Go through the subsequent junction as well, a wide one marked by a log bench, and in due time you should find yourself navigating a low bowl, one in which tulip trees, dogwoods, maples, and hollies grow branch-to-branch with oaks and laurels. Jog right at the succeeding fork (a post marks this corner), which delivers you to the opposite side of the depression, hemmed in here by thorny catbrier.

The Grand Tour veers to the right at the next full intersection (GPS: N40° 23.795' W73° 59.952'), but the straight option, to Battery Lewis and Rocky Point, is a worthwhile detour, especially for history buffs. In brief, the narrow path darts through a closely gathered cover of thorny vines, where wild roses and colorful violets thrive, hurtling left at the first fork, as you near a residential area. Tootle to the right at the Y, still gaining elevation, then left near the top of the hill, back among laurels. Dart left on hitting the pavement and steer to the right, toward the parking lot, when a green water tower comes into view. Battery Lewis is the high, weed-covered mound, straight ahead beyond the parking area. You may climb it, and enjoy superb views of the ocean and NJ 36 to the south, by passing through the concrete archway and swinging right at the wooden railings.

When you've finished exploring the ruins of the old coastal defense, return to the earlier turnoff, by the briar-cloaked bowl, and steer left. Marching uphill once more, keep an alert eye out for a glimpse of the Navesink through the trees off your port side, and for pileated woodpeckers throughout this part of the

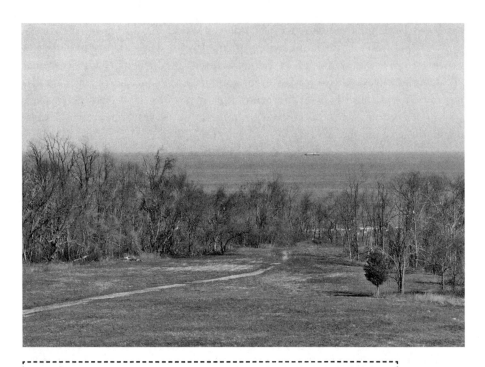

The vistas from atop Battery Lewis extend over the Atlantic, supporting its former role in defending the coast.

forest. In a short time, a log cabin (a group-rental facility) appears to the left of the path; just beyond you'll hit a T, with the hike hopping to the right.

Ten minutes of walking through a concentration of mountain laurels brings you to yet another fork. The right stem leads back to the trailhead, so unless you're feeling tired, head left into the Buttermilk Valley section of Hartshorne. This is another stretch of the LRT, though its namesake shrubs slowly give way to holly, oak, and birch as you climb the ridge. The Navesink is again visible from the crest, and then—too soon—it's back down the hill. The Claypit Creek Overlook spur, tucked among trees on your left, succeeds the next rise. The clay pit itself is hard to spot, but you will be rewarded, somewhat anticlimactically, with even better vistas of the Navesink as well as Oceanic Bridge.

From that 7-minute side trip, Laurel Ridge begins a steep slide downward. A short spell of level terrain ensues, and then the final 15 minutes of the hike flows by a residential neighborhood—with all the sights and sounds that entails.

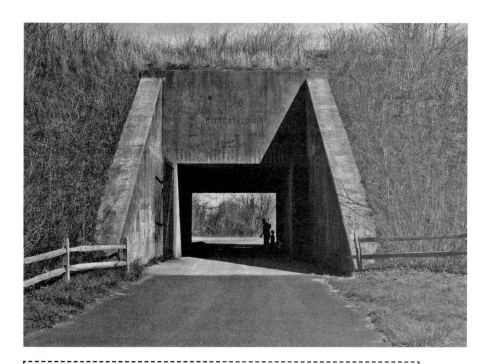

Battery Lewis was erected in 1942 as a strategic part of New York Harbor's defense in WWII.

## NEARBY ACTIVITIES

**Huber Woods Park,** in Locust, features 6 miles of trails that pass through a colorful grove of tulip trees, an extensive stand of oaks and hickories, as well as an open meadow that teems with wildflowers from late spring through early summer. In addition to partridgeberry and trailing arbutus, you may find pink lady's slipper orchids among the ground cover. Huber also shelters foxes and great horned owls. For further information, call 732-872-2670 or visit **tinyurl.com/huberwoodspark.**

Time now to go get some seafood! Cruise down Shore Drive or Bay Avenue in Highlands for a taste of the Jersey Shore.

# 50 JENNY JUMP GHOST LAKE LOOP

### KEY AT-A-GLANCE INFORMATION

**LENGTH:** 5.4 miles

**ELEVATION GAIN:** 1,241 feet

**CONFIGURATION:** Balloon

**DIFFICULTY:** Moderate

**SCENERY:** Dense deciduous forest, seasonal streams, upland swamps, a picturesque lake, stunning vistas

**EXPOSURE:** Shady canopy, except at vistas and by the lake

**TRAFFIC:** Generally light

**TRAIL SURFACE:** Dirt, rocks

**HIKING TIME:** 2.5 hours

**DRIVING DISTANCE:** 65 miles

**SEASON:** Year-round, sunrise–sunset

**ACCESS:** Free; pets on leash

**MAPS:** At park office; USGS *Washington*

**FACILITIES:** Latrine and water fountain by trailhead

**COMMENTS:** Hunting is allowed. The observatory site of the United Astronomy Clubs of New Jersey, within the park, may offer an otherworldly type of activity. Visit uacnj .org. Otherwise fishing, boating, skiing, or hunting will keep you busy. For further information, call 908-459-4366 or visit njparksandforests.org /parks/jennyjump.html.

## GPS COORDINATES

N40° 55.292' W74° 53.774'

## IN BRIEF

A scenic pond, colorfully framed by densely wooded hills, is just one attraction of this lightly trafficked circuit, a mildly arduous uphill–downhill grind into a beautiful forest. Also appealing are the colossal granite boulders and rocky uplift—reminders of the last ice age—that are naturally interwoven with a heavy helping of hardwoods, including oaks, beeches, maples, and tulip poplars. Bears range throughout these hills, as do wild turkeys and other birds.

## DESCRIPTION

To reach Jenny Jump State Forest, you will have to travel through some of the prettiest farmland in the entire Garden State. Moravian immigrants were attracted to this lush, fertile area, the Kittatinny Valley, in the latter part of the 1700s, probably because the rolling hills reminded them of the Old Country. Although a smallpox epidemic and financial difficulties led the group to disband in 1808, many of their solidly built limestone buildings (as well as a few of their sturdier wooden structures) still survive in the neighboring communities.

------------------------------------------

## *Directions*

Follow I-95 across the George Washington Bridge and take Exit 69 to merge onto I-80 West. Drive to Exit 12 and merge onto Hope Blairstown Road/CR 521. Drive 1.2 miles south and turn left on Millbrook Road/CR 611. Proceed 0.3 mile and veer left on Hope Johnsonburg Road/CR 519. Continue for 1 mile to Shiloh Road, make a right on it, and drive 1.1 miles to State Park Road. Go right and, after 1 mile, turn left and then quickly right to proceed to the trailhead parking, 0.1 mile ahead.

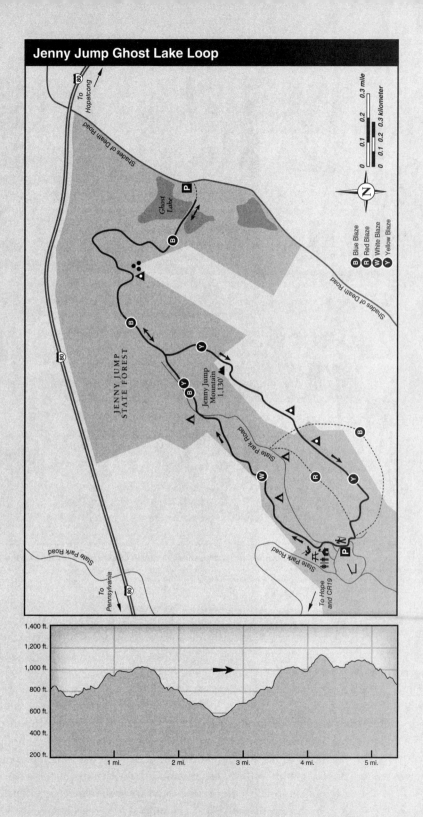

# Jenny Jump Ghost Lake Loop

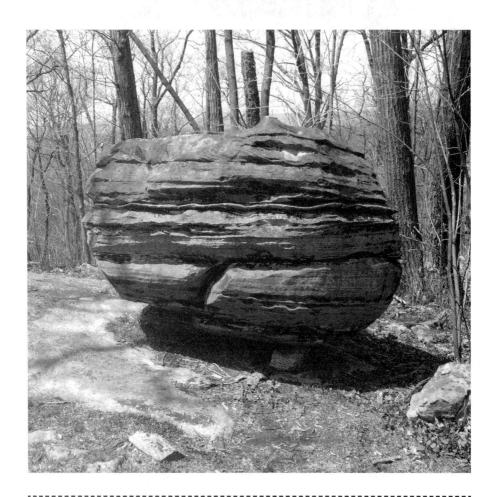

Twenty thousand years ago, the Wisconsin Glacier deposited this grooved boulder, not too far from the summit of Jenny Jump Mountain.

Also surviving is the legend of how this mountain range acquired its unusual name. In 1747, Sven Roseen, a Swedish missionary, recorded that a girl named Jenny was picking berries on a high ridge when a band of Lenape Indians approached. Her father, spying the natives and fearing the worst, called out to her to jump, which she supposedly did. Perhaps Jenny's tragic end is also responsible for how Ghost Lake came by its moniker, as well as Shades of Death Road, which leads to it. Rather than motor to the lake, though, we prefer to haunt the forest paths that go there and back, an effort that allows us to savor all the more both a picnic lunch by its appealingly rocky, grass-fringed shore and the rough, boulder-strewn, wilderness-like quality of this glacier-wracked woodland.

Leave your car in the small parking lot across from the stone-sided latrine and walk downhill, back toward the visitor center. Keep to the blacktop as you near the latter, swinging right and ascending the road toward the group camps and sites 15 to 27. Bear left at the first bifurcation, onto the dirt-and-gravel-surfaced access road leading to group camping site A. As it arcs downhill to the right, look for the white blazes of the Orchard Trail (OT) and continue heading east, down the alameda of white pines, past the outhouse, straight ahead even as the road bends right. A rich range of such trees as tulip, maple, birch, oak, and beech populates the upward-sloping forest to your right, while an open meadow is visible through a thin curtain of hardwoods on the left. By your feet, meanwhile, are, in addition to a great deal of rocky debris, Dutchman's breeches, violets, mayapple, meadow parsnip, anemones, and wild geraniums.

In a few toe-stubbing minutes, the single-file OT curves right and begins to climb the chunky slope, passing over a fern-fronded seasonal arroyo, rapidly reaching the paved camp road, where the white blazes end. Point your paws to the left, and in just 200 yards, near the end of the lane, shift right, back into the forest. Initially, this path, which follows an old forest road, is a union of the Ghost Lake and Summit Trails, blazed with blue and yellow, respectively. Listen closely and you may hear the shriek of hawks soaring over this undulating terrain, and there's a good chance you will also observe blue azure and mourning cloak butterflies flitting among the fair-size erratics. Shortly after the disused forest lane hops through a pocket swamp, you will arrive at a post, with the Ghost Lake Trail (GL, blue blazes) heading left and the Summit Trail (ST, yellow markings) breaking to the right. Hold to the left, now on the narrow GL, moving toward Ghost Lake.

The eye-popping outcroppings you see along this stretch, which grow increasingly impressive as you navigate your way toward the water, were deposited by the Wisconsin Glacier some 21,000 years ago, as it made its way down from Canada; of a far more recent vintage is the oxidized green of lichen speckling those formations. From the crest of this ridge (where we've spied a pair of Baltimore orioles and a scarlet tanager), the GL descends over a long-abandoned forest road, passing, as it does so, a short spur to the right. Scoot down that trace, to a lip of ledge where an old cabin once stood, and take in the far-reaching views to the west, which include the notch of the Delaware River Gap.

Back on the main path, the descent continues, intermittently picking up road noise from I-80 while twisting toward the west-northwest. The enormous fern-capped boulders and rocky protrusions to the left of the trail, as you near the bottom of the hill, endow the setting with an appealing aura of the antediluvian, which is only mildly softened by the presence, in spring, of lavender-flowering myrtle, trout lily, and Canada mayflower. The seasonal streams pouring off the steep hill to your right feed Ghost Lake, just ahead, and the surrounding hills themselves contribute a highly scenic backdrop to the waterside setting, once you cross the grassy berm that divides the Ghost into twin bodies of water. You'll find plenty of space on the rocks by the shore, among the yellow coltsfoot, violets, and ramps, to enjoy a sandwich or snack.

Once through with that repast, return the way you came, all the way back to the wooden post, where you should now swing left onto the Summit Trail. The scenery along this route is much the same as what you encountered on the GL, without the high drama of those remarkable rock formations. Nonetheless, this is a fun ramble from one ridge node to another, once you've put the straight streak upward to the first summit behind you. On reaching that initial crest, you may find the west-facing vista point a tad underwhelming. Take heart: the views grow increasingly fetching with each of the four peaks this trail hits. The second rise culminates in a delightful rock shelf, another fine spot in which to indulge in a snack or to contemplate a favorite volume of verse. Leap over the crossing with the Spring Trail (blue blazes), which occurs in the lull between this node and the succeeding one, and proceed to the third peak to enjoy what is arguably the best vantage spot, both toward the east as well as west.

From the fourth and final crest, which is lower than the others but holds the distinction of being adorned with a pair of picturesque erratics, the inevitable descent begins. A short trace to the left leads to a multitiered rock shelf that looks onto a rising bump of a hill just west of you—perhaps the one from which Jenny jumped. Moving onward, turn left at the subsequent intersection, where the ST joins the red-blazed Swamp Trail. Ignore the spur to the left, in another minute of strolling, and the one that succeeds it, both of which connect to walk-in campsites. The trail, bearing both yellow and red markings, now hooks sharply downhill over rocks and dirt, with the parking area—and hopefully your car—just ahead.

## NEARBY ACTIVITIES

In spite of being a major location for the filming of *Friday the 13th,* historic **Hope** radiates charm. Some stores and banks provide brochures for self-guided walking tours among the town's Moravian architecture. It is listed in the state and national registers of historic places.

The **Land of Make Believe** is an amusement and water park in the foothills of the Jenny Jump Mountains, ideal for cooling off after a hot summer hike. For further information, visit **lomb.com.**

# JOCKEY HOLLOW RUN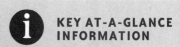

## IN BRIEF

*Ten-hut!* This short hike traverses the mountain ridge where the Continental Army weathered the hardships of a brutal winter, from 1779 to 1780. The undulating nature of the trail, which meanders from forest to swamp and back again, while passing by several historic structures, helps illustrate why George Washington chose this as defensible place to bivouac. *At ease!*

## DESCRIPTION

Normally, when you visit a national historic site you can expect to see statues, monument stones, and plaques aplenty. Morristown has all that, along with some fairly excellent hiking terrain. Doubtful? Bear in mind that one of the reasons that Washington chose this spot as a place for his army to bivouac, from October 1779 through June 1780, was its strategically defensible position atop a mountain ridge. His army may be long gone, but the rolling hills of Morristown remain, with 27 miles of trekking trails winding through Jockey Hollow alone.

- - - - - - - - - - - - - - - - - - - - - - - - - - - - -

### *Directions* ⟶

Follow I-95 across the George Washington Bridge and take Exit 69 to merge onto I-80 West. Take Exit 43A and merge onto I-287 South. Proceed to Exit 30B and turn right on North Maple Avenue, followed by a quick right on US 202 North/Morristown Road. Continue 1.8 miles and turn left on Tempe Wick Road. The park entrance is 1.4 miles ahead, to the right. Once there, follow the signs to the one-way tour road (Cemetery Road) and the visitor center. Follow Cemetery Road for 1.2 miles, then turn right on Grand Parade Road and proceed 0.6 mile to the parking lot.

## KEY AT-A-GLANCE INFORMATION

**LENGTH:** 5.1 miles

**ELEVATION GAIN:** 833 feet

**CONFIGURATION:** Loop

**DIFFICULTY:** Easy to moderate

**SCENERY:** Dense deciduous forest, grassy grounds, quiet streams, 18th-century soldier's huts, and a farm

**EXPOSURE:** Mostly shady canopy; Wick Farm and the soldiers' huts are exposed.

**TRAFFIC:** Generally light; some trails are shared with horses.

**TRAIL SURFACE:** Dirt, rocks, and grass

**HIKING TIME:** 2.5 hours

**DRIVING DISTANCE:** 47 miles

**SEASON:** Year-round, sunrise–sunset

**ACCESS:** No fee for the Jockey Hollow Unit; pets on leash

**MAPS:** At park office; tinyurl.com/morristownmap; USGS *Mendham*

**FACILITIES:** Restrooms and water at trailhead

**COMMENTS:** Park is closed during controlled hunts. For further information, call 973-543-4030 or visit nps.gov/morr.

## GPS COORDINATES

N40° 46.337'  W74° 31.690'

# Jockey Hollow Run

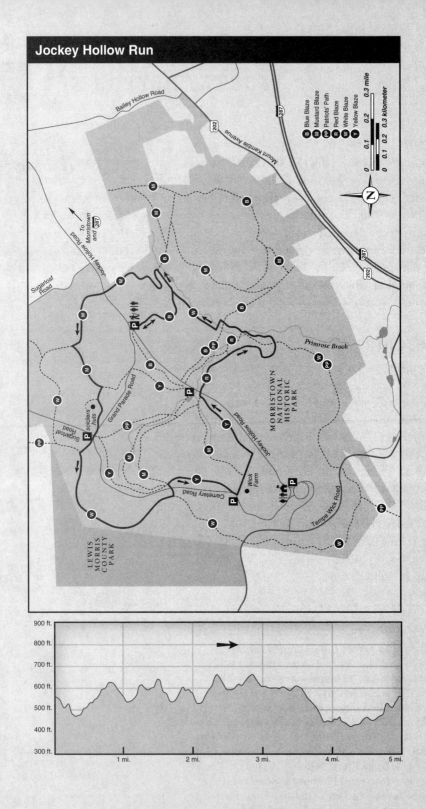

As you wend your way past historic structures and pad through secluded woodlands, you may learn something about the suffering of Continental Army during a winter so severe many considered it the "cruelest" of the Revolution. (So much so that most of the Pennsylvania volunteers mutinied, while nearly 200 soldiers from New Jersey attempted to desert.) What you probably will *not* hear about are the unsung heroes of this national park, the participants of the Civilian Conservation Corps. In Jockey Hollow, Franklin Roosevelt's "army of the unemployed" constructed the trail system, built the park road, and conducted archeological digs at the Soldiers' Huts, Guerin House, and Wick Farm, while also planting the garden and apple orchard at the last site. Here, as in so many parks around the country, theirs was a lasting contribution to the cultural and recreational wealth of our nation.

Your tour begins on the New York Brigade Trail (NYB), by the comfort station at the northeast end of Jockey Hollow Road. Pick up the blue blazes opposite the kiosk, behind the toilet pavilion, at the southeast end of the parking area. Once past the black metal gate, the wide, straight path enters into a dense forest of oaks, beeches, an occasional black walnut, and other hardwoods. This in itself stands in marked contrast to when the Continental Army was here. In need of shelter the winter of their encampment, the troops cut down most of the trees in the vicinity in order to build more than a thousand huts. Which makes the grove of aged tulip poplars you'll walk by on this route—some of the stoutest and tallest in the park—all the more impressive.

In 5 minutes or so, the NYB meets the Grand Loop Trail, merging with it to the left. The NYB shears off to the right rather soon, shortly after you pass the little pond (complete with bench), but instead of following it, bear left, remaining with the Grand Loop (GL, white blazes). As it narrows to single-file, the GL begins to gain elevation, hitting Jockey Hollow Road in perhaps 10 minutes of steady striding. The path crosses the pavement and initially descends, only to rise steeply yet again. During the course of that small effort, you'll come to an unblazed (but well-indicated) spur on the left that leads to the Soldiers' Huts site: take it. At the next intersection, leave this slightly overgrown cutoff for the Soldiers' Hut Trail (SH, yellow tags), turning right. The Huts site is 0.1 mile distant, with the dirt-surfaced SH approaching it from above, behind a double-wide cabin. The view as you emerge from the cover of birch and tulip trees is of a wide, sweeping meadow, with the nearby huts situated at the upper end of it.

Once finished with examining these historic recreations, resume the trail, sticking with the yellow blazes down the hill, all the way to the park road. Turn right on the pavement and make your way to the parking area, dead ahead at the confluence of Grand Parade and Cemetery Roads. At the left end of the parking lot is a connector trail (also bearing the blazes of the Patriots' Path): take it. Two minutes of hustling up this overgrown spur should return you to the white-blazed Grand Loop, where you swing left.

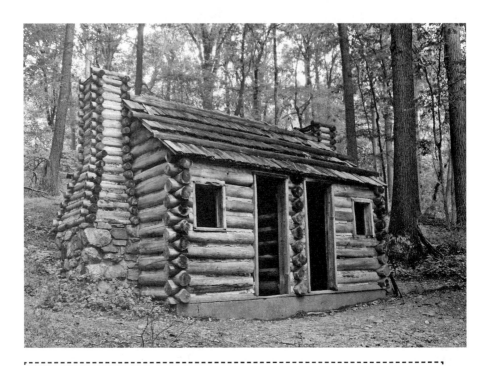

Soldiers of Washington's Continental Army built more than 1,000 simple log huts in Jockey Hollow, where they camped during the harsh winter of 1779.

Hang with the GL for the ensuing six-sevenths of a mile, as the two-person-wide track initially rises steeply, cresting by another grove of colossal poplars, then begins the inevitable descent. Here, as elsewhere in Jockey Hollow, the forest, while well treed, offers rather clean sight lines through an understory of lush grasses and pricker plants. About 3 minutes after passing a deer-proof enclosure, the GL bends to the right, while an unblazed spur branches left. Go left, cross Cemetery Road, and roll right at the subsequent junction, back on the yellow-blazed SH and now paralleling the pavement. Well, not *exactly* paralleling it, for in a few minutes the path returns to Cemetery Road, bringing you to the threshold of Wick Farm. Keep to the left at this Y-intersection, walking along the grass-covered lane in the direction of the farmhouse. When you reach the wood hut, at the corner of the apple orchard, look sharply for the yellow blazes of the Grand Parade Trail (GP), which begins here. The hike continues on this trail, but you may first choose to explore Wick Farm and check out its adjacent garden, which is sowed with Colonial-era crops (in season).

Initially, the GP shadows the apple orchard, with shagbark hickory, oak, and locust trees shadowing *it*. Keep right when a spur arises on the left; then, as the path bends from east to northeast, bear left—still on the GP—at the appearance of Jockey Hollow Road. In an additional 5 to 6 minutes, the GP passes the other end of the aforementioned spur, hops over a bridge, and once more meets the road. This time head directly across the asphalt and transfer to the red-blazed Primrose Brook Trail (PB), which hugs a slow-moving swamp stream in what is one of the lovelier stretches of the hike. To get the most out of this tranquil setting, and to close the circuit, bear left at the first junction, where the PB splits, and, after a brief uphill–downhill, hook right at the next one.

As you now hike east-southeast, the moss-sided trail hops over Primrose Brook via three fair-size rocks before meeting the Grand Loop Trail at a four-way intersection. Turn left onto the GL (which overlaps the Patriots' Path for now), and bear left again at the next junction, a crossing with the New York Brigade Trail. Once over the wide bridge, the white-blazed GL breaks to the right, away from the NYB (and the Patriots' Path). Take that right, and then, in about 6 minutes of persistent marching, lunge left, back on the stem of the NYB that began your hike. Follow the blue blazes, and in a few moments you will be face-to-face with the comfort station by the trailhead.

## NEARBY ACTIVITIES

History buffs will want to save time for the Morristown Unit of this splendid park, which can also provide a great introduction to your hike/tour. Both the **Washington Headquarters Museum** and the **Ford Mansion,** which was the home of George Washington during the infamous winter of 1779–1780, can be toured almost daily. For details call 973-539-2016, ext. 210.

For a change of pace, and an insight into completely different era of architecture and design, be sure to visit **Craftsman Farms.** Once the country estate of Gustav Stickley, best known for his Mission (a.k.a. Craftsman) furniture, Craftsman Farms offers guided house tours, a museum, walking trails, a pond, gardens, and more. There is an excellent website to stimulate your curiosity; visit **stickleymuseum.org.**

**52** LEWIS MORRIS LOOP

## KEY AT-A-GLANCE INFORMATION

**LENGTH:** 5.4 miles

**ELEVATION GAIN:** 817 feet

**CONFIGURATION:** Balloon

**DIFFICULTY:** Easy to moderate

**SCENERY:** Hardwood forest, swamps, several stream crossings, and a sizable lake

**EXPOSURE:** Tree-shaded, but very exposed in winter

**TRAFFIC:** Heavy on weekends and after work on weekdays

**TRAIL SURFACE:** Packed dirt, which can be muddy in spring; some roots; periodic stretches of loose stones

**HIKING TIME:** 2.5 hours

**DRIVING DISTANCE:** 40 miles

**SEASON:** Year-round, sunrise–sunset

**ACCESS:** Free; pets on leash not exceeding 6 feet

**MAPS:** At the park's Cultural Center; download from morrisparks.net /maps/iviewer/lewismorris.asp; USGS *Mendham*

**FACILITIES:** Restrooms, water, and much more near trailhead

**COMMENTS:** A multipurpose park with many activities to choose from, but to avoid the nonstop parade of bicycles, the best time to visit is weekdays before 5 p.m. Call 973-267-4351 or visit morrisparks.net /aspparks/lmmain.asp.

## GPS COORDINATES

N40° 47.344'  W74° 32.766'

## IN BRIEF

You won't require a bicycle to get the most out of this hilly hike, just a decent pair of walking shoes and a couple of hours' time. Part of the fun comes from trails that are hardly ever level yet seldom reach the steepness of more-rugged climbs, making this ideal for family outings. Several streams add to the natural flavor of the setting, and the healthy mix of hardwoods may make you feel like you're farther out in the sticks than you actually are.

## DESCRIPTION

George Washington brought the Continental Army to Morristown in 1777, and again for the notoriously bitter winter of 1779–80. History buffs have been making the same pilgrimage ever since, visiting Morristown National Historical Park in an effort to better understand the trials those men endured. While the role this locale played in the Revolutionary War is worth noting, there's more to Morristown than a memorial to monumental hardship, stoic determination, and bloody rag–covered feet.

------------------------------------------------

*Directions* ───────────────────➤

Follow I-95 across the George Washington Bridge and take Exit 69 to merge onto I-80 West. Drive to Exit 43A and merge onto I-287 South. Proceed to Exit 36, stay left on the ramp, and turn right onto CR 510 West/ Lafayette Avenue. Continue 0.4 mile and turn right on Morris Street/CR 510. Drive 0.3 mile and turn right on East Park Place, followed by a left on North Park Place/US 202 South and a right on Washington Street/CR 510 West/ NJ 24, which will eventually become Mendham Road. Stick with CR 510 West for about 3.7 miles to the park entrance, on the left.

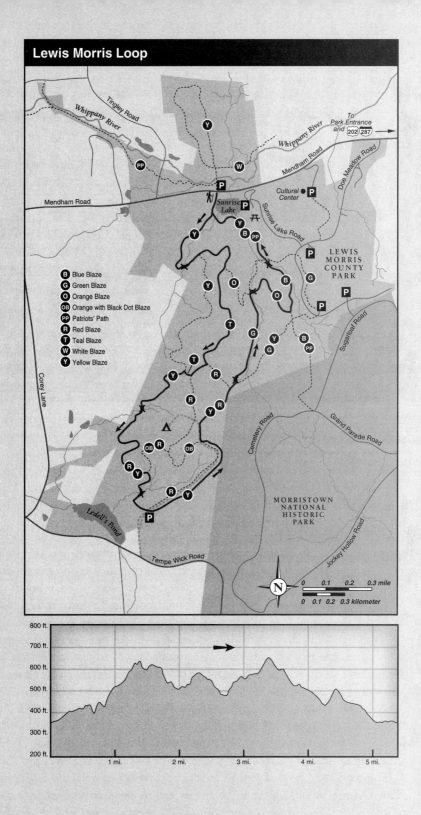

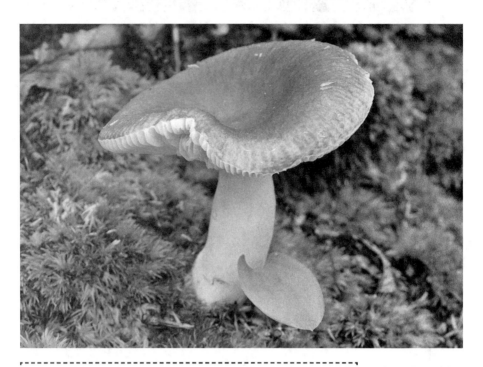

As the name suggests, the conspicuous vomiting russula is best left to slugs and red squirrels, which favor it.

Like, for instance, Lewis Morris County Park. Established 50 years ago as the county's first park, this 1,154-acre preserve was named in honor of Lewis Morris (1671–1746), New Jersey's first governor. In an age of high-handed royalists and backroom double-dealing, Morris lived for politics. When barely 21 years old, he was appointed judge in East Jersey while serving concurrently on Governor Alexander Hamilton's council. He enjoyed a similar position later, on the council of Lord Cornbury, governor of what were then the provinces of New York and New Jersey, but was dismissed for insubordination. Undeterred, Morris ran for, and was elected to, the assembly in 1707, from which post he continued his campaign against Cornbury, going so far as to file a protest with Queen Anne, who shortly thereafter canned the governor. If Morris had hoped to be named to replace the arrogant, corrupt Cornbury, he was disappointed in that ambition, at least temporarily, becoming instead, in 1715, chief justice of New York's supreme court. Years later, when he ran afoul of Governor William Cosby, summarily dismissing a case the latter had brought before the bench, the governor returned the favor by dismissing Morris from the judiciary. Lewis's response was to return to the assembly, using his position there to publicize his grievances against the chief executive; this time around, however, the Crown failed to take action on his complaints. Finally, in 1738, Lewis Morris attained his goal, being elevated to the governorship. In a classic case of "what goes around comes around," his tenure was notable for his contentious, quarrelsome relationship with the provincial assembly, which he argued lacked the authority to question his power.

We trust you'll find nothing contentious or quarrelsome in your own encounter with Lewis Morris. Its hilly contours make it fun to wander the woodland, even as it rolls up (to a peak elevation of 631 feet) and down several times, without ever being the lung-popper of more-sustained climbs. The hike begins opposite the parking area, across Mendham Road (CR 510). Follow the yellow-blazed trail (YT, which runs concurrently, at first, with the blue markings of the Patriot Path spur) along the gravel-surfaced road, strutting by Sunrise Lake on the left. Just as you leave the water behind and enter the shelter of oaks, pines, black birches, and many beech trees, the path forks. Bear right, breaking away from the Patriot Path spur, now treading uphill, with trout lily, ramps, and wild rose growing by the sides of the single-file track. Within 5 minutes, the YT widens, levels off, bends left, and crosses, via triple-wide duckboards, the stream which hitherto it had been paralleling. From there it arcs sharply to the east-northeast and begins climbing again, meeting, along the way, an orange-blazed trail on the left. Take that left option (you'll return to the YT later on), a rambling route that descends slightly in first aiming north, then gains ground as it circles around the head of the ridge in a southeasterly direction, showcasing, en route, great globs of quartz jutting out from the soil, along with an array of Canada mayflowers and ferns.

The roller coaster continues on switching to the teal-blazed trail, a right turn shortly after the track tacks south. First it's level, then it descends a tad, followed by a gradual climb, with the latter ultimately topping out at 631 feet, the highest point you'll attain on this hike. Naturally, an elevation loss ensues, and within very few minutes this teal-tagged stretch comes to a junction with a red-blazed trail, which merges from the right. Continue straight, and remain with the teal markings as the red-blazed path lumbers off to the left in roughly 30 strides. In roughly a minute or two you'll have descended from the silvery beech–dominated heights, at which point turn left, back on the well-beaten dirt track of the YT. Further meanderings ensue, trending generally uphill, with your next crest a relatively modest, and easily attained, 615 feet. Keep to the right at the unblazed intersection directly after that, still hanging with the YT, which soon delivers you to a skunk cabbage–festooned fen. Ignore the spur on the left there, but enjoy the great growths of artist's conk crusting off the bark of the tulip trees in this vicinity. Not content with any one direction, the path roams from south to southeast, crosses a short bridge, and snakes south, then north, east, and south again. Your third crest, at a less-than-rarefied elevation of 591 feet, is heralded not by any sense of thinning air, but rather the T-intersection that occurs there. That's your cue to slice right, on a stretch now blazed both red and yellow.

On climbing and descending yet again, the trail meanders through a pocket meadow bordered by two or three cedars, hooks east, and then passes a path on the left. Remain with the YT (which is still saddled with the red blazes), and in a couple of minutes of stomping downward over chunky, gravelly ground, it brings you to a swamp stream, prettily bordered by trout lilies. Ford that via the low bridge, and after further sinuousness, you'll arrive at a campers' parking area. Cut directly across the lot, to the far side of the dirt road, where the YT forges onward to the left (the red blazes, finally branching off, hold to the nearer side of the road). The YT flanks the road for several minutes, gradually drifting gently toward the grassy, rising slope on the right, where deer often graze. Then, abruptly, it shifts back to the west and recrosses the road, immediately reaching an intersection. You may think at first that the loop lopes onward, back into the forest. Think again: the YT shears off to the right, hanging with the dirt drive (and rejoining the red blazes). Fortunately, the only vehicles you're likely to encounter along this part of the hike are of the fat-tired, two-wheeled variety, though on weekends they're so numerous you may feel like you've stumbled upon a bicycle freeway. Heave to the right in 500 feet, when the downward-slanting road forks, and persist in that direction as the red blazes vault left onto the $O^2$ sidetrack. In a few scant seconds, and no more than 50 yards' distance, a green-blazed trail (GT) surfaces; bound left onto that, leaving the dirt road behind, and use the low bridge to ford the swamp stream.

This very appealing part of the hike involves a descent so gradual it almost seems like you're walking on level land, while the GT hugs the bank of a stream, colored green with the large leaves of skunk cabbage, through the elongated gully between two ridges. Saunter to the right, in 10 minutes of very easy strolling, when the orange-blazed trail merges from the left into the GT. Leave the latter in 30 yards, scuttling left with the orange path and hopping over the bridge, even as the GT continues straight ahead. A short uphill burst ensues, with the moss-sided track hitting its apex at 535 feet, amid a cluster of ill-looking laurel. On snaking your way down the other side of the ridge, you come to an intersection, where you rejoin the YT by turning left (note that it also bears the blue blazes of the Patriot Path spur). Other trails will intersect this one as it draws you by a cattail-rimmed pond and the picnic grounds adjacent to Sunrise Lake. Traveling clockwise around that body of water, plan to stick with the YT all the way back to the trailhead, by Mendham Road. And should you still be bounding with energy, well, you might continue on the YT north of your car for a mini-loop of a little more than half a mile.

## NEARBY ACTIVITIES

Still game for hoofing it through the woods? The aforementioned **Morristown National Historical Park**, adjacent to Lewis Morris County Park, offers 27 miles of horse and foot trails. General Washington twice chose Morristown as his winter base—its strategic position, between the Watchung Mountains and Long Hill, afforded protection against a sneak attack by the British while simultaneously allowing him to monitor the enemy's movements. Washington envisioned a "log-house city" to house the 10,000 soldiers under his command, and while 600 acres of hardwood trees were felled, an early snowfall kept most of the army in tents through February, 1780. For further details, call 973-543-4030 or visit **nps.gov/morr**.

# SANDY HOOK HIKING TRAIL   53

## IN BRIEF

Beach dunes, huge holly trees, saltwater marshes, coastal-defense ruins, a 19th-century fort, and even a historic lighthouse combine to endow this long, level jaunt with an interdisciplinary appeal. The icing on the cake comes in two flavors: a striking view of Manhattan from an observation deck near the Hook's end, and the many waterfowl and migratory birds that pass by at various times of year.

## DESCRIPTION

Of the 2.5 million people who visit Sandy Hook every year, less than a fifth of them ever make it off the beach. No question, this barrier peninsula is blessed with extraordinary ocean vistas along its 7 miles of sandy shore. But to limit yourself to sunbathing, salt spray, and splashing surf is to miss the greater part of what Sandy Hook is all about.

A unit of Gateway National Recreation Area, the 1,665-acre Sandy Hook is, essentially, an elongated sandbar that extends from the north end of New Jersey's coast up toward Coney Island. But what a sandbar! With salt marshes, a maritime forest—including one of the densest concentrations of American holly on the Atlantic coast—and great diversity of plant life, it is also a critical stopover point in

### KEY AT-A-GLANCE INFORMATION

**LENGTH:** 9.6 miles

**ELEVATION GAIN:** 68 feet

**CONFIGURATION:** Out-and-back

**DIFFICULTY:** Easy to moderate

**SCENERY:** Dunes, beaches, marshes, forests, historic lighthouse, and fort

**EXPOSURE:** Mostly exposed

**TRAFFIC:** Summer sees hordes of beach-lovers, but few visit the trail.

**TRAIL SURFACE:** Mostly sandy

**HIKING TIME:** 5 hours

**DRIVING DISTANCE:** 60 miles

**SEASON:** April–October, 5 a.m.–10 p.m.; November–March, 5 a.m.–8 p.m.

**ACCESS:** $15 beach parking Memorial Day–Labor Day; pets on leash

**MAPS:** At visitor center; USGS *Sandy Hook*

**FACILITIES:** Restrooms, water, and public phone at visitor center; seasonal restrooms in Fort Hancock area

**COMMENTS:** Be sure to come before 10 a.m. on summer weekends; when the parking lots fill, the park closes until space frees up. In spring and summer, parts of the beaches may be closed to protect nesting shorebirds. For further information, call 732-872-5970 or visit nps.gov/gate.

## Directions ──────→

Follow I-95 across the George Washington Bridge, drive south and take Exit 11 to merge onto the Garden State Parkway South. Proceed 10.8 miles to Exit 117 and merge onto NJ 36 East. Drive for about 12.9 miles, go across the Highlands Bridge to the park entrance, and then proceed 2 miles north to the parking lot by the Spermaceti Cove Visitor Center.

## GPS COORDINATES

N40° 25.615'  W73° 59.060'

# Sandy Hook Hiking Trail

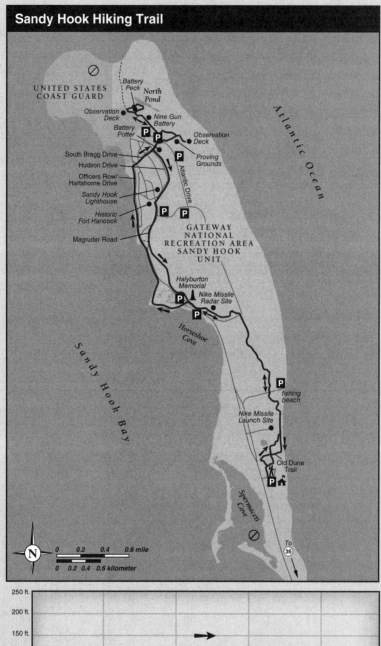

United States Coast Guard

Battery Peck
North Pond
Observation Deck
Nine Gun Battery
Battery Potter
Observation Deck
South Bragg Drive
Hudson Drive
Proving Grounds
Officers Row/ Hartshorne Drive
Sandy Hook Lighthouse
Atlantic Drive
Historic Fort Hancock
Magruder Road

GATEWAY NATIONAL RECREATION AREA SANDY HOOK UNIT

Atlantic Ocean

Halyburton Memorial
Nike Missile Radar Site

Horseshoe Cove

Sandy Hook Bay

fishing beach

Nike Missile Launch Site

Old Dune Trail

Spermaceti Cove

To 36

N
0   0.2   0.4   0.6 mile
0   0.2   0.4   0.6 kilometer

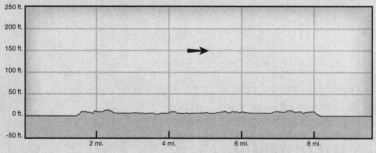

250 ft.
200 ft.
150 ft.
100 ft.
50 ft.
0 ft.
-50 ft.

2 mi.    4 mi.    6 mi.    8 mi.

the Atlantic Flyway, as birds of all feathers flock to it during spring and fall migrations. And because of Sandy Hook's strategic position at the mouth of New York Harbor, it has played a role in guiding ships and protecting the city since 1764. The lighthouse built then is still in use; it's our nation's oldest such beacon. Near it is Fort Hancock, an aggregation of dozens of gun batteries and buildings, which defended the harbor from 1895 through 1974.

This visually exciting linear hike takes in much of Sandy Hook's historic and natural attributes. It is level and easy, but the sun exposure for much of its 9- to 10-mile length is fairly extreme. Pick up a Fort Hancock walking-tour pamphlet at the visitor center and strike out on the Old Dune Trail (ODT) there. Right from the get-go, the peninsula's plant diversity is on display, with red cedar, holly, scrub oak, black cherry shrubs, bayberry, black gum, and even prickly pear cactus thriving in the sandy soil.

In a few minutes, the winding track opens up to a view of the ocean. Remain north across the first beach-access road, then hop over the paved multiuse path. The ODT soon soars through the four-way intersection, by the viewing platform, to post 11, which relates to the Nike missile site that was once within the nearby rusty chain-link fence. Turn left there, onto the Sandy Hook Hiking Trail, running along the right side of the fenced-in Nike compound, which now shelters a pair of old dumpsters and a derelict trailer. To the right is the ocean, where tankers and other ships often cruise the waves farther out.

The path flows along the tops of the dunes, first cutting through the fragile grass (try to walk gently so as not to damage the plants) and then settling onto the beach sand. Once past another fenced-in depot, the trail swings away from the giant clamshells and driftwood of the beach and back into a cedar grove—be alert for the gray post marking this turnoff (GPS: N40° 26.153' W73° 59.001'). In a few hundred yards, it scoots by a paved access road to South Beach, with a pillbox and bunker to the right—leftover defenses from World War II.

The subsequent stretch is one of the few shady points of the walk, slipping through a thick, junglelike entanglement of vines, very tall holly, sumac, catbrier, and phragmites. Bear left at the sandy fork, and in 5 to 8 minutes a fenced-in bunker appears, succeeded by additional ruins a few paces later. At the next paved access road, dogleg left and then right to stay with the path. Keep an eye out for the blue-blazed gray posts (or *white,* as the blue of most has been bleached by the sun), which run the length of this hike.

Had enough of military ruins yet? Let's hope not, since many more compounds await along the loamy ground. Moments after merging to the right with the paved bike path, another fenced compound comes into view, this one being a Nike radar station used to track Soviet jets. Only a series of elevated platforms remains of the former, with three of them decorated with mock-up machinery. Be sure to check out the informative signboard on the installation's west side before continuing along the bike path to the grassy pocket-park memorial for James

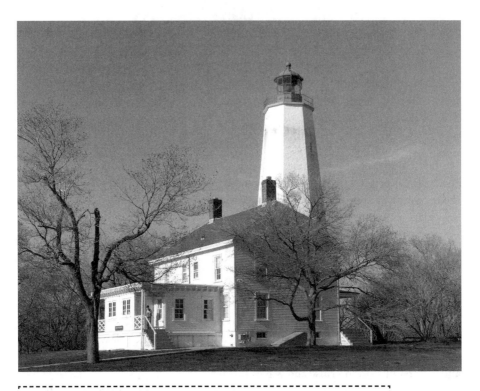

Forget Cape Hatteras! The Sandy Hook Lighthouse is reportedly the oldest such beacon still functioning in the country.

Champion and Hamilton Halyburton, British naval officers who died in a blizzard in 1783 while trying to apprehend a pack of deserters.

From their memorial mast, return to the paved path and, in 300 yards, at the diminutive parking lot, hook left across the road and pick up the walkway, wending west, out to Horseshoe Cove and an overlook of the salt marsh. If you don't see an abundance of cavorting waterfowl here, you'd better have your eyes checked! Move north by the rotting pilings of an old pier and, also to your left, the cement foundations of the shipyard (as well as an appalling amount of litter that was not all left, alas, by a capricious Neptune); the trail proceeds just right of that latter ruin, approaching and passing between two more monoliths. The track then jogs to the right, past a third concrete hulk, finally splashing down on sand.

Enjoy this peachy patch of beach, for soon you'll climb up to the park road, turn left, and remain with pavement, bearing left at the entrance to Fort Hancock, marching due north. Although the military has used the Hook since the War of 1812, most of the sand-colored brick buildings of the fort date from the early 1900s. Stroll up the west side of Officers Row to the Rodman Gun, where Hartshorne Drive meets South Bragg, and strut right onto the latter. The next blue-blazed post is 200 yards ahead, on the north side of the road. Canter two blocks farther from there and take a right on Atlantic Drive, then cross the road and enter the proving ground, where cannons were tested, or "proofed," before being put into action.

This spur flows for perhaps 150 yards by a number of old foundations, then veers left, just as the lane arcs right, and leads to a gravel parking area. Before proceeding to the latter, mosey to the right and climb the steps to the top of the observation deck. Not only are the views of the ocean spectacular, but you'll also be rewarded with an extended panorama of the Manhattan skyline. Back at the turnoff, swing right, then quickly left, a maneuver that should have you walking first along the east side of the parking lot and then the cordoned-off Nine Gun Battery, a ghostly concrete structure with a labyrinth of rooms and cells. The trail continues at the north end of the lot, past similar batteries. When you reach the interpretive sign about warblers, by Battery Peck, go right and struggle through the sand dunes to a rail fence, then loop left to the observation deck. From atop that post, which overlooks North Pond, you can clearly see the Verrazano-Narrows Bridge and, just beyond, the Manhattan skyline. (The Coast Guard facility nearer at hand is off-limits to the public.) From the base of the observation deck, shift left to rejoin the trail and retrace your steps to South Bragg Drive. Before doing so, however, you might venture out on the Fisherman's Trail (1 mile round-trip) to the end of the Hook.

Back by South Bragg, head left onto Hudson Drive, passing Battery Potter and the brick power plant, one of the oldest edifices of the fort. As the street angles to the right, it runs smack dab into the lighthouse. This tower was originally built on the tip of the peninsula, but an accumulation of tide-swept sand over the years has extended Sandy Hook more than a mile northward. Who knows, someday it may reach Staten Island. Pick up Magruder Road at the lighthouse and stick with it to the Nike missile site at the fort's entrance. Branch left onto the bike path, moving south, and return from there to your earlier route. Go left at post 11 on the Old Dunes Trail, drifting along the beach to complete the loop.

## NEARBY ACTIVITIES

In addition to testing the surf, you can also tour a few buildings inside the park. The Sandy Hook lighthouse, the lighthouse keeper's quarters, the Nike missile site, the Fort Hancock Museum, and the History House are all open to visitors. For further information, call 732-872-5970 or visit **nps.gov/gate/planyourvisit /sandy-hook-hours.htm.**

The illuminating **Twin Lights of Navesink Light Station,** in Highlands, was designated a National Historic Landmark in 2006. The double lighthouse features a commanding view from its north tower, and its museum documents the works of inventor Guglielmo Marconi and the U.S. Life-Saving Service. For details, call 732-872-1814 or visit **twinlightslighthouse.com.**

# 54 SOURLAND MOUNTAIN TRACK

## KEY AT-A-GLANCE INFORMATION

**LENGTH:** 5.4 miles

**ELEVATION GAIN:** 724 feet

**CONFIGURATION:** Loop

**DIFFICULTY:** Easy to moderate

**SCENERY:** Lush second-growth hardwood forest, bisected by a few streams and the Texas Eastern Pipeline, boasts fantastic boulders and discreet vernal ponds.

**EXPOSURE:** Mostly shady

**TRAFFIC:** Light to moderate; can be busy on weekends

**TRAIL SURFACE:** Dirt, roots, and many rocks and boulders

**HIKING TIME:** 2.5 hours

**DRIVING DISTANCE:** 63 miles

**SEASON:** Year-round, sunrise–sunset

**ACCESS:** Free; pets on leash

**MAPS:** At trailhead kiosk; tinyurl. com/sourlandmap; USGS *Rocky Hill*

**FACILITIES:** Emergency phone near parking lot

**COMMENTS:** For further information, visit somersetcountyparks.org.

## GPS COORDINATES

N40° 28.429'  W74° 41.653'

## IN BRIEF

Are you familiar with that kids' game, Scissors, Paper, Stone? This hike abbreviates that to "Stones." You'll be stepping over egg-size stones, fist-size stones, stones like boccie balls, and some that are larger than cantaloupes— really *big* cantaloupes. Don't worry . . . boardwalks and bridges carry you over the worst of those, preventing this from becoming a prolonged exercise in ankle-aching agony. Meanwhile, the many winding streams, bird-filled stands of cedars, and a pair of thrilling boulder cataclysms add up to an excellent, memorable outing.

## DESCRIPTION

If you have spent any time in the Watchung Mountains, the geology of Sourland Mountain should seem familiar: both are made up of an unusual gray diabase known as traprock. Sourland is so flush with it that the locale once boasted a quarry, with much of its substrate being carved out and paved into roads or crushed for use as railroad gravel. Sourland is also rich in history; during the Revolutionary War, John Hart, who had signed the Declaration of Independence, successfully eluded British troops in these hills. The German immigrants

----------------------------------------

### *Directions*

Follow I-95 across the George Washington Bridge and drive south to Exit 22. Merge onto I-78 West and continue to Exit 29. Merge onto I-287 South and proceed to Exit 17, onto US 206 South. Drive about 7.8 miles, then head right, or west, on Amwell Road/CR 514. After 3.1 miles, turn left onto East Mountain Road. Continue for 1.9 miles to the park entrance on the right. The parking area is straight ahead.

# Sourland Mountain Track

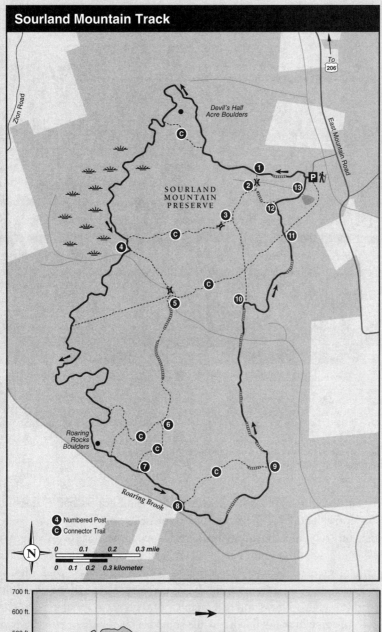

**Zion Road**

*To 206*

*Devil's Hall Acre Boulders*

C

SOURLAND
MOUNTAIN
PRESERVE

**East Mountain Road**

1
2
13
12
3
C
11
4
C
5
C
10

*Roaring Rocks Boulders*

6
C
C
7
C
9
8

*Roaring Brook*

**4** Numbered Post
**C** Connector Trail

N

| 0 | 0.1 | 0.2 | 0.3 mile |

| 0 | 0.1 | 0.2 | 0.3 kilometer |

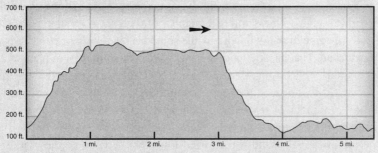

700 ft.
600 ft.
500 ft.
400 ft.
300 ft.
200 ft.
100 ft.

1 mi.  2 mi.  3 mi.  4 mi.  5 mi.

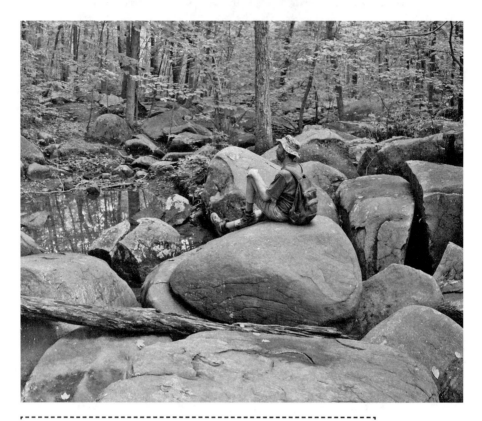

In a summer drought Roaring Brook can be rather quiet, but its boulders remain an impressive sight year-round.

who later farmed this region, though, were responsible for its name, dubbing the mountain "*Sorrel* land," for the russet-red color of its soil.

After you stub your toe a few times in this wilderness of rocks, you may feel that "*Fels* land" or "*Stein* land" would have been more appropriate monikers for an area where the surface stones appear to occupy more space than the topsoil. Don't let the thought of a bruised big digit deter you from visiting this Somerset County park, though—unless you're a member of the Barefoot Hiking Club. Hikes, like ice cream, come in many flavors; while some prefer vanilla or chocolate, others enjoy rocky road. It is in large part the rocky road of so many boulders and rocks that makes Sourland Mountain Preserve such a fascinating—and exciting—place in which to walk. Most of its 2,600 acres are undeveloped, but intrepid bushwhackers will find a number of traces branching away from the main loop that lead to enchanting boulder fields, secluded streams, and upland swamps.

The hike begins beyond the covered kiosk at the edge of the woods. Head into the forest, where maple, oak, beech, and tulip trees compose the canopy and bittersweet, barberry, chokeberry, rue anemone, jack-in-the-pulpit, garlic mustard, violets, and mayapple compete for root room among the litter of stones. A boardwalk helps in fording a boulder stream and seasonal water flow, and in a couple of minutes, by post 1, the path swerves over a bridge. Rather than cross that span, however, bear right (straight, actually), striking uphill on a well-designed zigzag of a track that gains about 300 feet in elevation in just a few minutes. The trail into this part of the preserve has only recently been developed, though it is surprisingly well delineated and navigable (all rocks being relative), with square white blazes indicating the way. As you approach the ridgeline, note the impressive boulders to the left, covering the crown of the mountain. The path eventually meanders through the heart of those colossal stones, which are known collectively as the Devil's Half Acre, before circling south, back toward the main section of Sourland. Along the way, you may notice a number of C-blazed spurs, connector trails that can be used to shorten the outing. Several traces have also been worn into the diabase by intrepid mountain bikers, but only skilled bush-whackers should venture far afield on those, as the forest grows thicker and the rocks more numerous the deeper you delve into the backcountry. If you're search-ing for a reason to extend your adventure beyond the Devil's Half Acre, though, we've seen a handful of the rare and beautiful *Orchis spectabilis* flowering about 100 yards to its west, in the middle of a secluded swamp.

Eventually, the white blazes lead sinuously back to marker 4, where you cruise right, toward the south. Take the next spur, blazed with a red circle, which surfaces, in a minute, on the right. This is a newer trail that meanders through a more remote section of the upper preserve—a gorgeous, boulder-filled nook pop-ulated by giant tulip poplars and, occasionally, trout lily. Eventually, the path emerges under the open sky of a forest cut for the Texas Eastern Pipeline (yes, you read correctly). The trail soars across it diagonally to the right, then lurches back into the cover of trees.

The red-blazed route's final descent passes among a clutch of jumbo rocks, oblong and dramatically fractured, ending at a junction with the main white trail. Head right, and in a few minutes step through the derelict chain-link fence. Next up is Roaring Rocks, a tremendous cataclysm of boulders concen-trated around Roaring Brook, a habitat that nurtures such amphibians as wood frogs, gray tree frogs, and spotted salamanders—and is a popular party spot for local teens.

From this rousing setting, continue along the trail (still white-blazed), com-ing to a T, in about 2 minutes, by a pyramidal cairn and post 7. Go right, descend-ing over rocky ground, and, once more slipping through the chain-link fence, go right again at post 8. Carrying on from there, the forested mix evolves from dominating tulip poplars to beech and birch to a smattering of cedars. Continue straight at post 9, immediately after the appearance of an old dam wall to your left. As you stroll over the ensuing series of boardwalks, listen attentively for melodious birdcalls. You may not see the flickers, rufous-sided towhees, red-bellied and pileated woodpeckers, wood thrushes, bluebirds, and mockingbirds that nest in these trees, but you can't miss their rich range of twitterings, tubular notes, and

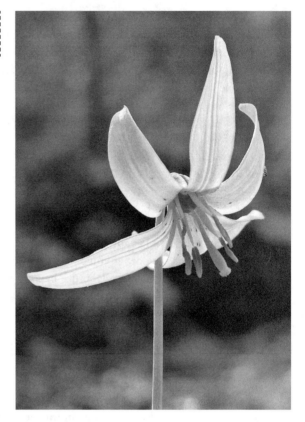

In April, sprawling patches of yellow trout lily carpet the preserve's forest floor.

deep vibratos. Glide right at post 10, descending first over chunky ground, succeeded by more wooden spans. Cross the clear cut of the pipe break, just after post 11, and hang a right at post 12. The path terminates on the far side of a diminutive pond (where the frog population surges in summer), with the parking area to the left.

## NEARBY ACTIVITIES

The **Delaware & Raritan Canal State Park,** at Blackwell Mills, attracts lovers of history as well as the outdoors. In the 19th century, steam tugboats and mules delivered freight along this corridor, and many historic buildings, bridges, and locks still exist. For further information, call 609-924-5705 or visit **njparksandforests.org /parks/drcanal.html.**

The **Old Dutch Parsonage** and the **Wallace House,** both state historic sites in Somerville, may slake your appetite for history with their wide array of period furnishings and architecture. For information, visit **tinyurl.com/olddutchparsonage.**

# WATCHUNG SIERRA SAMPLER

## IN BRIEF

Don't be put off by the overdeveloped nature of this county park. With several miles of trails, you have plenty of opportunities to lose yourself among the hardwoods and conifers that flavor so much of the domain. A couple of ponds, a long, narrow lake (where oddly shaped erratics decorate its shoreline), and the well-preserved remnants of a mill town–cum–resort community contribute to the delights of the hike. Other highlights include the diverse bird populations that thrive around water holes, and herds of deer that chomp through the woods.

## DESCRIPTION

*Gesundheit!* That, in a word, is the response we hear most often on bringing Watchung into a conversation. In fact, *Watchung* is actually a corruption of *wachunk,* a Lenape Indian word for "high hills," and there are two soaring ridges of the Watchung Mountains running the length of the park, with a bubbling brook

------------------------------------------

## *Directions* ⟶

**Follow I-95 across the George Washington Bridge and drive about 15 miles south to Exit 22. Merge onto I-78 West and continue to Exit 43. Take a right onto Diamond Hill Road/CR 655, followed by another right—at the traffic light—on McMane Avenue/CR 640. At the next traffic light, in 0.8 mile, turn left onto Glenside Avenue/CR 527, and in 1.4 miles hang a right into the reservation, on W. R. Tracey Drive/CR 645. Proceed 1.3 miles, past Lake Surprise and a picnic area, to the traffic circle. Take the first right on Summit Lane, and in 0.4 mile go right again on New Providence Road, which leads in 0.2 mile to the trailhead, on the left across from the Trailside Nature & Science Center parking lot.**

---

### KEY AT-A-GLANCE INFORMATION

**LENGTH: 5.7 miles**

**ELEVATION GAIN: 659 feet**

**CONFIGURATION: Loop**

**DIFFICULTY: Easy to moderate**

**SCENERY: Gently rolling terrain boasts mixed forests, lake, bogs, abandoned village, and some exceptionally tall tulip trees.**

**EXPOSURE: Semi-shady**

**TRAFFIC: Can get really heavy on summer weekends**

**TRAIL SURFACE: Dirt, roots, rocks**

**HIKING TIME: 3 hours**

**DRIVING DISTANCE: 39 miles**

**SEASON: Year-round, sunrise–sunset**

**ACCESS: Free; pets on leash**

**MAPS: At Trailside Nature & Science Center; download from tinyurl.com /watchungresmap; USGS *Roselle***

**FACILITIES: None along trail, but Trailside Nature & Science Center has restrooms, water, and public phone.**

**COMMENTS: The Trailside Nature & Science Center, on New Providence Road, is a great educational resource, with exhibits on taxidermy, animal life, fossils, and energy, as well as a planetarium and various gardens for herbs and wildflowers. For further details, call 908-789-3670 or visit tinyurl.com/trailsidesc.**

## GPS COORDINATES

**N40° 40.965'  W74° 22.386'**

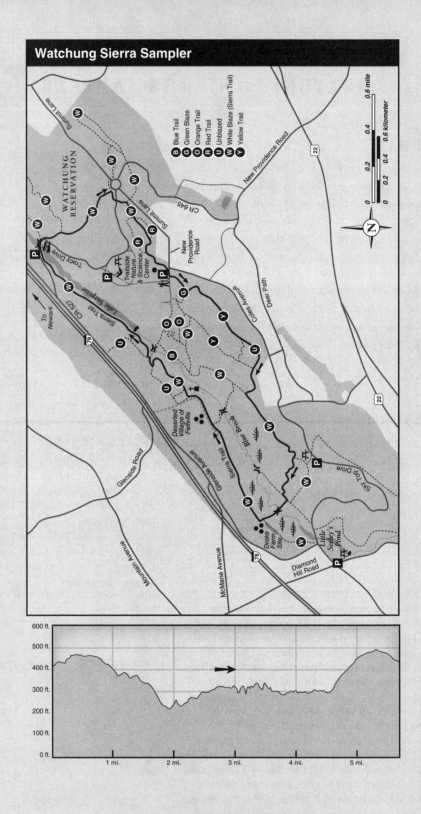

# Watchung Sierra Sampler

**Legend:**
- **B** Blue Trail
- **G** Green Blaze
- **O** Orange Trail
- **R** Red Trail
- **U** Unblazed
- **W** White Blaze (Sierra Trail)
- **Y** Yellow Trail

WATCHUNG RESERVATION

Summit Lane

Summit Lane

CR 645

New Providence Road

New Providence Road

Coles Avenue

Deer Path

22

22

Tracy Drive

Trailside Nature & Science Center

Sierra Trail

Lake Surprise

CR 527

To Newark

78

Deserted Village of Feltville

Glenside Avenue

Blue Brook

Sierra Trail

Sky Top Drive

Drake Farm Site

Little Seeley's Pond

Glenside Road

Mountain Avenue

McMane Avenue

78

Diamond Hill Road

0.6 mile

0.6 kilometer

N

**Elevation profile:**
600 ft.
500 ft.
400 ft.
300 ft.
200 ft.
100 ft.
0 ft.

1 mi.  2 mi.  3 mi.  4 mi.  5 mi.

and Lake Surprise nestled in between. Even so, hoofing it through Watchung is hardly a rugged wilderness experience. On the contrary, this is a highly developed park that features a playground, greenhouse, various gardens, a riding stable, ball fields, Scout camp, picnic area, trailside museum—even a planetarium. There are also several well-preserved buildings from a 19th-century company town and the ruins of its mill.

Considering all that, the hiking in Watchung is pretty darn good. An intricate network of trails covers almost every inch of the reservation's 2,000 acres, with the Sierra Trail (ST, white blazes) circling the perimeter for a total of 10 miles. The following trek overlaps a large segment of the ST and provides a fine introduction to the varied topography of the largest preserve in Union County's park system. Note that not all trails are blazed, muddy conditions are common in early spring, and distances on the park map vary in scale.

Start at the southwest corner of the parking lot and stride west over the paved road to the archway entrance of the Nature Trail. The path, blazed with both green and white swatches, descends swiftly, passing via a bridge over a rocky arroyo, then cuts upward by a bench and a couple of birdhouses. Two more seasonal streams follow, as well as some ups and downs. Just as you begin to wend to the right, a yellow-blazed spur appears to the left; take it. Yellow gains ground and meanders into an overgrown forest of maples, oaks, and tulip trees, with sassafras sprinkled throughout and ramps, a savory wild leek, abundant in midspring.

Leave Yellow in 5 minutes for the unblazed stem to the left (more of a straight, actually). Ignore all the side traces and increase your pace, as this route brushes against a residential neighborhood, picking up such native noises as barking dogs and lawnmowers. Hang a left at the T onto the ST, then slide through the succeeding junction in about 5 minutes. A series of enjoyable undulations ensues as Sierra descends slightly, snakes upward past beech trees, then drops once more through a couple of gentle switchbacks before yielding to another gradual climb. The grass-sided track finally tilts downhill, colliding with a bridle path, where you swerve left.

In less than a minute, the level, dirt-surfaced trail meets another junction, with the ST veering left and a wide, unmarked gravel path spurting right; go right, toward Blue Brook. Hop over the bridge and press onward, bypassing the left toward a boardwalk and Little Seeley's Pond. The next right is yours, but before turning on it, stroll a few more steps up-trail to the ruins of the Drake Farm Site, where a large pine now hangs over the stone and concrete foundations. If you enter the ruin in warm weather, remember that rattlesnakes occasionally doze unseen by the cool base of such walls.

The ST now travels northeast, evolving meanwhile into a somewhat wilder stretch of trail. The ground slants steeply downward from west to east, and a couple of streams sluice through the path as the surrounding forest, highlighted by white pines, cedars, and locust trees, is slowly being swallowed by vines; you

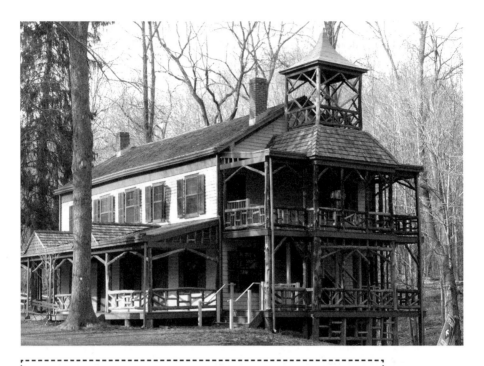

Ten buildings are all that remain of Feltville, a once-thriving mill town now listed on the National Register of Historic Places.

may have to scramble over several fallen trees here. Don't be drawn off the ST by the miscellaneous side trails; the Deserted Village of Feltville lies directly ahead.

No, that's not the title of a new Stephen King horror flick. Feltville originated as a company mill town in 1845, though the remaining buildings were modified when the property was later converted to a resort community. The resort was eventually abandoned, and in 1980 the site was placed on the National Register of Historic Places. Off-white with green trim, the houses look invitingly intact and well maintained. Look more closely, though, and aside from three that are still inhabited, most are in various stages of decay and may be dangerous to approach. White-tailed deer like to graze in this area.

Stick with the paved road as it leads from Masker's Barn past three houses and a trail to the right that cuts by the old mill site. Another pair of houses (with a second duo down below them) follows, and then the road starts to bend to the left. There is a turnoff to the right for the cemetery just as the pavement reaches the old church and store, a massive pale-yellow structure trimmed in red. Go with that spur (on the near side of the church) to the pocket graveyard. Contrary to what the five headstones suggest, the small fenced plot is believed to hold something like two dozen bodies. The only original stone is on the far right, and supposedly none of the five marks the correct grave. Maybe there's a Stephen King angle to this place after all.

Pick up the white blazes of the ST by the front end of the cemetery as it nudges northeast back into the forest. Bear left at the Y, then bolt right at the T, joining a wide bridle path; as the trail arcs downhill, lurch left with the white markings and scuttle right in another eight steps, onto the narrow conduit between two towering tulip trees. This lush, swardlike setting gives way to Lake Surprise, where ducks often bob on the jade-green surface. In traversing the lakeside clockwise, note the large erratics, the first rocks of any significant size up to now.

As you continue along the lake, the Sierra and the bridle path join for a kiss, then diverge again, with your route running to the right. Now it gets tricky. On reaching CR 645, keep to the right shoulder, pass over the bridge, then cross to the left side of the road. Bear left on the cinder driveway, just a few paces beyond the bridge, but turn right at the first intersection, momentarily leaving the ST. Skip the spur that surfaces in 30 yards, and in a couple of minutes the Watchung stables will appear, roughly 200 yards through a clutch of tulip trees. The ST reunites with the track from that direction, but shears off to the left near the road, 1 minute after passing a wide bridle path on the left. Steer to the right on the cinder track, cross the road, then jump left at the first fork and right at the second, as the ST once more joins the path. Remain with the ST all the way back to the nature center and the parking lot.

## NEARBY ACTIVITIES

West Orange is less than 20 miles north and well worth a stop for the **Edison National Historic Site.** The self-guided Laboratory Complex and the Glenmont Estate mansion and greenhouse (vehicle pass required) are open again after a lengthy period of renovations. For more information, call 973-736-0550, ext. 11, or visit **nps.gov/edis.**

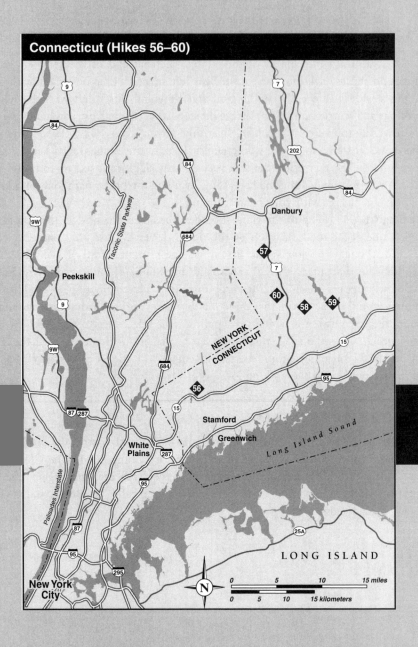

Connecticut (Hikes 56–60)

# CONNECTICUT

# 56 BABCOCK CIRCUMFERENCE TRAIL

### KEY AT-A-GLANCE INFORMATION

**LENGTH:** 3.5 miles

**ELEVATION GAIN:** 382 feet

**CONFIGURATION:** Loop

**DIFFICULTY:** Easy

**SCENERY:** Gently rolling terrain in a hardwood forest containing laurel groves, a small pond, many fieldstone walls, and seasonal bogs

**EXPOSURE:** Good canopy cover throughout summer

**TRAFFIC:** Light, except on weekends

**TRAIL SURFACE:** Packed dirt with scattered rock crossings and root networks

**HIKING TIME:** 1.5 hours

**DRIVING DISTANCE:** 29 miles

**SEASON:** Year-round, sunrise–sunset

**ACCESS:** Free; pets on leash, no bicycles

**MAPS:** Large map with blazed trails on entrance kiosk; USGS *Glenville*

**FACILITIES:** None

**COMMENTS:** The dogwoods and mountain laurels explode with blossoms from late May to early June. Cross-country skiing is a popular winter activity. Horseback riding for Greenwich Riding and Trails Association members is allowed on designated trails. For more information, call 203-622-7814 or visit tinyurl.com/babcockpreserve.

## GPS COORDINATES

N41° 6.174' W73° 37.908'

## IN BRIEF

Only ogres and elves are missing from this enchanting hike, which threads by bogs, boulders, and fallen trees along several meandering trails. Stone walls and catbrier carpet the undulating forest floor, making this charming preserve seem far larger than it actually is.

## DESCRIPTION

The Babcock Preserve is a fairy-tale example of conservation overcoming Grimm development. Once upon a time, the 297-acre tract was owned by the local water company. After the Merritt Parkway was built nearby, the Hobbit-size hollow was acquired by Charles and Mary Babcock. Their heirs later donated part and sold this land to the town of Greenwich, leading to the creation of a wild, shady park that seems, magically, far larger and more remote than it really is.

More than 30 years ago, excavators found evidence of an American Indian presence dating back to 2,500 B.C. More recently, through the 1700s and much of the ensuing century, the trees were cleared and the land used for farming. Today it is densely forested once more, and all that remains of that latter era is a series of stone walls that run almost haphazardly among the vast stands of birch, beech, maple, and mixed oaks, over a rolling landscape spiced with boulders and bogs.

------------------------------------------------

### *Directions*

**Follow the Hutchinson River Parkway North, which becomes the Merritt Parkway/CT 15 North. Drive to Exit 31 and turn right at the end of the ramp, onto North Street. Proceed for 0.5 mile to the preserve entrance and parking area, on the left. The trailhead is by the west side of the lot.**

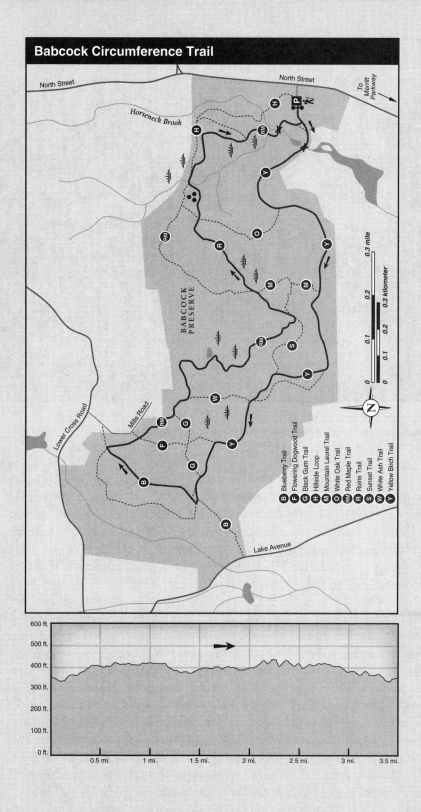

# Babcock Circumference Trail

North Street
North Street
To Merritt Parkway

Horseneck Brook

BABCOCK
PRESERVE

Lower Cross Road
Mills Road

Lake Avenue

0.3 mile
0.2
0.1
0
0.3 kilometer
0.2
0.1
0

**B** Blueberry Trail
**F** Flowering Dogwood Trail
**G** Black Gum Trail
**H** Hillside Loop
**M** Mountain Laurel Trail
**O** White Oak Trail
**RM** Red Maple Trail
**R** Ruins Trail
**S** Sunset Trail
**W** White Ash Trail
**Y** Yellow Birch Trail

600 ft.
500 ft.
400 ft.
300 ft.
200 ft.
100 ft.
0 ft.

0.5 mi.   1 mi.   1.5 mi.   2 mi.   2.5 mi.   3 mi.   3.5 mi.

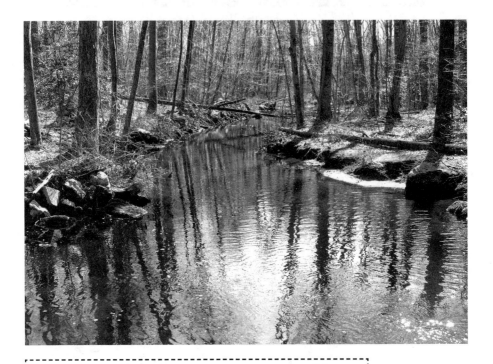

Early mornings, cavorting otters may disrupt the tranquility of Horseneck Brook.

To fall under the spell of this bewitching domain, try a 3.5-mile stroll around its perimeter, basically following the Yellow Birch Trail (YBT) on the way out and the Red Maple Trail (RMT) on your return. Begin at the kiosk in the parking lot, walk west on the dirt drive, and cross over the bridge, sticking to the yellow blazes along the old access road. Proceed by a turnoff to the right, about 200 yards beyond the bridge, as the YBT narrows, levels off, and passes into a moist, marshy zone. A bench to the side of the track beckons invitingly, with black birch and shagbark hickory trees flanking it. The main path then falls and rises over undulating ground, heading by the Mountain Laurel Trail (MLT) on the right. Ignore three succeeding left turns, as well as the orange-blazed Sunset Trail on the right, and walk straight ahead, through a dense patch of laurel, only swinging left after you have crossed a rusty chain-link fence, still with the YBT.

Forty yards farther, the path becomes rockier, at times feeling like a well-eroded streambed. You'll quickly bottom out by a small bog and, once through there, face two successive spurs to the right, the second being the Flowering Dogwood Trail (like the earlier MLT, the latter's worth walking along when the trees are in bloom). The next option, also to the right, is the Black Gum Trail (BGT); it joins the YBT for a few paces before breaking off again to the right, at a junction marked by the convergence of two rock walls. Bear left, still on the YBT, and in a scant 20 yards the path dead-ends at the Blueberry Trail, where you roll to the right.

Steer to the right at the next fork in the trail, then bend left in a few paces, where the BGT emerges from the right. Stay with Blueberry as it slowly rises over a more open ridge, until a huge eyesore of a house looms left of the path, after maybe 300 yards. Shift to the right there onto the RMT (red blazes), and stay with it as it passes the Flowering Dogwood's far end. After grazing over a granite debris field, just after a lichen-choked pond, and the BGT's reappearance, Red Maple bears to the left, drifting unpromisingly toward another house.

Fortunately for one's aesthetics, that vision proves a case of misdirection, as the red-blazed trace veers away from the house and into an overgrown patch of catbrier and fern-encrusted boulders. The RMT bends left at the next fork, threading through what is for now a less eye-appealing part of the forest. The scenery improves markedly, though, as you step once more through the chain-link fence (GPS: N41° 6.372' W73° 38.613') and the Red Maple drops down over a broad stone shelf into a rocky, roiling setting. This is one of the more rough-hewn parts of the preserve, a rock-pocked marshy area where you may need to rely on root- and rock-hopping to keep your boots dry—at least during periods of wet weather.

In the span of about 10 minutes, you will pass a trio of trails to the right, the first being the Sunset Trail (often flooded at this end) and the third being the MLT. Directly after that last, take a right onto the well-marked Ruins Trail (aqua blazes), which is also rather ragged and rocky. In a few minutes, you'll skip through a four-way intersection, still moving along the Ruins route, while the claws of catbrier climb closer on this increasingly narrow channel. (Long pants are advisable for this passageway.) As you drift by the overgrown wall that borders the left side of the path, look closely through the Japanese barberry for a pair of crumbly foundations, measuring roughly 7 by 10 feet (GPS: N41° 6.383' W73° 38.171'). Go ahead and enter the second; just keep an eye out for rattlesnakes.

A few yards beyond, the Ruins Trail rejoins the RMT; swing right, through the break in the wall, and stick with the latter all the way back to the parking area. Forget about the slight spurs you'll encounter on the way there, but do stop, if it's not too buggy, by the wooden and stone bridges in the swamp to look for frogs and animal tracks in the mud. The path to the left, just after you've ascended the erosion-control steps, is a shortcut to the trailhead.

## NEARBY ACTIVITIES

The **Greenwich Audubon Center** offers educational walks, workshops, school and group programs, and many exhibits for all ages, along with 7 miles of trails and a Leatherman's Cave on the grounds. Call 203-869-5272 or visit **greenwich .audubon.org** for information.

Thirsting for something of a cultural nature? Try the **Bruce Museum**, in downtown Greenwich. Its focus is on art, science, and natural history. Call 203-869-0376 to learn about the current and upcoming exhibits, or visit **brucemuseum.org**.

# 57 BENNETT'S POND AND BEYOND

## IN BRIEF

What's not to like about wandering a densely forested woodland, complete with a couple of ponds (one of which is patrolled by swans and beavers), where you are more likely to encounter wildlife than other hikers? The only thing we can think of is that eventually—after several heart-thumping climbs to boulder-filled ridges, with a few scenic swamps in between— you will have to leave this wonderful park.

## DESCRIPTION

Bennett's Pond State Park is yet another in a too-short-but-growing list of properties saved from the bulldozer of "development." It didn't just "become" a state park in 2002—Bennett's Pond was set aside only after years of protracted legal skirmishes and complex negotiations. All of which was put in motion back in 1997, when corporate giant IBM sold a 650-acre plot of pristine woodland to a developer. As word got around that said developer was considering using the space to build several hotels and conference centers, an 18-hole golf course, and hundreds of condominiums, a coalition of conservationists and community-minded citizens stirred into action. A petition drive, largely spearheaded by Ellen Burns, president of Ridgefield's Open Space Association (and owner

### *Directions* ———→

**Follow the Henry Hudson Parkway North, which becomes the Sawmill River Parkway North. Drive about 30 miles and merge onto I-684 North. Proceed 10.4 miles to Exit 9E and merge onto I-84 East. Continue 6.4 miles to Exit 3 and merge onto CT 7 South. After 3.9 miles turn right on Bennett's Farm Road. The parking lot is 0.7 mile ahead, on the right.**

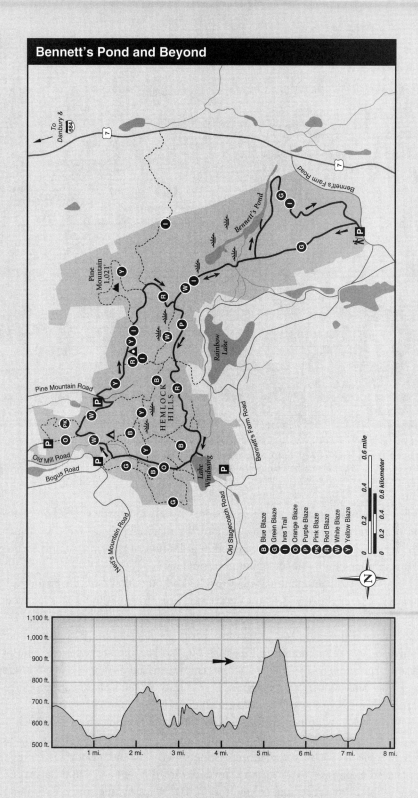

# Bennett's Pond and Beyond

To Danbury & 684

7

7

Bennett's Farm Road

Bennett's Pond

Pine Mountain 1,021

Pine Mountain Road

HEMLOCK HILLS

Old Mill Road

Bogus Road

Ned's Mountain Road

Rainbow Lake

Bennett's Farm Road

Lake Windwing

Old Stagecoach Road

P — Parking

**Ⓑ** Blue Blaze
**Ⓖ** Green Blaze
**Ⓘ** Ives Trail
**Ⓞ** Orange Blaze
**Ⓟ** Purple Blaze
**Ⓟᴷ** Pink Blaze
**Ⓡ** Red Blaze
**Ⓦ** White Blaze
**Ⓨ** Yellow Blaze

0    0.2    0.4    0.6 mile

0    0.2    0.4    0.6 kilometer

N

1,100 ft.
1,000 ft.
900 ft.
800 ft.
700 ft.
600 ft.
500 ft.

1 mi.   2 mi.   3 mi.   4 mi.   5 mi.   6 mi.   7 mi.   8 mi.

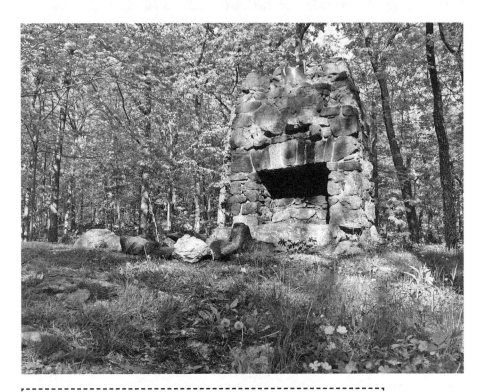

Louis D. Conley, a retired New York City businessman, built his estate on this hilltop. The crumbling chimney may be a remnant of his 34-room mansion.

of Books on the Common, a local bookstore), sought to convince the town to acquire the property via eminent domain. Eventually, that campaign—and a settlement of $12 million on the developer—resulted in a division of the land, with the northern 458-acre tract gaining the designation of state park.

As you stroll among the ancient maples and pines that flank the main trail into the park, you might consider how appropriate it is that this land was saved from the wrecking ball of modernity. About a century ago, it (along with hundreds of surrounding acres) was known as Outpost Farm. Established in 1914 as the home of Louis Conley, an aluminum-foil magnate, it also became known as the one of the largest plant nurseries on the East Coast, employing scores of workers while supplying shrubs and trees to Yale, Harvard, Franklin Roosevelt's Hyde Park property, the Berlin Turnpike, and many other companies and communities.

Conley's 34-room mansion, which was later turned into a boys' school, is long gone, having been razed to the ground in 1974. And few but trained arborists will be able to identify the more distinguished descendants of his cultivations among an expansive forest often crowded with the hemlocks and hardwoods so commonplace to our region. No matter, for the pleasures and surprises of Bennett's Pond have less to do with its history than with the tranquil retreat it offers from civilization, and from one of the more densely populated corners of Connecticut.

The 8-mile hike described below travels through a vast hemlock grove, passes among dramatic outcroppings, crests by the ruins of a cabin believed to have been owned by composer Charles Ives, and concludes near Bennett's Pond, a 56-acre expanse of water often patrolled by graceful swans. If, along the way, you failed to observe wild turkeys, coyotes, foxes, deer, or beavers, well, you must not have been trying very hard.

From the car lot, walk east to the park sign and a dirt path that leads directly to a kiosk, where trail maps are posted. This hike begins with the Green Trail (green blazes), which goes both straight and left. Take the left leg, which overlaps an unpaved forest road, a wide, pebble-surfaced track that descends gently into the forest, devolving into chunky rubble as it does so. After about two-thirds of a mile, the path arcs to the right and arrives at a somewhat over-grown junction, where cattail reeds and poison ivy thrive. Green continues straight here, but you should swing left, now on the White Trail (white blazes). (Alternatively, if you are only up for a short outing, remain with the Green Trail as it leads to the shore of Bennett's Pond and then circles back to the kiosk, shaving the hike down to a 2.1-mile sprint. Skip down nine paragraphs to resume the narrative.)

If you are still with us on the White Trail, be assured that the better part of the hike still awaits. Ignore the many social trails along this stretch of trail, as you walk among sheep laurel and wild azalea (lovely pink blossoms in spring), while drawing closer to the water. In a few minutes, the dirt-packed trail (more of a muddy morass after heavy rainfall) jogs left through a gap in an old stone wall, yielding an improved view of Bennett's Pond as it climbs slightly to higher ground. Padding along White, which soon passes over a bridge and then swings to the right, remember to scan the pond for swans and beavers. At the very least you should be able to spot the latter's lodges and, if the weather is warm, hear the distinctive call of red-winged blackbirds.

In 10 minutes or so of hiking in near-proximity to the pond, you may observe bull lilies and foam flowers giving way to sedge grass and skunk cabbage, as the water thickens to a swampy consistency. The White Trail then pulls away from what's left of Bennett's Pond, for a short time paralleling a tributary stream, its banks well colored by such springtime bloomers as trillium, bloodroot, and jack-in-the-pulpit. Skip the subsequent spur (and numerous social trails) and follow the white blazes to the left at the next intersection, where a bridge lies to the right (you will be returning via this second trail in a few hours).

A rapid ascent ensues, bringing you, in a couple of minutes of huffing, to a T. The white markings head right, while you should turn left, on the purple-blazed path. The climb persists, drawing you deeper into a mature forest of impressively large tulip trees, as well as a smattering of maples and oaks. Skip the spur to the left, as the main track bends toward the right, threads through a notch of lichen-specked granite, and proceeds to zigzag by a few antediluvian erratics. After several minutes of meandering in this undulating, attractively wild setting of oversize rocks and boulders, the purple trail comes to a T: go left, now following red blazes.

This next stretch of trail is great fun, displaying a fair amount of sinuosity in traveling through a granite-rich landscape colored with laurels, hemlocks, maples, and—at certain times of the year—an amazing array of mushrooms popping up from among the moss-coated rock debris. Stick with the red-blazed route even as several unmarked spurs surface, first on the left, then, in perhaps 10 minutes, on the right, and, once the inevitable descent begins, two more (connecting the Pine Mountain ski loop) to the left. Finally, with the imposing bluffs now behind you, replaced by a seasonal stream and slow-moving swamp, the suddenly wide trail emerges from under tree cover by the edge of Lake Windwing.

Both the Red Trail and the hike proceed to the right, but you may first want to rest for a spell on a sun-struck rock, soaking in a waterside vista. If so, swing left, cross over the bridge by the concrete dam, and make yourself at home. Once back on the main circuit, however, you will have all of about a minute before the switch to your next trail—to the right, blazed orange. This path pitches sharply uphill initially, passes a blue-tagged spur, and then levels off. Stay with orange, straight onward, at the imminent junction with an unpaved forest road, and likewise ignore the appearances of green-, yellow-, and blue- blazed routes that appear in somewhat rapid succession on your left, right, and left again as you stride along this wide, easy lane.

Your departure from the Orange Trail comes just after an unmarked spur on the right, when you meet the White Trail (white blazes), also on the right. Take White as it leads you into a denser part of the forest, dropping off the ridge and, once by a blue-blazed turnoff on the right, bending left and paralleling a swamp stream. On crossing that swamp, White next passes first an orange-blazed path, then a pink-blazed one (both on the left), crosses a short bridge, and, on ascending an earthen dam, meets yet another blue-tagged trail (forking left). Take the right option, still with White, as the moss-sided track scoots between some imposing slabs of granite (look for pink lady's slipper orchids if you happen to be here in mid-May). White ends at a junction with the Yellow Trail, where you turn left.

When Yellow hits Pine Mountain Road, a few moments later, step around the steel gate and lurch left on the pavement. Keep an eye out for the yellow blazes, first on a telephone pole on the left side of the road, then on a utility pole on the right side. Shortly after the latter, Yellow resumes its forested route, on the right. Now forging uphill, this commences what is perhaps the most strenuous part of the hike, and also one of the more subliminally appealing. Plan to remain with Yellow for the next mile or so, ignoring the many spurs and side trails that crop up as the track first surmounts the craggy slope, then courses along the lush, grassy ridge. The apex of your effort, shortly after the Ives Trail (red blaze on yellow, overlain with a musical clef symbol) merges with Yellow from the right, is a granite plateau fringed with pitch pines, oaks, and one or two dogwoods.

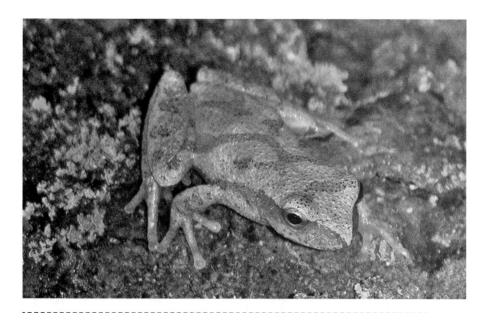

If you're hearing "Jingle Bells" three months after Christmas, it means spring peepers are out.

From that lovely perch, which is blessed with an expansive view of the southern hills, Ridgefield direction, the undulating trail skips by the start and end of the short Pine Mountain Loop (yellow blazes) before cresting at the ruin of what some believe was Charles Ives's cabin. All that remains is the fieldstone chimney, which is slowly, sadly being picked apart by vandals intent on using its stones for their own improvised fire rings. Wandering farther along the pristine ridge, the track soon comes to a kiosk, where the Ives Trail breaks off from Yellow. Turn right, following the Ives, and turn right again, in roughly 100 yards, at the junction with the red-blazed Bennett's Pond Trail (BPT). At the conclusion of this precipitous descent, the BPT crosses a wooden bridge and rejoins the white trail of earlier, closing one of your loops.

Veer left on the White Trail and retrace your earlier steps all the way back to that overgrown junction by the cattail reeds, where you initially turned off the Green Trail. Swing left on Green, and in the course of 15 minutes the path will draw you close to the pickerelweed-rimmed edge of Bennett's Pond. By all means, take the short spur to sit on a waterside rock; just keep an eye out for poison ivy. Green eventually breaks to the right, away from the pond, slicing through a stone wall and rolling to the right when it hits a forest lane. On departing that wide track, Green then undertakes a two-stage uphill burst, emerging at the perimeter of an open field of knee- to waist-high grass. The trail keeps to the north-northeast side of the meadow, dips briefly back into tree cover, and, at the subsequent small clearing, arrives at an asphalt turnaround, part of an old driveway, with an ancient maple growing in middle of it. Stay with Green to the right of the park kiosk, and in a minute you should reach the entrance kiosk, where you can pick up the path back to the parking lot.

As for the remaining 155 acres of Bennett's Pond's original tract, the parcel that *wasn't* turned into a state park? It lies across the road to the south, still in limbo, as the developer persists in its drive to turn the wild, wooded land into 300 or so townhouses.

## NEARBY ACTIVITIES

Just a little north, in Danbury, is elegant **Tarrywile Mansion,** with attractively landscaped gardens, easy trails, a greenhouse, and several outbuildings. It is listed in the National Register of Historic Places as an outstanding example of Shingle-style Victorian-era architecture. Visit the mansion, or hike the trails, after consulting **tarrywile.com** or calling 203-744-3130.

# DEVIL'S DEN CONCOURSE  58

## IN BRIEF

The extensive trail system of this sanctuary offers something for every level of walker, from tyros of turf to foot-hearty highlanders. It slices through a rich variety of woodland habitats, showcasing a large pond and numerous streams, a rocky ravine, several granite-wracked gorges, high plateaus with expansive views of the surrounding hills, and even the ruins of a 19th-century lumber mill. Wild turkeys and white-tailed deer teem through these woods, and moist weather brings an intoxicating mix of mushrooms.

## DESCRIPTION

No one knows for certain how Devil's Den came by its sinister sobriquet. The Great Ledge viewpoint isn't guarded by a three-headed Cerberus, its streams don't flow with molten lava, and not a whiff of sulfur taints its air. On the contrary, when your lug soles start padding through the varied terrain, you will find yourself treading in hiker's heaven. Which isn't to say you'll feel like an angel at the end of this 8-mile hike. But with more than 1,700 acres to the preserve, encompassing hundreds of varieties of trees and wildflowers, dramatic ridgetop views, the ever-popular Godfrey Pond, a rocky ravine bisected by a picturesque

### KEY AT-A-GLANCE INFORMATION

**LENGTH:** 7.8 miles

**ELEVATION GAIN:** 811 feet

**CONFIGURATION:** 2 connected loops

**DIFFICULTY:** Easy to moderate

**SCENERY:** Rolling woodlands, wetlands, gorge with gentle cascade, rocky ledge with disappearing view of Saugatuck Reservoir, and several relics of lumber mills

**EXPOSURE:** Mostly shady, except for a few ledges and Godfrey Pond area

**TRAFFIC:** The farther out you go, the fewer people you encounter.

**TRAIL SURFACE:** Packed dirt with rocky, rooty, and muddy stretches

**HIKING TIME:** 4 hours

**DRIVING DISTANCE:** 51 miles

**SEASON:** Year-round, sunrise–sunset

**ACCESS:** Donation suggested; no pets, no bicycles, no motorized vehicles

**MAPS:** At the entrance kiosk; download from tinyurl.com/devilsdenmap; USGS *Bethel*

**FACILITIES:** None

**COMMENTS:** The Den promotes passive recreation like hiking, birding, and nature study, while cross-country skiing and snowshoeing are permitted in winter. For information, call 203-226-4991 or visit tinyurl.com /devilsdenpreserve.

## Directions ──→

Follow the Hutchinson River Parkway North, which becomes the Merritt Parkway/CT 15 North. Drive to Exit 42, and turn right on CT 57 North/Weston Road. Stay with it for 5 miles, and turn right (east) on Godfrey Road. In 0.6 mile steer left onto Pent Road (the preserve is signposted), which—in about 0.4 mile—leads to the parking lot.

## GPS COORDINATES

N41° 14.224'  W73° 23.766'

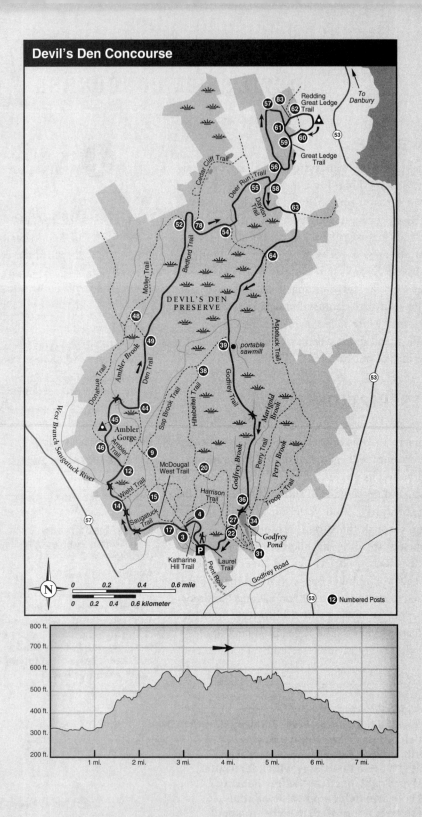

cascade, and several scores of bird species, there's more than enough to elevate the spirits of even the most downtrodden of trekkers.

Numbered posts at most intersections simplify trail-hopping while minimizing the chance you'll get lost. Just remember to pick up a map at the kiosk before leaving the dogwood-, beech-, and hemlock-fringed parking area. We like to warm up briskly by starting with the Katharine Hill Trail to the right of the kiosk, a short but steep stretch that climbs past a multitude of mountain laurels before cresting on a rocky knob. This brief burst is by no means the only such ascent in the park, but it may be the most strenuous.

From that lichen-spattered granite aerie, the path drifts left, descends sharply over stone-studded turf, and bottoms out by a boggy stream. Follow the fern-flecked, granite-scarred gully for a few minutes to the trail's end at post 4. Turn left, and in a couple dozen steps hang a right onto the McDougal West Trail, at marker 3. If you happen to be on this lush, marshy track in summer, look along the slick sides of the stream for cardinal flowers, some of the Den's more colorful bloomers. As chunks of granite start to supplant the swamp, you'll turn left onto the Saugatuck Trail, by post 17.

A series of short boardwalks helps to ford a few of the swampier spots along this relatively level course, which, incidentally, tends to be prime mushrooming territory in early autumn—black chanterelles and cinnabars being among the choice specimens. The latter part of the track slants downward toward a more glacial, rocky environment, with oaks and birches pressing in upon the scene. Dawdle a moment on the bridge that shifts the path from the left side of the West Branch of the Saugatuck River to its right bank: the clear-flowing water often teems with trout.

Having set aside your figurative fishing rod, angle past post 14 (the Wiehl Trail tacks back to McDougal there) and across yet another bridge to marker 12, where you'll change over to the Ambler Trail (AT). Here commences a mildly arduous ascent past laurels (we once spotted a dozen wild turkeys feeding nearby), only to level off by an eye-catching escarpment to the right that rises 15 to 20 feet off the ground. Swing right at number 46, where you meet—and shun—the Donahue Trail, and enter directly into an even denser mass of mountain laurels, punctuated by an increasingly impressive display of granite. A brief side trip at post 45 leads to a blueberry-bordered vista point, with the rock shelf making a fine spot on which to pause and catch your breath.

Back on the AT, your ankles are in for a minor stress test as the route traverses a fair amount of shale and angular stones in one of the preserve's more enjoyable rock-scrambling spots. No sooner have you reached the ridgeline than the trail begins trending downward again, reaching a scenic climax at Ambler Gorge. The great, gray-granite walls and rockslide of this ravine are truly sensational, and the seasonal cascade flowing through is sweet music for the eyes as well as ears. If you are a quiet hiker, you may find downy woodpeckers,

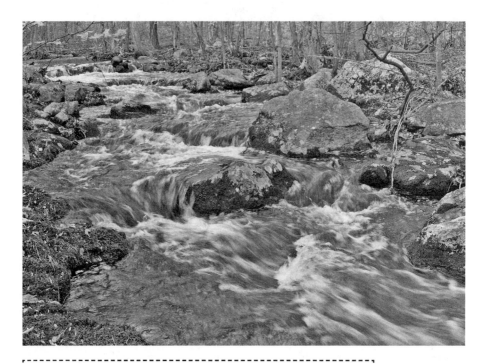

Last one in ... after heavy rainfall, the otherwise docile Saugatuck River looks like a whitewater-rafting paradise.

yellow-shafted flickers, and other birds bathing in the water. In any case, remain vigilant for the elusive trail blazes here, as well as for slick rocks near the stream.

The AT ends at pole 44, as you move left onto the Den Trail, which in turn morphs seamlessly after a while into the Bedford Trail. It is 1.4 miles from that last number to post 54, where you should vault left onto Deer Run, a grassy area frequented by wild turkeys, as well as its namesake four-legged ruminants. Keep right at marker 55, in 0.3 mile, and then swing left in another 5 minutes at pole 58. In four steps you'll come to a fieldstone wall, with a left turn at marker 56 just beyond that.

This begins the first of two mini-loops that reach a pinnacle at the Great Ledge, with its fabulous views over the Saugatuck Reservoir and surrounding hills. (Note that you'll want to adhere to the white blazes throughout these circuits—the large yellow slashes date from an earlier era and are no longer valid.) At 0.35 mile, you'll take the right fork at post 57, just beyond a tumbledown rock wall, an area where, if you hike here in late summer, when the sedge grass is tall and the shagbark hickories have dropped their nuts, you're likely to see more deer and squirrels than hikers. Shuffling onward, roll left at number 61, the straighter of two options, then right at marker 83, 0.1 mile later. Make a left in about 10 paces, at post 62, and in approximately 30 yards you'll have to scramble over some rocks and roots and past some hemlocks before finally reaching, in a small knoll of oaks

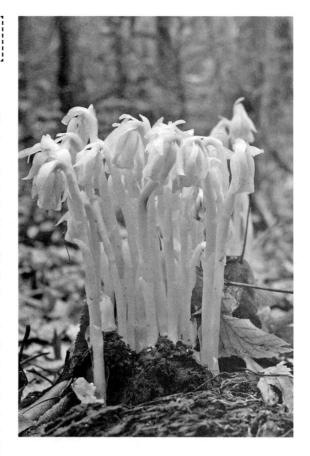

Once summer starts, clusters of Indian pipe poke their heads up through the dirt.

and white pines, the Great Ledge, with its panorama toward the east. This appealing, rocky plateau, which extends for 25 feet and also features a lower, smaller ledge, makes an ideal picnic spot, though you'll probably have to share it on most weekends. Look for pink lady's slipper orchids here in early June.

With the laurel canopy increasing in density as you mosey along the ledge to the south, you may have trouble finding the white blazes. Aim toward the south-southwest, over the rocky, mossy surface, until you reach post 60, down the hill. Bearing left there, descend further into a marshy zone, where horned toads huddle among the ferns and mud. Keep left again at pole 59, as the rocky path snakes uphill among oaks, laurels, and pines, peaking atop a moss-covered dome. The view isn't so splendid, but the laurels, oaks, and pines lend an enchanting air to the spot.

Stay left a few minutes later on picking up post 56 again, and do the same at number 58. In 0.3 mile, transfer from the Dayton Trail onto Godfrey (GT), to the right. What starts as a subtle downward direction becomes, in roughly 40 yards, a rather steady descent into a beech-bespeckled swampland. The next post, 64, appears in 5 minutes, with the GT the middle of three options. Remain on that for another 0.6 mile, passing marker 39, until you reach the old sawmill site, notable for its rusty remnants of a 19th-century steam boiler and flywheel. Near the woods is the well-preserved foundation of a shed that may have housed the mill's boiler.

On concluding your explorations of the ruins and miscellaneous unblazed traces in this locale, return to the GT and proceed for another mile, sauntering right at post 36. With Godfrey Pond straight ahead, glide right at the T and spring over the bridge, which is notable for a crackling cascade that plunges through the rocky gorge in springtime. A short uphill detour at post 27 showcases a high stone ledge: its recessed pockets were used as shelters by Paleolithic hunters as early as 3,500 B.C.

Back by Godfrey Pond, continue counterclockwise and step up to the edge of the water when you reach the spill-off stream, near marker 26. Take a breather by the bench—and maybe a photo or two of the picturesque pond. Then go on to post 25 and turn right, moving down the graded slope to a bridge. Head left at number 24 and travel straight on until you reach the Laurel Trail, at post 22, loping left there. The parking lot lies ahead, past a spot where a charcoal kiln formerly stood—one of 40 such sites that once existed in the Den. The production of charcoal—used among other things for gunpowder, paint and ink, iron forging, and medicines—was a big business in these parts during most of the 19th century. Considering the volume of cut timber necessary for such endeavors, it seems a minor miracle that the Devil's Den is the wooded paradise we find it today.

## NEARBY ACTIVITIES

The handsome town of Ridgefield has a true gem on Main Street in the **Aldrich Contemporary Art Museum,** the only establishment of its kind in Connecticut that is devoted to contemporary art. In addition to the award-winning new museum building, there is also a small sculpture garden. For information, call 203-438-4519 or visit **aldrichart.org.**

A registered National Historic Landmark, the 62-room **Lockwood-Mathews Mansion Museum,** in Norwalk, is a fine example of a Second Empire–style country house, abundantly furnished with period antiques and bibelots. For details, call 203-838-9799 or visit **lockwoodmathewsmansion.com.**

# TROUT BROOK VALLEY CIRCUIT  59

## IN BRIEF

This handsome, hilly preserve has more ups and downs than a bipolar roller coaster. That's part of the fun in hiking through terrain that alternates from hardwood forests to mossy hemlock hamlets, from swampy streams to great granite ravines. An old reservoir, largely overgrown, is a fertile setting for wildflowers in spring and summertime, and there's also an orchard where you can pick blueberries and apples.

## DESCRIPTION

The name Trout Brook Valley conjures images of a fisherman's paradise, the sort of place where you have no sooner baited a hook than a brownie or rainbow is wriggling on the end of your line. But if snuggling into hip-waders and switching a fly over the water is truly what makes your outdoor experience one to savor, a trip to Trout Brook will hold all the allure of a dive into a deer tick–loaded leaf pile. Maybe even less. The reality is that of the many streams coursing through this 1,003-acre preserve, few reach depths much beyond one's ankles, and none that we're aware of contain trout, or any other fish for that matter. True, there used to be a picturesque pond

### KEY AT-A-GLANCE INFORMATION

**LENGTH:** 8.6 miles

**ELEVATION GAIN:** 1,294 feet

**CONFIGURATION:** Loop with spur

**DIFFICULTY:** Moderate

**SCENERY:** Dense hemlock forest, beech grove, stream crossings, extended swamps, and an orchard

**EXPOSURE:** Largely shaded

**TRAFFIC:** Light on weekdays before mountain bikers descend after work

**TRAIL SURFACE:** Moss, dirt, stones

**HIKING TIME:** 4 hours

**DRIVING DISTANCE:** 56 miles

**SEASON:** Year-round, sunrise–sunset

**ACCESS:** Free; no bicycling January 1– April 30; bridle trails

**MAPS:** In box just beyond the trailhead and posted at all major trail crossings; download from tinyurl .com/troutbrookmap; USGS *Botsford*

**FACILITIES:** None

**COMMENTS:** Hunting is allowed in parts of the preserve. In summer, visitors are allowed to pluck a modest amount of blueberries in an orchard bursting with wildflowers. Visit aspetucklandtrust.org/17213 for further information, or call 203-331-1906.

## Directions

**Follow the Hutchinson River Parkway North, which becomes the Merritt Parkway/CT 15 North. Drive 27 miles to Exit 44, turn left at the end of ramp, and then left again onto CT 58. Proceed under the parkway overpass and drive 5.1 miles, turning left on Freeborn Road. Continue for 0.7 mile and veer right on Elm Drive. Park in the circle at the end of the road, in 0.2 mile.**

## GPS COORDINATES

N41° 14.762' W73° 20.007'

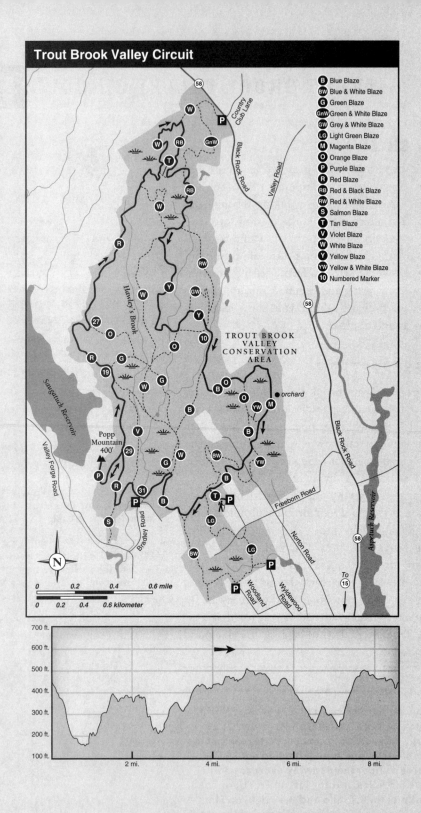

# Trout Brook Valley Circuit

**Blue Blaze**
**Blue & White Blaze**
**Green Blaze**
**Green & White Blaze**
**Grey & White Blaze**
**Light Green Blaze**
**Magenta Blaze**
**Orange Blaze**
**Purple Blaze**
**Red Blaze**
**Red & Black Blaze**
**Red & White Blaze**
**Salmon Blaze**
**Tan Blaze**
**Violet Blaze**
**White Blaze**
**Yellow Blaze**
**Yellow & White Blaze**
**Numbered Marker**

TROUT BROOK
VALLEY
CONSERVATION
AREA

orchard

Popp
Mountain
400'

Saugatuck Reservoir

Hawley's Brook

Country Club Lane

Black Rock Road

Valley Road

Valley Forge Road

Bradley Road

Freeborn Road

Norton Road

Woodland Road

Wyldewood Road

Black Rock Road

Aspetuck Reservoir

To 15

N

0        0.2        0.4        0.6 mile
0    0.2    0.4    0.6 kilometer

700 ft.
600 ft.
500 ft.
400 ft.
300 ft.
200 ft.
100 ft.

2 mi.        4 mi.        6 mi.        8 mi.

here, part of a vast reservoir system that provided drinking water to lower Fairfield County, and no doubt it contained fish. That's gone now, however, drained into swampland and overgrown by weeds and wildflowers. While that may sound like a minor tragedy, it is in fact just the opposite, the happy result of long-running efforts to preserve the land—great glacial ridges rimmed with granite outcroppings, scenic swamps and rocky rivulets, antediluvian groves of ancient hemlocks lined with spongy beds of moss—from the demolition ball of "development." The largest piece of this sizable parcel, amounting to 758 acres, was acquired from the Bridgeport Hydraulic Company in 1998, after considerable lobbying by the Aspetuck Land Trust, which now maintains the property, and such area activists as actor Paul Newman, who helped persuade the governor and legislature to set aside the funds for its acquisition. Given the possible alternative, even a diehard angler should appreciate those efforts.

From the parking circle, follow the "tan"-blazed trail into the forest, picking up a park map as you pass the box behind a tree. Turn left in a few moments, when this spur ends at a T. Although the network of trails and blazes can be rather confusing in this part of the park, plan to stick with the blue markings for the next half-mile, even as other blazes and trails merge and shear off. If you listen carefully as you walk, by the way, you may notice the high-pitched chirping of downy woodpeckers, which, in addition to wood thrushes, inhabit this area of the hemlock-dominated forest. The rocky path crosses a narrow stream, tilts steeply downhill, and then comes to a break in the tree cover, and another stream crossing, one of many in this water-logged preserve; such wildflowers as toothwort, jack-in-the-pulpit, and bloodroot, with showy white blossoms, add to the aesthetics here in early spring. As the path bends toward the right, or north, you come within range of the old reservoir, with pebbles now underfoot and a flush of ferns lining the way. Continue straight onward when you arrive at one of the dam works, bypassing the well-beaten spur to the left. A few seconds later the trail shifts left, glides over a couple of duckboards, and hits a wide woods road. Hoof it to the left there, trading the blue blazes for green-and-white ones.

Remain on the unpaved road until, nearing another parking area, you come to a post with the number "31" on it, right by the old dam. Turn right there, crossing over the dam. The reservoir, to your right, is largely overgrown, with goldenrod and other wildflowers flourishing around its perimeter. Here begins one of the more enjoyable stretches of the hike, as you stick with red blazes for the next 3.4 miles. From a setting of tulip trees, oaks, and a clutch of poplars, the track circles to the left, scooting past a lavender-marked spur to the right, and begins threading through a modest rockslide on its way to the top of the ridge. The prolonged ascent is broken at several stages by brief level stretches, as the environment changes to one of hemlocks, moss-draped granite outcroppings, and many fallen trees, their rotting trunks slowly turning to mulch. We once saw a yellow-billed cuckoo in this part of the preserve, as well as a young rat snake that somehow managed to climb a hemlock sapling on our approach. The tree marked

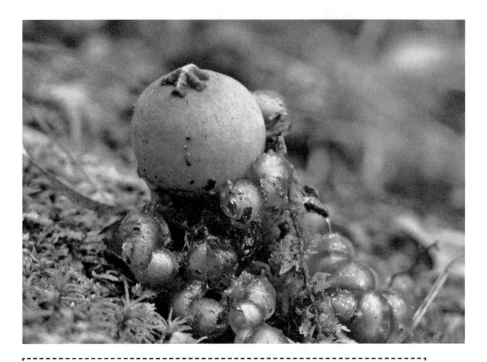

Pretty mouth (or stalked puffball-in-aspic) isn't toxic, but you're better off sticking to trail mix.

with a "29" indicates a purple-blazed spur, on the left, to Popp Mountain, a worthwhile side trip, even if there's less mountain to that Popp than its name suggests. Although the end point is a scant 0.4 mile off the main circuit, the secluded setting, with a screened view of the Saugatuck Reservoir, feels like a hidden oasis out in the deepest woods. Few people bother to take this trail, making it a great spot in which to enjoy lunch or a quiet bit of meditation.

Having put that respite behind you, double back to the main trail and resume the tour, heading north, or left. Several minutes later, the path merges to the right onto a woods road (the large dam work of the Saugatuck is visible up the hill to the left) and then runs into, and briefly overlaps, a green-tagged track. Bear left, still sticking with the red (and green) blazes, and use the wooden planks to get by the patch of mud. In roughly a hundred yards, by a tree marked with a "19," the two colors diverge, with red spurting to the left, uphill. For a time the trail clings to the cleft between two ridges, an area in which hemlocks are gradually being supplanted by oaks, beeches, and maples, and the ground is dappled green with ferns. You'll negotiate another swath of swamp on descending from that high turf and then encounter a forest road, by a tree bearing a "27." Cross over the road, ignoring the orange blazes (which can appear reddish in low light) to the right. This more luminous part of the preserve appears to be a vestigial riverbed, with the jumble of rocks underfoot serving as a stress test for your stability and sense

Multiple stretches of duckboard in this preserve help keep your boots mud-free when you hike after a downpour.

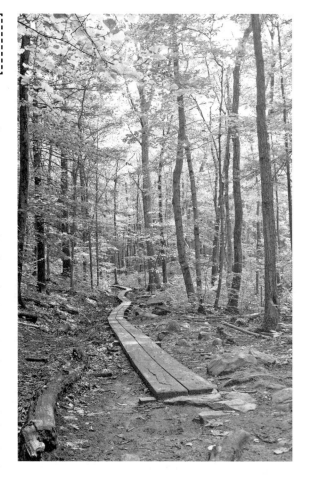

of balance. On reaching the stream (all that remains of that ancient river?), make use of the plank bridge tucked off to the right, an easy span to overlook. From there, the track wends up another low ridge, where it ends at a junction with a white-blazed trail. Cruise left onto the latter, and stay straight with the white markings when you come upon the "tan"-colored cut-through, in a little less than a quarter-mile.

For the next several minutes, the path zigzags from one series of rocky uplift to another, a fun romp over roly-poly terrain that provides insight into why mountain bikers flock to this park like pigs to peanuts. That ends when you reach an intersection with a red-and black-marked path, which you take to the right (GPS: **N41° 16.422' W73° 20.301'**). Hang with this segment for about a mile, all the way to its end, ignoring first a "tan" trail, on the right, then a green-and-white-colored one, on the left, and, also on the left, a red-and-white-blazed trail, finally scooting left on a white-blazed connector. In just 1 minute of walking you'll jump left on Ruth's Trail (yellow markings), as white proceeds to the right. Ignore all other side trails, as Ruth passes by a vernal pond, whose inky water teems with frogs in summer, cuts through additional swampland, leaps (via stepping-stones) over a stream, and brushes by the base of a fairly impressive escarpment, ending, finally, by a tree sporting the number "10." Turn left at that junction, now treading on an orange-blazed trail.

Having made use of a bridge to ford the rock-filled stream, the path swings right and parallels the water, steadily losing elevation. In spring, the stream bank to your right is ruffled green with the shoots of ramps (a kind of cross between scallions and leeks, much-prized by gourmets) as well as flowering red trillium.

Shortly after stepping over a negligible stream, you'll observe the orange markings cutting left with blue ones, uphill, while the blue tags also continue straight ahead. Go left, and in 5 minutes this trail meets a magenta-colored spur to the left. That latter leads to an orchard where hikers are invited to pick blueberries in late July and apples in autumn. Even if that seems a fruitless side trip, the wildflowers that bloom there throughout the warm months, including oxeye daisies, Queen Anne's lace, soapwort, cow vetch, and violets, make it a fine detour.

Should you decide to skip the orchard, proceed as you were on the orange-and-blue-blazed trail, remaining with the blue markings all the way back to the "tan" spur (GPS: **N41° 14.794' W73° 20.107'**) that leads to the parking circle. Otherwise, switch to the magenta-marked path, bear right when it forks (the left branch is for equestrians), cross the bog, and enter the fenced field. Farther down the deer fence, on the right, is the access gate to your return route, still colored magenta. Proceed along that track all the way to the magenta leg's termination, at a junction with a yellow-and-white-blazed path. Take the left fork (basically straight) and switch to blue, bearing left, when the latter merges from the right a few minutes later. Remain with the blue blazes till you reach the starting spur, noted with the GPS coordinates above.

## NEARBY ACTIVITIES

The walking is easier—but no less appealing—at **Collis P. Huntington State Park**, a short drive to the north, in Redding. The former estate of a railroad tycoon was donated to the state in 1950, and its old carriage roads continue to be the basis for most of the wide, graded trails that meander through this 878-acre property. Lake Hopewell is near the parking area, but it's possible to extend your loop to 5 miles or more. For further details, call 203-938-2285 or visit **tinyurl.com/huntingtonsp**.

# WEIR POND AND SWAMP LOOPS 60

## IN BRIEF

While not on the level of Walden, the beech-and-laurel-rimmed Weir Pond is historic in its own right, with a small trickle of a cascade, a rocky bog, and a colorful boulder-filled forest all part of the compact package. Feel free to bring your easel or sketchpad to this former haunt of American Impressionists, and to learn about them at the National Historic Site that is part of this parcel.

## DESCRIPTION

You don't have to be a big fan of American Impressionist paintings to enjoy Weir Farm's easy 2-mile woodland hike. If the names Julian Alden Weir, Childe Hassam, and John Henry Twachtman are tantamount to Tom, Dick, and Harry, it won't detract a whit from your pleasures by the pond or the serenity of the swamp. Still, Weir Farm, Connecticut's sole national park, offers a unique opportunity to learn about an important period in American art history, to visit an artist's studio, and to tour a 19th-century farm, while also getting in a decent little hike. Talk about having your cake and eating it, too.

J. Alden Weir bought his namesake farm in 1882. He summered there for the next 37 years, until his death, while the bucolic beauty of the locale, reflected in its forests, pond,

### KEY AT-A-GLANCE INFORMATION

**LENGTH:** 2.1 miles (from parking lot)

**ELEVATION GAIN:** 233 feet

**CONFIGURATION:** Double balloon

**DIFFICULTY:** Easy

**SCENERY:** Peaceful woodlands surrounding lily pond, bog, and hidden cascadette

**EXPOSURE:** Mostly shady

**TRAFFIC:** Busy on summer weekends, very light otherwise

**TRAIL SURFACE:** Dirt and exposed roots, some rocky stretches

**HIKING TIME:** 1 hour

**DRIVING DISTANCE:** 52 miles

**SEASON:** Year-round, sunrise–sunset

**ACCESS:** Free; no dogs, no bicycles

**MAPS:** At visitor center; download from tinyurl.com/weirfarmmap; USGS *Bethel*

**FACILITIES:** Portable toilets near visitor center, no water

**COMMENTS:** To learn more about early American Impressionism, take a leisurely ranger-led tour of the grounds, free. For more information, visit nps.gov/wefa.

---

## *Directions* ———————➤

**Follow I-95 North to Exit 15 and go north on US 7. Drive 8.7 miles, then turn left on CT 102 (after the Branchville Station). In 0.3 mile make a left on Old Branchville Road, followed by another left, in 0.5 mile, on Nod Hill Road. Parking is available on the left side of the road in 0.7 mile, across from the visitor center.**

## GPS COORDINATES

N41° 15.389'  W73° 27.363'

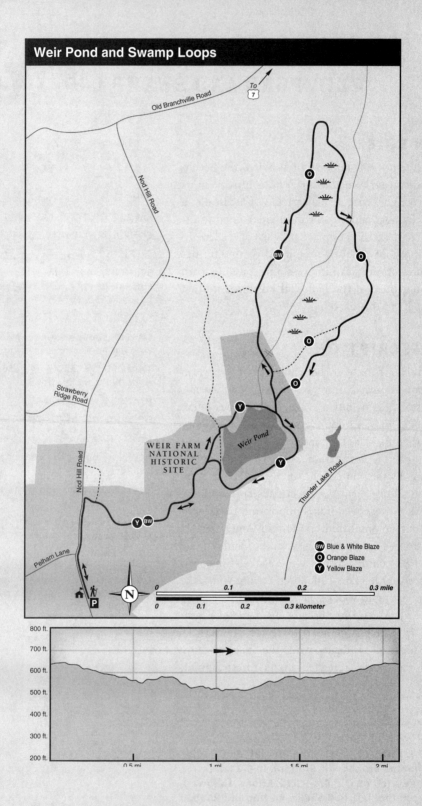

# Weir Pond and Swamp Loops

**BW** Blue & White Blaze
**O** Orange Blaze
**Y** Yellow Blaze

rock walls, and open fields, became the subject of many of his and his colleagues' paintings. Pressures from suburban development by the late 1970s led to a grass-roots drive to protect the property, with the result that the 60-acre Weir Farm was designated a National Historic Site in 1990.

The visitor center, across the road from the parking lot, is open only on select days, but the grounds are accessible throughout the week. Views of the pond are best from late fall through early spring, when the water level of its streams and swamp is also greater. That is balanced, of course, against the fact that the many private dwellings besieging the park are more visible then. To reach the pond, turn right on leaving your car and follow the road to the next corner, where Pelham Lane meets Nod Hill and the Weir house sits catty-corner across the street. Pass through the gap in the wall (GPS: N41° 15.455' W73° 27.381'), directly opposite the red farmhouse, and, at the bottom of the granite steps, swing left onto the path. Look for Asiatic daylilies, butter-and-eggs, tick trefoil, and other wildflowers as you stroll along the edge of the small, overgrown meadow; then bear right at the fork, just after crossing the small footbridge. Turn right again in 25 yards, and stick with this bark-covered Pond Path (white blaze bisected by a vertical blue line) as it wends into the woods, highlighted at this stage by oaks, maples, black birches, and shagbark hickories.

As is typical in these parts, a labyrinth of old walls courses through the forest, and you'll see a part of that near a short boardwalk over a fern-flecked patch of bog as you gradually descend toward the water. Ignore the trace to the right, which appears within a couple of minutes: that's your return route. On reaching the bottom of this slight slope, swing to the left side of the pond, descend the stone steps, and rock-hop over the runoff. A duckboard fords the next pour-off and brings you to the rim of the pond, where skimmers, damselflies, various frogs, scarlet gilia, and goldenrod thrive.

A sign at the northeast corner of the pond points the way to the Waterfall Trail (orange blazes), on the left. To reach that "waterfall," which is really more of a trickle cascading over a series of stones, keep left again when the path forks. Minimalist waterfall notwithstanding, this secondary loop is an excellent, bite-size dip into a cooler, wilder habitat, largely one of marshland and glacial ridges. The path is less maintained, with initially a good—or *bad*—number of rocks underfoot. Before you know it, in perhaps 80 yards, you'll be past the dribbling flow that passes for a waterfall (GPS: N41° 15.654' W73° 27.068') and heading toward a towering mound of granite that comes to a dull point, like an eroded pyramid, 35 feet off the ground. The track, now moss-covered, moves to the left of that, drifting among many ferns, beeches, and poplars en route to a junction. Continue to the right on the Rock Walk, marked with blue-line-over-white blazes as well as orange ones.

As the trail moseys downhill, you'll notice a series of 3-foot-high white poles spaced in a staggered line through the forest. Keep your eyes peeled for a right fork in this area; it's not well marked. Following that, the descent becomes

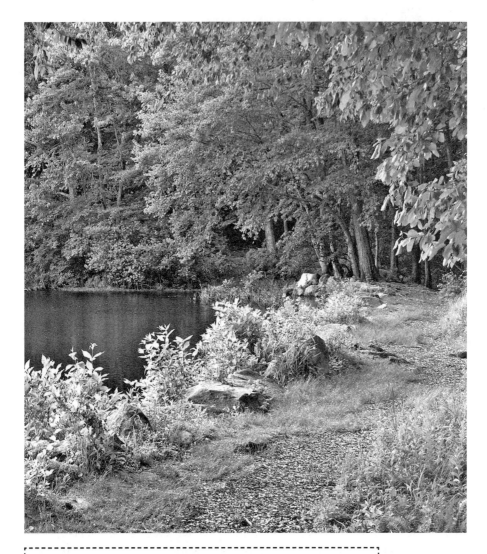

Lovely Weir Pond lies hidden in the middle of successional hardwood forests and is circled by a gently meandering trail.

rockier, delivering you finally to the bottom of an appealing shelf of angular granite. For the next few minutes, the circuit negotiates a fine line between this buttress on the left and a fetid, fecund swamp to the right. Then—presto!—you veer east by a couple of stone cairns (and a couple of unwelcoming NO TRESPASSING signs), leaving the granite-graced ground behind. There are two seasonal streams to rock-hop over—you may see (or hear) frogs here—after which it's back southbound toward the pond.

Oaks and laurels shade this high ground route—but not enough, alas, to shield from view the steady series of private homes to the left, just beyond the boundary of the park. These hallmarks of "civilization" remind us, of course, to be grateful for such conservation efforts as those that helped preserve Weir Farm. Still, you may want to direct your gaze toward the right, across the unsullied expanse of forest and bog. In due time, a turnoff to the right surfaces, which leads back to the Waterfall Trail and Nod Hill. Skip that, and in a few minutes the trail ends by the pond. Turn left, now sticking with yellow blazes, to resume the previous loop. Circle the pond clockwise to its southwest corner, then lope left up the dozen or so stone stairs to a rocky shelf that overlooks the pond (though in summer it is pretty well screened-in by trees). From that picturesque vantage point, follow the trace back to the main path, turn left, and retrace your steps back to the parking lot.

## NEARBY ACTIVITIES

You can extend your hiking by about 3 miles at the **Weir Preserve**, a Nature Conservancy property abutting Weir Farm (access is via the Burlingham Barn, just past the visitor center). Trails cut through a successional forest, open fields, a secluded stream, and laurel-covered hills. For more information, visit **tinyurl .com/weirpreserve**.

Another short hike worth considering is a tour through the **Leon Levy Preserve**, a 386-acre parcel that was established in 2005 through a joint effort by the town of Lewisboro and the Westchester Land Trust. Several blazed trails have since been created that showcase much of the preserve's beauty, including a second-growth forest, swamplands, dramatic rock outcroppings, even a 25-foot-high ravine. The trailhead is just south of NY 35 on NY 123, in the town of Lewisboro, marked by a sign on the west side of the road. For further information, call 914-241-6346 or visit **westchesterlandtrust.org/leon-levy**.

Lewisboro also has the precious **Frederick P. Rose Preserve**. Woods, wetlands, wildlife, and ruins attract hikers and equestrians. For details and a map, visit **westchesterlandtrust.org/rose-preserve**.

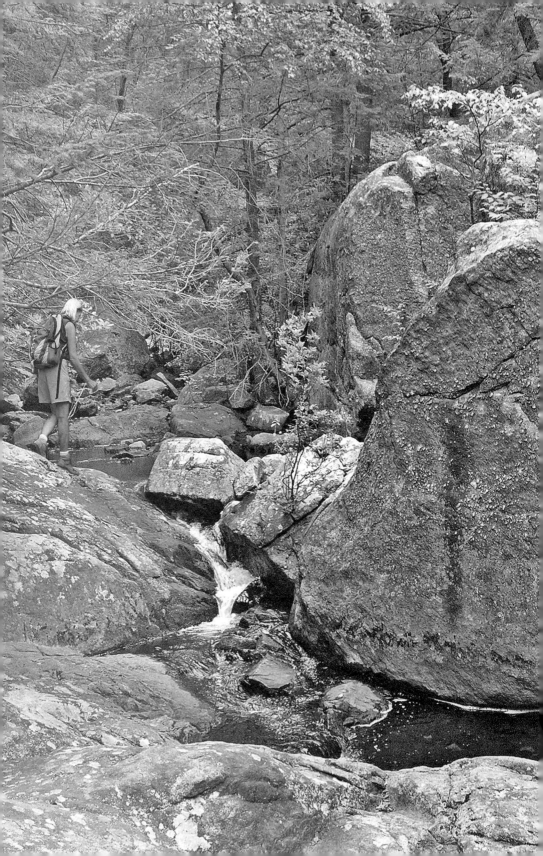

# APPENDIX A:
## OUTDOOR STORES

**CAMPMOR**
campmor.com
810 Route 17 N.
Paramus, NJ 07652
201-445-5000

**RAMSEY OUTDOOR**
ramseyoutdoor.com

**Paramus Towne Square**
240 Route 17 N.
Paramus, NJ 07652
800-699-5874, 201-261-5000

**Ramsey**
835 Route 17 S.
Ramsey, NJ 07446
201-327-8141

**Roxbury Mall**
281 Route 10 E.
Succasunna, NJ 07876
973-584-7798

**TENT AND TRAILS**
tenttrails.com
21 Park Pl.
New York, NY 10007
800-237-1760, 212-227-1760

« Harriman's Ga-Nus-Quah Rock (Hike 20)

# APPENDIX B:
## TRAIL-MAP RESOURCES

**CAMPMOR**
campmor.com
810 Route 17 N.
Paramus, NJ 07652
201-445-5000

**DeLORME**
delorme.com
2 DeLorme Drive
P.O. Box 298
Yarmouth, ME 04096
800-561-5105

**DIGITAL MAP STORE**
digital-topo-maps.com

**4X4BOOKS**
gpsnow.com

**HIKER CENTRAL**
hikercentral.com/maps

**NEW YORK–NEW JERSEY
TRAIL CONFERENCE**
nynjtc.org
156 Ramapo Valley Road
(NJ Route 202)
Mahwah, NJ 07430
201-512-9348

**RAMSEY OUTDOOR**
ramseyoutdoor.com

**Paramus Towne Square**
240 Route 17 N.
Paramus, NJ 07652
800-699-5874, 201-261-5000

**Ramsey**
835 Route 17 S.
Ramsey, NJ 07446
201-327-8141

**Roxbury Mall**
281 Route 10 E.
Succasunna, NJ 07876
973-584-7798

**U.S. GEOLOGICAL SURVEY,
EASTERN REGION**
usgs.gov

**USGS National Center**
12201 Sunrise Valley Dr.
Reston, VA 20192
800-228-0975, 703-648-7075

**WILDERNET**
wildernet.com

# APPENDIX C:
## HIKING CLUBS AND ORGANIZATIONS

**ADVENTURES FOR WOMEN**
adventuresforwomen.org
15 Victoria Ln.
Morris Township, NJ 07960
973-644-3592

**AMERICAN HIKING SOCIETY**
1422 Fenwick Ln.
Silver Spring, MD 20910
800-972-8608

**APPALACHIAN MOUNTAIN CLUB, NEW YORK–NORTH JERSEY CHAPTER**
outdoors.org/chapters/newyork
 -northjersey-chapter.cfm
381 Park Ave. S., Ste. 809
New York, NY 10017
212-986-1430

**APPALACHIAN TRAIL CONSERVANCY**
appalachiantrail.org
P.O. Box 807
Harpers Ferry, WV 25425-0807
304-535-6331

**AUDUBON NEW YORK**
ny.audubon.org
200 Trillium Ln.
Albany, NY 12203
518-869-9731

**CHINESE MOUNTAIN CLUB OF NEW YORK**
cmcny.org

**GERMAN-AMERICAN HIKING CLUB OF NEW YORK AND NEW JERSEY**
gah.nynjtc.org

**HARRIMAN HIKERS**
harrimanhikers.org
973-471-0492

**JEWISH OUTDOORS CLUB**
jewishoutdoorsclub.com/joc.aspx

**LONG ISLAND GREENBELT TRAIL CONFERENCE**
hike-li.com/ligtc

**MORRIS TRAILS PARTNERSHIP**
morristrails.org
P.O. Box 1295
Morristown, NJ 07962-1295

**MOSAIC OUTDOOR MOUNTAIN CLUB OF GREATER NEW YORK**
mosaic-gny.org
212-502-0820

**NASSAU HIKING AND OUTDOOR CLUB**
nhoc.org

**NEW JERSEY AUDUBON SOCIETY/ WEIS ECOLOGY CENTER/ WEIS WYANOKIE WANDERERS**
njaudubon.org
150 Snake Den Rd.
Ringwood, NJ 07456
973-835-2160

**THE NEW YORK CITY HIKING MEETUP GROUP**
hiking.meetup.com/3

**NEW YORK HIKING CLUB**
nyh.nynjtc.org

**NEW YORK–NEW JERSEY TRAIL CONFERENCE**
nynjtc.org
156 Ramapo Valley Rd.
(NJ Route 202)
Mahwah, NJ 07430
201-512-9348

**NEW YORK RAMBLERS**
nyramblers.org
212-260-4879

**SCENIC HUDSON**
scenichudson.org
1 Civic Center Plaza, Ste. 200
Poughkeepsie, NY 12601
845-473-4440

**SIERRA CLUB**
newjersey.sierraclub.org/outings.asp
newyork.sierraclub.org/midhudson
newyork.sierraclub.org/outings

**URBAN TRAIL CONFERENCE**
urbantrail.org
P.O. Box 264
Bronx, NY 10463-0264
718-652-9075

**WESTCHESTER TRAILS ASSOCIATION**
westhike.org

**WILD EARTH ADVENTURES**
wildearthadventures.com
845-357-3380

# APPENDIX D:
## GREEN-SPACE
## ORGANIZATIONS

**NATIONAL PARK SERVICE,
NORTHEAST REGION**
nps.gov/nero

**NATIONAL WILDLIFE REFUGES**
refuges.fws.gov

**THE NATURE CONSERVANCY**
nature.org

**Connecticut Chapter**
55 Church St., Floor 3
New Haven, CT 06510-3029
203-568-6270

**Eastern New York Chapter**
265 Chestnut Ridge Rd.
Mt. Kisco, NY 10549
914-244-3271

**Long Island Chapter**
250 Lawrence Hill Rd.
Cold Spring Harbor, NY 11724
631-367-3225

**New Jersey Chapter**
200 Pottersville Rd.
Chester, NJ 07930
908-879-7262

**NEW JERSEY DEPARTMENT OF
ENVIRONMENTAL PROTECTION
(NJDEP)**
nj.gov/dep
401 E. State St., 7th Floor, East Wing
Trenton, NJ 08625-0402
866-337-5669, 609-777-3373

**NJDEP GREEN ACRES PROGRAM**
nj.gov/dep/greenacres
501 E. State St.
Station Plaza Building 5, Ground Floor
Trenton, NJ 08625
609-984-0500

**NEW JERSEY DIVISION OF PARKS
AND FORESTRY**
njparksandforests.org

**NEW YORK STATE DEPARTMENT OF
ENVIRONMENTAL
CONSERVATION**
www.dec.ny.gov
625 Broadway
Albany, NY 12233-0001
518-402-8013

**NEW YORK STATE OFFICE OF PARKS,
RECREATION AND HISTORIC
PRESERVATION**
nysparks.com
625 Broadway
Albany, NY 12207
212-866-3100

**OPEN SPACE INSTITUTE**
osiny.org
1350 Broadway, Ste. 201
New York, NY 10018
212-290-8200

**PALISADES INTERSTATE PARK
COMMISSION**
njpalisades.org/pipc.htm
Administration Building
Bear Mountain, NY 10911-0427
845-786-2701

**SIERRA CLUB, ATLANTIC CHAPTER**
newyork2.sierraclub.org

**New York City Field Office**
116 John St., Ste. 3100
New York, NY 10038
212-791-3600

**Northeast Field Office**
85 Washington St.
Saratoga Springs, NY 12866-4105
518-587-9166

**LAND TRUST ALLIANCE**
landtrustalliance.org
1660 L St. NW, Ste. 1100
Washington, DC 20036
202-638-4725

**WESTCHESTER LAND TRUST**
westchesterlandtrust.org
403 Harris Rd.
Bedford Hills, NY 10507
914-241-6346

# INDEX

**DEAR CUSTOMERS AND FRIENDS,**

**SUPPORTING YOUR INTEREST IN OUTDOOR ADVENTURE,** travel, and an active lifestyle is central to our operations, from the authors we choose to the locations we detail to the way we design our books. Menasha Ridge Press was incorporated in 1982 by a group of veteran outdoorsmen and professional outfitters. For many years now, we've specialized in creating books that benefit the outdoors enthusiast.

Almost immediately, Menasha Ridge Press earned a reputation for revolutionizing outdoors- and travel-guidebook publishing. For such activities as canoeing, kayaking, hiking, backpacking, and mountain biking, we established new standards of quality that transformed the whole genre, resulting in outdoor-recreation guides of great sophistication and solid content. Menasha Ridge continues to be outdoor publishing's greatest innovator.

The folks at Menasha Ridge Press are as at home on a white-water river or mountain trail as they are editing a manuscript. The books we build for you are the best they can be, because we're responding to your needs. Plus, we use and depend on them ourselves.

We look forward to seeing you on the river or the trail. If you'd like to contact us directly, join in at www.trekalong.com or visit us at www.menasharidge.com. We thank you for your interest in our books and the natural world around us all.

**SAFE TRAVELS,**

*Bob Sehlinger*

**BOB SEHLINGER**
**PUBLISHER**